Managing Pharmacy Practice

Principles, Strategies, and Systems

Convienent

CRC PRESS
PHARMACY
EDUCATION
SERIES

Managing Pharmacy Practice

Principles, Strategies, and Systems

EDITED BY
Andrew M. Peterson

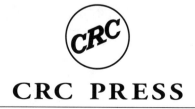

CRC PRESS

Boca Raton   London   New York   Washington, D.C.

Library of Congress Cataloging-in-Publication Data

Managing pharmacy practice : principles, strategies, and systems / [edited by]
    Andrew M. Peterson.
          p.   cm. — (CRC Press pharmacy education series)
    Includes bibliographical references and index.
    ISBN 0-8493-1446-1 (alk. paper)
    1. Pharmacy—Practice. I. Peterson, Andrew M. II. Series.
    [DNLM: 1. Pharmaceutical Services—organization & administration. 2.
    Pharmacy—organization & administration Qv 737 M2656 2004]
    RS98.M36 2004
    615′.4′068—dc22   2003065420

Visit the CRC Press Web site at www.crcpress.comwww.com

© 2004 by CRC Press LLC

No claim to original U.S. Government works
International Standard Book Number 0-8493-1446-1
Library of Congress Card Number 2003065420
Printed in the United States of America 1 2 3 4 5 6 7 8 9 0
Printed on acid-free paper

Dedication

This book is dedicated to my wife, Hanna. Without her never-ending patience, support, and love, this book would still be in the recesses of my mind. Thank you.

Preface

This text is designed for students in the professional years of their pharmacy curricula. The purpose of this book is to introduce students to a variety of managerial issues facing pharmacists presently and in the future. Throughout the text, references are made to changes occurring both internally and externally to the profession. Much of the material applies to all settings of pharmacy practice — community, hospital, industry, ambulatory care, and long-term care. Readers should not confine themselves to one area of practice; rather, when a particular setting is used as a platform for discussion, they should also see how the issue manifests itself in another setting. The concepts and skills underpinning the management of human resources, drug distribution systems, formularies, and drug use evaluations are transferable among the variety of practice settings.

The chapters are written by contributors within and outside pharmacy practice. As such, the style of writing and presentation of information will vary among chapters. This diversity of contributors, as well as the diversity of writing styles, should not be considered a distraction, but rather a reflection of the complexity of management in pharmacy settings.

The text is organized into three sections. The foundations of management section discusses some of the more pertinent managerial issues facing pharmacists. Starting with a background in basic management theories and a detailed discussion of systems theory, the section will help readers develop a foundation on which to analyze other managerial systems encountered in pharmacy practice. The systems approach will allow students to understand the contextual relationships among seemingly disparate concepts. For example, the discussion of professionals and their roles in society is juxtaposed with discussions of organizational designs and power. Understanding and applying good leadership and motivation strategies will enhance the professional's ability to resolve conflict and recruit and retain valuable employees.

In the second section, human resources discussions are followed by other traditional chapters on accounting, inventory control, and purchasing. These chapters begin the foundation for developing profession-specific concepts, such as drug formularies, P&T committees, DUEs, and disease management. How technology can help in the flow of products and information related to drugs and drug use is the basis for the chapter on eHealth. This section is designed to help the reader use these systems and solutions to improve the quality of care through reduced medication errors and improved medication use.

All of these topics serve as the groundwork for the final section, which describes major business and policy changes affecting the profession. The section begins with an overview of the current U.S. health care system, including how managed care and pharmacy benefit managers influence practice. It also involves a discussion of pharmaceutical care as a system and how this practice philosophy can operate within current and future practice models. These topics are complemented by discussions of organizations affecting pharmacy. Chapters are dedicated to accrediting agencies and regulatory bodies, professional organizations, and corporate compliance. Lastly, time is dedicated to social trends affecting pharmacy, such as the diminishing workforce, consumerism, and other health policy decisions impacting the practice.

The overarching intent of this text is to give students of pharmacy a broad overview of the complexities and intricacies inherent in managing systems in pharmacy. Regardless of students' practice settings, knowledge of these principles and strategies will aid them in their transformations to competent and confident practitioners.

Acknowledgments

I acknowledge the following individuals for their assistance in the development and production of this book: Mike Brown for originally believing in the concept; Steve Zollo for his continued belief and support in the project; Pat Roberson, Barbara Uetrecht-Pierre, and Allison Taub for their patience during the manuscript development and production phases; and, finally, the contributors for their diligence and patience as this project progressed. Without them, there would be no book.

Editor

Andrew M. Peterson is associate professor of pharmacy at the Philadelphia College of Pharmacy, where he teaches management and managed care pharmacy practice. Before Dr. Peterson joined the University of the Sciences in Philadelphia in 1996, he was assistant director of pharmacy and clinical services at Thomas Jefferson University Hospital. Prior to that, he was associate director of pharmacy, drug information, and clinical services at Crozer-Chester Medical Center. He currently is a senior consultant for Besler, Inc., in New Jersey. He is a board-certified pharmacotherapy specialist (BCPS) through the American College of Clinical Pharmacy.

Dr. Peterson has concentrated his years of research in pharmacy management, managed care pharmacy, pharmaceutical care, and medication adherence. His more recent scholarly publications include "A Survey of the Extent of Electronic Prescribing as Perceived by MCOs" and "A Meta Analysis of Interventions to Improve Medication Adherence." He has coauthored a book on therapeutics for mid-level practitioners entitled *Advanced Pharmacotherapeutics: A Practical Approach.*

Dr. Peterson is a member of several pharmacy organizations, including the American Society of Health-System Pharmacists, Academy of Managed Care Pharmacy, American College of Clinical Pharmacy, and the Pennsylvania Society of Hospital Pharmacists.

Contributors

David A. Ehlert
Director of Clinical Pharmacy
Practice
McKesson Medication Management
Muskego, Wisconsin

Victoria E. Elliott
Executive Vice President
Pennsylvania Society of Health-
System Pharmacists
Philadelphia, Pennsylvania

Ellen Fernberger
Deputy Director of Human
Resources
Community College of Philadelphia
Philadelphia, Pennsylvania

Harold Glass
University of the Sciences in
Philadelphia
Philadelphia, Pennsylvania

James M. Hoffman
Fellow in Outcomes Research and
Drug Policy
University of Wisconsin Hospital
and Clinics
Madison, Wisconsin

Jaime B. Howell
Department of Health Policy
Thomas Jefferson University
Philadelphia, Pennsylvania

Brian C. Isetts
Department of Pharmaceutical Care
& Health Systems
University of Minnesota, College of
Pharmacy
Minneapolis, Minnesota

Patricia C. Kienle
Medication Safety Manager
Cardinal Health Pharmacy
Management
Laflin, Pennsylvania

Katherine K. Knapp
Professor and Director of the Center
for Pharmacy Practice Research
and Development
College of Pharmacy
Western University of Health
Sciences
Pomona, California

Jennifer H. Lofland
Department of Medicine
Department of Health Policy
Thomas Jefferson University
Philadelphia, Pennsylvania

Christy-Lee Lucas
CVS Pharmacy
Warrington, Pennsylvania

Alan Lyles
University of Baltimore
School of Public Affairs, Health
  Systems Management
Baltimore, Maryland

Jacob Mathew
Rutgers University
Piscataway, New Jersey

Diana Papshev
Advanced Concepts USP
University of the Sciences in
  Philadelphia
Philadelphia, Pennsylvania

Andrew M. Peterson
Associate Professor of Clinical
  Pharmacy
Philadelphia College of Pharmacy
Philadelphia, Pennsylvania

Laura T. Pizzi
Department of Health Policy
Thomas Jefferson University
Philadelphia, Pennsylvania

Barbara J. Plager
University of the Sciences in
  Philadelphia
Philadelphia, Pennsylvania

Glenn Rosenthal
University of the Sciences in
  Philadelphia
Philadelphia, Pennsylvania

Steven L. Sheaffer
Associate Professor and Vice Chair
  for Experiential Learning
Department of Pharmacy Practice
  and Pharmacy Administration
Philadelphia College of Pharmacy
University of the Sciences in
  Philadelphia
Philadelphia, Pennsylvania

Susan Skledar
Assistant Professor
Department of Pharmacy and
  Therapeutics
Director, Drug Use and Disease
  State Management Program
University of Pittsburgh Medical
  Center
Pittsburgh, Pennsylvania

Joshua J. Spooner
Manager, Health Outcomes
  Research
Health Core, Inc.
Newark, Delaware

F. Randy Vogenberg
Aon Consulting, Life Sciences
  Practice
Wellesley, Massachusetts

Robert J. Votta
University of the Sciences in
  Philadelphia
Philadelphia, Pennsylvania

Table of Contents

chapter one

Introduction to management

Andrew M. Peterson

Contents

Introduction

The world of pharmacy management is changing rapidly. The myriad changes in the health care system, including managed care, long-term care, and assisted living facilities, require students of pharmacy to have a broad understanding of how the profession fits in the current and future health care delivery systems. Along with health care system changes, the traditional concepts of leadership, mentoring, organizational design, and behavior have also changed in pharmacy. The conventional notion of a pharmacist working in a retail or hospital pharmacy is no longer applicable: pharmacists are assuming a greater responsibility for the outcomes of patients by using newer technologies, such as electronic prescribing, robotics, and automation, coupled with more direct patient care activity. In addition, today's consumers are more interested in self-management, fueled by the Internet and 24/7 information availability. This age of consumerism clearly poses new challenges to pharmacists of the future.

The practice of management is key to the successful performance of professional responsibilities. Managing people, information, and systems allows the creation of an environment suitable to carry out the mission of providing pharmaceutical care. Often considered a second-rate subject by pharmacists, management is considered by students to be less important than traditional topics such as pharmacology or pharmacotherapeutics. However, without the organizational structures and wherewithal of management, it would not be possible to carry out professional duties. Given that, this text is organized to help students understand how and where management fits in their daily lives as practicing pharmacists.

Management theories

The theory of management takes a variety of forms. Classical management deals with the traditional five responsibilities of a manager: planning, organizing, directing, coordinating, and controlling. This is coupled with the science of management, which deals with studying the impact of people and systems on productivity, or output. In pharmacy, this typically involves studying how to minimize waiting times for customers or to increase the number of prescriptions processed without increasing staff. Behavioral management, in contrast, deals with organizational and individual responses to situations. Instead of considering workers as machines and attempting to improve productivity through improving processes, behavioral management looks at environmental, interpersonal, and group interactions and their impacts on productivity. Systems management involves taking a holistic approach to all aspects involved in the process of producing a product or a service. This theory not only looks at processes and human or environmental influences but also focuses on interactions and how they affect the organization. The different management theories are discussed in this chapter, and the concept of systems theory is further addressed in Chapter 2.

Management skills

Managers must possess specific skills in order to effectively manage people, systems, and processes. These skills are technical, interpersonal, and conceptual. Technical skills relate to a manager's knowledge of the day-to-day operations of the organization. For example, a pharmacist has the technical skills necessary to process a prescription or make an intravenous solution. However, in the course of the day, the pharmacist also needs interpersonal skills to communicate with patients regarding how the medication should be used, with technicians on how best to prepare the medication, or with physicians and nurses regarding drug therapy. Lastly, pharmacists must be able to conceptualize their roles within the entire health care system. Pharmacy is but one part of how patient care is delivered. For example, a director of pharmacy within a hospital must understand, conceptually, how the entire

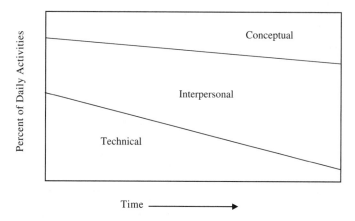

Figure 1.1 Manager skill changes during career.

pharmacy department integrates with other departments in the complex operation of a hospital.

As a pharmacist's career progresses, the percentage of time spent on technical, interpersonal, and conceptual skills changes. There is a need for growth in the interpersonal and conceptual skills, while the time needed for technical skills decreases (Figure 1.1).

Classical theory of management

The process of management

Henri Fayol believed that management was a process consisting of five different functions. He saw a manager's job to include the processes of planning, organizing, directing, coordinating, and controlling. These five functions are part of classical management theory and are at present important components in the daily functions of a manager.

Planning

The planning process is designed to help the organization minimize uncertainty in the future. Planning helps determine future success as well as anticipate potential pitfalls. Planning also helps to maximize efficiency. When an organization understands where resources, people, and money are to be deployed, it can make the best use of them to accomplish its goals. Planning includes considering monthly as well as annual budgets and anticipated profits. This involves recognizing the potential revenue an organization expects at that point of time and in the future, as well as expenses associated with current and future operations. Along with the budgeting process, planning also entails identifying and preparing for the appropriate mix of staff (pharmacists, technicians, ancillary personnel) and the hours of operation of the current and future pharmacy.

Table 1.1 Steps in the Process of Planning

- Assess the situation.
- Determine the organization's
    strengths.
    weaknesses.
    threats.
    opportunities.
- Review (or develop) the organization's mission.
- Determine the vision for the organization.
- Develop objectives in concert with the mission and vision.
- Develop implementation plans through measurable objectives, budgets, schedules, and marketing.

A manager engages in several types of planning on a daily basis. First, strategic planning is the process of charting the course for the organization. This type of planning considers the strengths and weaknesses of the organization in light of the opportunities and threats that the organization may face in the future. Typically, strategic planning attempts to plan three, five, or ten years into the future. Once the overall direction of the organization is planned through this process, tactical planning — plans that carry out the strategic plan — occurs. Typically, these plans come in the form of long-term objectives, which are measurable achievements by which the organization and all its members can benchmark progress. For example, a retail pharmacy's strategic plan may include an initiative to become a leader in diabetes care within the next three years. To accomplish this plan, long-term objectives are needed to support the initiative. These objectives could include having all pharmacist-certified diabetes disease managers, constructing a patient counseling area supporting patient education, and redesigning the work flow to allow pharmacists to perform this function. Short-term planning involves planning for activities within the upcoming year or sooner. Typical short-term objectives include determining hours of operation, marketing plans, and monthly and annual budgets. The process of planning, in particular strategic planning, incorporates the steps listed in Table 1.1.

Organizing

Organizing is the second function of a manager. It encompasses assigning responsibilities to employees and determining how and when things are to be accomplished. One of the primary organizing functions is to determine the organizational chart. This chapter reviews briefly some basic organizational theories; the ins and outs of organizational charts are discussed in greater detail in Chapter 3.

Most organizations today are based on the scientific management theory, yielding the bureaucratic model. The bureaucracy is the typical organizational structure, which is founded on the principles of logic, order, and legitimate authority. The characteristics of a bureaucratic organization include a clear division of labor, job specialization, a hierarchy of authority implemented through a system of formal policies and procedures, fairness in applying rules, and a career ladder by which individuals have the opportunity for promotion based on merit and accomplishments within the organization. Bureaucratic organizations are typically considered mechanistic in nature.

Modern theories of organizations suggest that one organizational design is insufficient and that flexibility in organizational design is important. There should be little hierarchy, or, if it does exist, it should be fluid. There should also be fewer policies and procedures and more overlap in job responsibilities. This flexibility is characteristic of organic structures and considers the size of the organization, its purpose and function within society, and important external variables (e.g., market forces) that may influence the organization. Both bureaucratic and organic organizations, with examples, are further discussed in Chapter 3.

Directing

One of the most important functions of a manager is directing — leading, delegating, and motivating employees to accomplish their jobs. This function relies primarily on the interpersonal skills of a manager because directing involves dealing with people. Further, this function includes recruiting and retaining employees. How a manager interacts with employees, or prospective employees, sets the tone for the culture of an organization. Related to this is the concept of power within an organization. Various organizational structures lend themselves to granting more or less authority to an individual manager, but how the manager uses that power is key in directing employees to carry out job responsibilities. Chapter 4 discusses in more detail power and its relationship to organizational design and authority.

One of the primary tasks in the directing function is issuing orders or directives to employees. *What* is to be ordered stems from the scientific aspect of management and *how* it is to be ordered is the art of management. One can directly give orders, or one can delegate the authority to accomplish a task to a subordinate as a means of directing. The risk of delegating is that the job may not be accomplished exactly as the manager expected — sometimes the result is worse than expected and sometimes it is better than expected. For delegation to operate effectively, the manager must consider how to motivate and lead the employee. These concepts are further deliberated in Chapter 5.

Coordinating

Synchronizing activities is the hallmark of coordination. Within a department, many functions take place simultaneously or in sequence to accomplish an objective. The function of the manager in this respect is to bring these activities together in an efficient and effective manner to produce the desired output. Coordinating activities include corrective actions, in which adjustments to a process need to be made to bring about the outcome; preventative actions, which prevent problems from occurring; and promotive actions, in which relationships are developed within and among departments and personnel.

A key aspect of the coordinating function is managing conflict. Conflict arises on a daily basis in organizations. Not all conflict is bad. At times, conflict is a means of identifying problems and presents an opportunity to improve. However, poorly managed conflict can have serious consequences for employee morale and customer satisfaction. One way to manage conflict is using teams or committees to identify and resolve problems between an organization's units. Chapter 10 discusses further means of managing conflict.

Controlling

The controlling function of a manager is regulatory in nature, by which the manager assures that the functions of the department are progressing in accordance with predefined plans. The manager reviews the plans developed, determines the performance measures needed to assure progress toward the goal, compares the results of these measures with the standards set in the plans, and attempts to make adjustments, through one of the other functions, to ensure congruency with the desired outcome.

The idea of management control can be considered in a variety of settings. For example, the manager compares the actual performance of a system to the planned performance, and if there is a mismatch takes corrective action so that the actual performance meets the planned performance. Depending on what the manager wants to control, a variety of control devices can be used, such as budget reports, performance appraisals, or opinion polls. These varied devices provide a measure of performance — profits or expenses through budget reports; productivity of workers through performance appraisals; and consumer satisfaction through opinion polls. Several of these control devices are discussed in later chapters.

The science of management (aka Taylorism)

Until the early 1900s, managers used intuition and past experiences to manage people and processes. However, F.W. Taylor revolutionized the process of management through his publication of "Scientific Management" in 1911. In his proposal, Taylor suggests that workers underperform primarily because of how work is organized and how it is supervised and directed by management. Taylor taught that there is only one method of work that maximizes efficiency, "and this one best method and best implementation can only be discovered or developed through scientific study and analysis." The main thrust of his treatise focuses on breaking tasks down into smaller, repetitive activities that can be accomplished by well-trained workers. These tasks should be standardized and placed in the most efficient order that would take the least amount of time to produce the desired output. Lastly, workers should be motivated to produce more through a system of rewards based on productivity and output. This theory led to the development of the assembly line process used within many organizations today.

Behavioral theory of management

Also known as human relations theory, behavioral theory developed as a consequence of the application of the scientific theory. In the late 1920s, Elton Mayo conducted individual productivity experiments at the Hawthorne Works plant of the Western Electric Company (Reshef, *Elton Mayo & the Human Relations Movement*). By varying environmental conditions such as lighting, rest breaks, and lengths of workdays, Mayo attempted to determine which conditions were conducive to the most efficient productivity. The experiments failed to determine which conditions were best because productivity improved in all conditions. Later studies showed that group dynamics influenced the output; that is, when coworkers put pressure on others to decrease or increase output, the group norm took precedence. Further, when supervisors were watching workers or when individuals were singled out to perform tasks at a higher level, productivity improved. This "Hawthorne effect" demonstrated that productivity is influenced by the situation and not necessarily by the rewards or conditions of the job.

These findings led to the development of Douglas McGregor's Theory X and Theory Y management. Theory X, a basic assumption of bureaucratic organizations, assumes that people inherently dislike work, must be coerced and threatened to do the job, avoid responsibility, and have few career ambitions. Theory Y, in contrast, looks at workers as individuals willing to work and accept responsibility and as capable of self-direction and control. It also considers that the expenditure of mental and physical energy at work is the same as at play.

When managers subscribe to either of McGregor's theories, the Hawthorne effect comes into play, thus creating a self-fulfiling prophecy. If a manager believes that workers must be directed and coerced into performing duties, then the workers will conform to those expectations. On the other hand, if a manager assumes a Theory Y stance, then the workers will also respond accordingly.

Further investigations stemming from the psychological literature surround the motivational aspects of management. Abraham Maslow (1943) developed the theory of human needs and helped spur an abundance of thoughts around motivation and work productivity. His theory focuses on two basic principles: a satisfied need is not a motivator and the complexity of needs increases as prior ones are satisfied, i.e., needs change. Maslow identified five basic needs of all humans: physiologic, safety, social, esteem, and self-actualization. His theory suggests that as physiologic needs are satisfied (e.g., food and water), safety needs become the primary motivators for individuals. As these needs are satisfied, social needs take precedence. It makes sense that managers should help employees satisfy needs and remove barriers to employee self-fulfillment. All this must be considered within the context of the organization and an understanding of other motivational factors. Chapter 5 discusses how to use this theory and others derived from the human relations management movement.

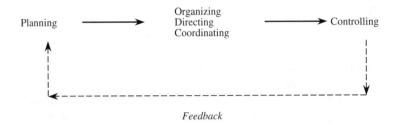

Feedback

Figure 1.2 Relationship between the classical theory and the systems theory.

Systems theory of management

Systems theory provides a model in which a manager can understand the interactions among various components of an organization. In contrast to scientific management which analyzes processes by breaking them into smaller parts, systems theory contends that the product of a system is due to the interactions of its parts — if the parts are separated, the system no longer produces the desired output. Systems theory takes a holistic approach instead of an analytical approach to better understand the factors affecting the desired output. If one of the components of the system falters, then the desired output is not achieved. A good manager understands both the task-oriented processes as well as the behavioral aspects that affect production.

Systems in pharmacy management involve people, drug products, information, and money. All these factors are related to one another in some way; and the care delivered by pharmacists is in some way affected by the behaviors or actions of each system and each system affects the behaviors and actions of others. Further, the classical theory of management, in terms of the functions, can be depicted as an interrelated system (Figure 1.2). The concept of systems theory is further discussed in Chapter 2.

Conclusion

The theories of management form the foundation for our workforce today. Pharmacy is a complex series of technical, interpersonal, and conceptually integrated processes in which drugs are produced and distributed, and information regarding proper use and monitoring is key to the success. As a basis for understanding how managers should function, one can look at the classical theory of management, in which the day-to-day and long-term operations of a pharmacy can be planned, organized, directed, coordinated, and controlled. The subsystem of drug dispensing can be viewed in terms of the scientific theory of management, in which processes are broken down into discrete functional tasks that could be performed by robots or automated dispensing devices and overseen by pharmacists and technicians. The art of leading and motivating pharmacists and technicians is embodied within the behavioral management theories. Lastly, systems theory allows managers to conceptualize how different subsystems integrate with one another to produce the desired output. In the case of pharmacy, the desired output is not merely the dispensing of a drug product; rather, it is the caring of patients, in which both product and information are integrally related.

Bibliography

Anon. Theory X and Theory Y. Net MBA Business Knowledge Center. http://www.netmba.com/mgmt/ob/motivation/mcgregor/, accessed December 29, 2003.

Liebler JG, McConnell CR. *Management Principles for Health Professionals*. Aspen Publishers, Gaithersburg, MD, 1999.

Longest BB. *Management Practices for the Health Professional*, 3rd ed., Reston Publishing Company, Reston, VA, 1984.

Maslow AH. A theory of human motivation. *Psych. Rev.* 1943; 50:370–396. As listed on Green, CD. Classics in the History of Psychology [online resource]. http://psychclassics.yorku.ca/Maslow/motivation.htm, accessed December 29, 2003.

Reshef Y. Elton Mayo & the human relations movement: 1880–1949. http://courses.bus.ualberta.ca/orga417-reshef/mayo.htm, accessed December 29, 2003.

Taylor FW. The principles of scientfic management, 1911. As listed on Halsall P. Modern History Sourcebook [online resource]. http://www.fordham.edu/halsall/mod/1911taylor.html, accessed December 29, 2003.

Tootelian DH, Gaedeke RM. *Essentials of Pharmacy Management*, Mosby, St. Louis, MO, 1993.

chapter two

Systems theory and management

Glenn Rosenthal

Contents

Chapter 1 looked at the history of management and discussed how various researchers attempted to understand it by scientifically analyzing each step in the process of management. This chapter looks at systems theory and discusses how it is used in modern business planning and action.

The pervasiveness of systems

Discussions of new principles or theories sometimes seem more complicated than they really are. Systems thinking is actually the most common and natural way of understanding the world. On a very large scale, our solar system is a group of planets surrounding the sun, each exerting some influence on the others. Earth is a very intricate system, depending on the sun for its existence and made up of interacting forces such as weather, plate tectonics, oceanic currents, and temperatures that interact and influence all the myriad forms of life on the planet (Figure 2.1). Archaeological discoveries

0-8493-1446-1/04/$0.00+$1.50

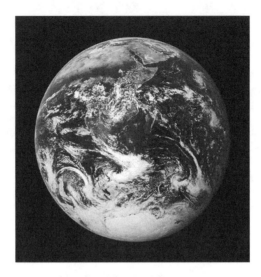

Figure 2.1   Earth is a complex system.

from Great Britain, Central America, Egypt, and the Far East have shown that ancient humans understood natural systems and were quite sophisticated in measuring and calculating from them. Stonehenge, on the plains of Salisbury, England (Figure 2.2), and other similar structures spread throughout England, Europe, and the U.S. have been demonstrated to be sophisticated astronomical calendars pinpointing the positions of the sun and moon at various times of the year. The Great Pyramids of Egypt (Figure 2.3) have been shown to line up perfectly with various stars and planets at specific times of the year. Agrarian societies from ancient times to the present have had such a symbiotic relationship with nature that the awareness of the cycles of the seasons and natural occurrences was normal and expected, and people saw themselves as part of the system of the natural world.

Another system that is so close to us that we seldom think of it as such is the human body. We refer to the circulatory, respiratory, or limbic systems,

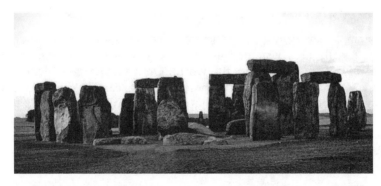

Figure 2.2   Stonehenge appears to have been an astronomical calendar. (Copyright Philip Baird, www.anthroarcheart.org.)

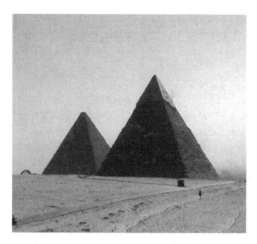

Figure 2.3 The pyramids line up with certain astronomical events. (Copyright 2000 by Joel A. Freeman, Ph.D., www.returntoglory.org.)

for example, without really picturing in our minds that they are intricately bound systems. Each system part is completely dependent on the others, feeding back information that constantly keeps the system parts in equilibrium, both within the particular system and in relation to the others.

In psychoanalytic theory, Carl Jung discussed the concept of archetypes, natural occurrences so common to human experience that their knowledge is inborn and instinctual; for example, every higher organism has a mother, so there is a "mother" archetype. Our awareness of systems, relationships among things, events, and symbols, is archetypal in the same sense. Events or things like those mentioned have been around since, quite literally, the beginning of time and exist for virtually every living thing on the planet. Seasons, in most parts of the globe, have followed such a regular pattern that life forms, including most plant life, have developed inborn responses to most conditions. Humans instinctually look for connections among events or things in order to make sense of them from the moment of birth, and probably before. Newborns immediately make connections between sights and sounds in a feedback loop; they cry when hungry or uncomfortable and stop when a need is satisfied. These systems form patterns or archetypes of systems that are readily recognizable in much of human and organizational behavior. However, the complex subsystems we all exist, compete, and live in are so ingrained in us that we scarcely take conscious notice of our interactions with our families, neighbors, towns, regions, countries, continents, and the world. And yet, writing in June 2002, as recent world events have made very clear, what happens in other parts of the world has more effect on us than do mere changes in the weather.

Therefore, the concept of systems and feedback loops, which is the core of systems thinking, is a very natural one for all life on Earth. Why is it then that we need to "study" systems thinking as though it were a recently

discovered phenomenon that, as the latest management theory, will provide
new and enhanced understanding of business?

Systems theory

Systems theory provides a model of a mindset, or a way of looking at things.
A system can be closed or open, but it is basically a group of things or a set
of circumstances that are related in some way and whose behaviors or actions
influence behaviors or actions of other members of the group or other sets of
happenings or circumstances. If a system is closed, then a finite number of
members or circumstances influence one another and no new ones are introduced. Because the system is closed, expected behaviors occur, expected patterns are seen, and we react to our surroundings more or less subconsciously.
If a system is open, then external influences are constantly introduced.

Birnbaum (1988) has developed two analogies that illustrate open and
closed systems. A closed system is like a pool table. It has rigid boundaries
with a simple, definable input, the cue stick. The cue stick hits the cue ball,
which then moves in a more or less predicted path. We can see where and
how the input — the cue stick hitting the ball — impacts the ball's final
position, the outcome. Birnbaum maintains, "Closed systems are linear; the
system parts do not change and cause and effect can be predicted with great
accuracy. Success comes from playing by the rules." (p. 34). The rules for
human behaviors are not like the rules of the game of pool, but rather are
like expected patterns or structures of behaviors that may be archetypal —
they occur so frequently. In an open system, which Birnbaum likens to a
college or a company, the boundaries are permeable. Input comes from all
directions and must be sorted through, decisions are complex, and the rules
are fluid and sometimes hard to discern. He notes that "open systems are
dynamic and nonlinear" (pp. 34, 35).

Additionally, Birnbaum describes closed systems as deterministic
whereas open systems are probabilistic. In a closed system, represented by
the pool table and cue balls, the simple action of the cue stick hitting a ball
can be seen and followed directly from input to output (the final resting
place of each ball on the table) and the actions of each ball can be seen. By
describing open systems as probabilistic, Birnbaum means that although the
inputs and the outputs may be known or measurable, what caused the inputs
to become the exact seen or measured outputs is unknown and can only be
inferred. This can occur for many reasons. For example, the output may be
separated from the input by a great deal of time, or there may be additional
unforeseen or unknown inputs at different stages during the transition from
the original input to the final output whose effects are unknown to a particular participant.

A problem for managers is that they may see their environments as
closed when, in fact, they are quite open. This deterministic viewpoint sees
a simple input with hard boundaries instead of acknowledging the open
system where many, if not most, of the actions on an input cannot be effec-

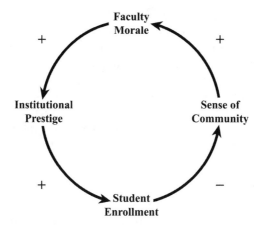

Figure 2.4 A feedback loop relating faculty morale to enrollment. (From Birnbaum, R., *How Colleges Work: The Cybernetics of Accdemic Organizations and Leadership*, Jossey-Bass, San Francisco, 1988. With permission.)

tively determined. The awareness of the probabilistic nature of the open environment allows for more complex management decision making. Birnbaum gives an example of a simple open system to illustrate the potential enormity of the options open to a manager (Figure 2.4). This system indicates that if faculty morale increases, as indicated by the "+" sign between faculty morale and institutional prestige, then prestige should increase. If institutional prestige increases, then student enrollment should increase. As enrollment increases, however, the sense of community present on a smaller campus decreases. But the sense of community is important to faculty morale in this system, and for faculty morale to increase, so must a sense of community. Decreased faculty morale would lead to decreased prestige, decreased enrollment, and eventually to an increased sense of community as enrollment returns to previous lower levels.

As in this simple example, the same flow of actions occurs in community neighborhoods, within companies, and with products and services. A retail store in any particular neighborhood may see its fortunes rise and fall as a result of the neighborhood it is in, the types of employees it can attract, the brand recognition of the store (e.g., a chain store vs. a local family-owned store), and other factors, many of which are beyond the immediate control of the proprietor. The implications for a manager in making decisions within this system would certainly include determining some level of equilibrium for each factor. In the educational example, equilibrium occurs at the point where faculty morale is maximized so that institutional prestige is high enough to ensure maximum enrollment, which ensures that the sense of community is maintained at an appropriate level. Standard marketing texts would have the manager believe that there is some "plan" that, if followed, would allow the resolution of this situation when in fact there is no right or wrong set of actions, only options to try. For the retail store manager, although factors well beyond the store itself might dictate success or failure of the enterprise, being aware of the possibilities and factors affecting performance are vital to successfully coping with the changing retail environment.

A number of writers have attempted to make systems theory more scientific by introducing postulates determining who or what can be included as an influencer or a respondent (see Schoderbek et al., 1985, pp. 34–44), but that is not the focus of this chapter. Rather, the chapter focuses on how systems theory can be used by managers or potential managers to help them perform their jobs better. To start, some history is reviewed.

The rise of systems theory

Following Darwin's observations in the 1850s that evolution is the natural order of life and that the world is not a static thing prescribed by God and described in the Bible, the industrial and scientific revolutions of the late 19th century led to increased interest in scientifically analyzing everything from manufacturing processes to religion. Frederick Taylor analyzed the work involved in bricklaying and developed a step-by-step procedure that demonstrated that economy of movement led to increased productivity: more bricks were laid in a day when extraneous steps were minimized or eliminated. His goal, to scientifically analyze a process, was one of the first applications of the new scientific method to business.

The scientific study of feedback loops or mechanisms began in World War II (see Burke, 1997) when artillery gunners needed to plot trajectories of increasingly faster moving planes and missiles. Calculations of anticipated speed, distance, and position needed to be constantly updated to increase accuracy when firing shells. Thus, it was important to monitor feedback of current position, speed, and so on as quickly as possible. Computers developed at the University of Pennsylvania and other institutions would soon compute fast enough to provide real-time information.

After the war, business practices began to be scientifically analyzed in newly developed business schools and programs around the country, and studying feedback loops became a legitimate field of study. One of the legacies of this analytical process, in the late 20th and early 21st centuries, is that people are taught to scrutinize things in a hierarchical manner. Business schools have taught marketers that planning follows a series of well-defined steps; if one follows the sequence of steps, plans will be successful. In the planning stage, the marketer develops strategic plans, which are then implemented. Implementation is carefully controlled, evaluated, and adjusted as necessary in what becomes a very mechanistic feedback loop. These steps seem to work well when the job is computer-driven and the task is a controlled industrial process. But whenever humans are involved in any of these steps, experience and common sense indicate that the results are often unexpected or unintended. As Peter Drucker (1972) noted, the new generation of U.S. workers would not be dominated by blue-collar tasks; they would be "knowledge" workers whose output would be more cerebral than manual. Given this transformation in the U.S. work-force, an employee's and a manager's focus had to be more systems-oriented than single-task-oriented; that is, they had to be concerned with how their output affected a larger customer base rather than just the next worker in line.

Systems theory is one of the solutions applied to business that went in a direction opposite to the stepwise analysis of Frederick Taylor and his successors. Instead of analyzing each individual step in a task, systems theory focuses on analyzing the whole process within its context and environment. The question that led to this change of focus was: How could one understand what was happening in any given situation without understanding the whole context within which the event is happening? Looking at a problem in a linear, mechanistic fashion does not work well for many issues in business, in part because many decisions do not see results for weeks, months, and, in many cases, years. Many times the original decision makers are not even in the same position, function, or company when the results of their decisions become apparent.

Systems analysis provides a tool to help understand the nature of feedback and the environmental impacts on many business decisions. Systems analysis is being taught as a "new" field of study because many researchers are attempting to scientifically analyze the concept and practice of this way of looking at business, exactly as Frederick Taylor did with manual labor. Recent texts (Schoderbek et al., 1985; Liebler and McConnell, 1999) attempt to quantify systems analysis as a mechanistic process, as though it followed a step by step, logical format.

Some writers prefer to look at systems within a single organization, studying how processes within that organization interact. For example, Hammer and Champy wrote several well-known business books on reengineering in the early 1990s (*Reengineering the Corporation* and *Reengineering Management*), examining, just as Frederick Taylor did, each process and method of work flow to minimize the steps needed to complete a task. Liebler and McConnell (1999, p. 44) discuss departments best suited to systems analysis, including cybernetics (the science of communication and control); data-processing systems; rheochrematics (the science of managing material flow); network analysis; and administrative systems. They simplify the concept of a system to include three steps: (1) inputs, (2) some throughput or action performed on the inputs, and (3) the resulting output. Looking at a system in this manner can be very useful while designing or redesigning a department or process within a department. It is important for managers to understand both *that* their work contributes to every other department and task within an organization and *how* their work contributes to those other areas. Liebler and McConnell also describe the tools of systems thinking as input analysis, throughput determination, and output analysis, which is nothing more than a rehash of the standard marketing viewpoint of (1) planning, (2) implementation, and (3) control or evaluation, except that the managers' worldview, the way they see a problem or department, and their understanding of their parts in the larger organization is important. If managers focus strictly on their own tasks and on their parts in the system, then they are looking at their work or groups as closed systems, with strong, easily recognizable boundaries.

But to be useful to a practitioner, systems theory must center on the study of increasingly complex feedback loops, meaning a much more open system. An open system implies a borderless, variable environment, impacting, and being impacted by, influences that may sometimes be quite hard to perceive. Thus, for the manager, learning to approach the organization or problems in this way can be quite formidable. Schoderbek et al. (1985, pp. 60, 61), in a discussion of the implications of systems theory for organizations, state:

> *In the process of conceptualizing goals, structure of tasks, regulatory mechanisms, environment, interdependencies of components, boundaries, subsystems, inputs, and their transformation into outputs, all begin to take on more significant meaning. Indeed, it is only through such conscious recognition of the organization as a system that one can begin to realize the full complexity that must be managed.*

One of the problems with this statement is that although it is important to consider all the things the authors describe, how does one human being actually do them? Schoderbek et al. paint the picture of a manager sitting alone in a room cogitating, making plans, studying the connections in an organization, and passing judgments without actually doing anything. This is why it is so important for the manager to get out of the office, to be a working member of several different teams, and to be constantly in a learning mode. Humans can rarely get their heads around large, complex problems without thorough knowledge of available resources and good interpersonal relationships.

John Kotter, in a series of studies on effective managers, highlighted the actual practices of managers he defined as successful. One of the more important findings was that managers actually spent a great deal of time with others: As Kotter noted: "They use their many personal assets to create agendas for their areas of responsibility, and networks of cooperative relationships with all those upon whom the job and their emerging agendas make them dependent." Additional time was spent "discussing a wide range of subjects, often in short, and disjointed conversations that are not planned in advance in any detail, in which the [manager] asks a lot of questions and seldom gives orders" (Kotter, 1986, p. 133). If this is the reality of managers' daily routines, then they intuitively act as though they think of their jobs as part of a system. To be useful, again, to managers, systems theory must be practical and answer practical needs. These practical needs center on three things: (1) how managers use systems thinking to improve their performance; (2) how managers help create an organization or department that can use systems theory to develop better departmental interrelationships; and (3) how managers use systems theory or thinking to help solve problems.

Using systems thinking to become a better manager

A useful analogy when thinking about the benefits of systems theory for managers is to imagine the difference between two scenarios. In the first, imagine you are driving down a major limited-access state highway. Your view of what is going on around you is limited to what you can see ahead of you, what you can see in the rearview mirror, and what you can see off to the sides. You are driving to a very important meeting and need to get there within the next 45 minutes, and at the rate you are going you will make it with time to spare. One mile ahead, the road curves off to the right so that you cannot see around the bend. You have no idea of conditions ahead and what you might be facing, but the weather is nice, traffic is moving well, including traffic coming in the opposite direction, and so you are not concerned. However, unbeknownst to you, a major accident has just occurred a mile past the bend up ahead. If you knew that by getting off at the next exit you could get around the accident with minimum delay, you would do so. But because you have no idea that an accident just occurred and everything appears to be going well, you do not act and you get caught in a major traffic jam as police and emergency equipment are called to the scene. You miss your business meeting and all the potential opportunities that might have come from the meeting.

In the second scenario, the same accident happens, but you are in a traffic helicopter and can see 50 miles in every direction from 8000 feet in the air. You see the accident, the cars before the bend in the road, the traffic in the other direction starting to slow down to look at the scene of the accident, and alternative routes that drivers might take to get around the accident. In short, your view of the whole scenario is greatly expanded. The bird's-eye view gives you the equivalent of a system-wide perspective that allows you to see and follow how people are reacting, from all directions, to this emergency. You may not be able to influence much, if any, of it, but you can see it all. Your knowledge of the situation and of many ramifications or alternative courses of action are greatly increased. If you were broadcasting the traffic report, you could alert people coming up on the bend in the road, suggesting they get off the highway while they can, but only if they are tuned in to your report.

A manager looking at things from a large enough perspective can frequently influence a great deal of what goes on in a positive way. If information is limited by what is immediately available, as in the case of the driver with only a two-dimensional point of view, then the manager will have a fairly limited perspective on what is actually happening. The options to act or to influence the situation will also be limited. Being experienced in looking for connections among events, or having the mindset that what one is experiencing is inherently part of a larger system of events including actions and counteractions, and counteractions to the counteractions, is very important to a manager's success. Slumping sales in a retail pharmacy may not simply be due to shortages from a supplier or allocation of shelf space, but may reflect new medical practices, new treatments, or new medical practitioners moving into the area. These factors may be affected by the changing demographics of the neighborhood, which in turn may be affected by political actions in another region of the country or even by political and economic realities in other countries. Managers employing systems thinking in their planning can examine their sales against such factors to better plan their stores' growth.

Creating a systems-thinking-oriented department or company

Managers perform a number of functions. They interact with people to gather information so that they can make decisions, help their subordinates develop their own skills so that they too can someday become managers, and bring their skills and experience to help address both opportunities and problems. Managers who practice systems thinking will serve as mentors for their subordinates, who need to develop skills in recognizing and seeking underlying systems. Peter Senge, in *The Fifth Discipline*, lobbied for the creation of what he called "learning organizations," groups, departments, or whole companies that are in a constant learning mode, looking for systems and their patterns, the systems archetypes that he maintained exist (Senge, 1990).

Managers can help develop the culture of the group for which they are responsible. For Senge, the fifth discipline is the ability to see things from a systems perspective, and it underlays the other four disciplines: personal mastery, developing mental models, having a shared vision of what you want the company to be and do, and team learning. By calling these factors "disciplines," Senge implied that managers, in addition to performing the tasks they were paid to do well, strove for personal development. This includes inviting changes to long-held mental models of the world, developing and sharing an energizing vision of their work, and encouraging the development of each member of the team. To do this, Senge maintained, managers must understand systems thinking and be able to see the interrelationships among people, departments, companies, actions, and their causes and effects.

Using systems thinking as an approach to problem solving

Beyond merely understanding the interrelationships that make up a system under study, the manager practicing a systems approach to problem solving must find the points of leverage in the system. Points of leverage are those aspects of the system where a change will impact the entire system. A point of leverage is where change is occurring and affecting the manager, but both the change and the result are removed enough that the average manager, thinking in a linear fashion, misses the connection completely.

An excellent example of this is found in a study by Leape et al. (1995), which is referred to in greater detail in Chapter 12. The study found 264 preventable adverse drug events (ADEs) for which 16 major systems failures were identified as underlying causes of the errors. Of these 16 systems failures, 7 were responsible for 78% of the errors and were due to poor information systems. Thus, assigning blame to an individual or a certain procedure would have missed the cause entirely, which was likely the way that information was disseminated in the institution. Only by approaching the analysis from a systems perspective would it be possible to correct the real cause of the errors.

For Senge, problem solving within systems thinking meant "seeing circles of influence rather than straight lines ... By tracing the flows of influence, you can see patterns that repeat themselves, time after time, making situations better or worse. From any element in a situation, you can trace arrows that represent influence on another element" (1990, p. 75). Senge developed several archetypal "circles of influence," which were different kinds of feedback loops, each representing an underlying structure to many types of problems. Analyzing them, he felt, would allow the manager to quickly recognize the type of system a problem represents and help develop solutions (see Senge, 1990, Ch. 5). In a circle of influence, one action influences another, which in turn influences another and so on, until a pattern emerges. It is that pattern, the structure underlying individual actions, that is the important part of real problem solving. When a problem emerges, if one addresses only the immediate cause of the problem, then the problem will frequently recur. The action that caused the problem to arise is only one part of the circle of influence. That action was derived from some other action, which in turn was caused by something else. Studying problems from a systems perspective can lead to a very different, more complete understanding, resulting in different ways of developing solutions to problems rather than just solving the immediate issue that arose. Just as in the two scenarios presented earlier (seeing things from the ground level in a two-dimensional way, or being up in the helicopter and seeing things from a three-dimensional perspective), systems thinking provides a much better picture of what is actually going on.

Thinking about and perceiving systems

As we made our way through the school system, from elementary through high school and into college, most of us were taught to think scientifically — in a very ordered, hierarchical manner — when approaching a problem. Two examples given here illustrate systems thinking: the first for self-practice if one is so inclined and the second an actual example from business.

To begin to get practice in systems analysis, start with something simple — a thought experiment such as those Einstein loved. Say you are sitting on your porch or patio on a pleasant summer evening and you glance over at a nice 50-year-old oak tree in your backyard. Stop for a moment and visualize the systems that tree is a part of — not only the natural systems of Earth, sky, and ground, but how the tree impacts you as well. What are some things you could do to affect the tree both directly and indirectly? Start with free association, thinking about things such as expiration, inspiration, sunlight, animals, and words such as *shade, shelter, food, wind, poetry, beauty,* and *construction.* Look for connections between that single tree and its immediate environment, how it impacts its immediate environment, and how the local environment is impacted by it. What are some of the many ways you can impact the tree, and all the systems it is part of, by any one of a myriad of actions you could do to it?

It is important that you practice seeing the connections: what influences what and where each influence leads. If this is hard for you to do, then understand that you will need practice in applying systems thinking to your business problems. It is not easy to relearn a new approach to problem solving. And I say *relearn* because, as stated at the beginning of the chapter, systems thinking is probably one of those archetypal ways of thinking that is instinctual. It was programmed out of us in school.

A fine example of systems thinking as applied to real business problems was reported by Pierre Wack in a series of articles in the *Harvard Business Review* in Fall 1985 (Wack, 1985a,b). As head of the Business Environment Division of the Royal Dutch/Shell Group Planning department in the early 1970s, Wack was instrumental in helping Shell Oil develop realistic scenarios that, alone among the top oil companies, prepared it to meet the rising cost of oil caused by the formation of Oil Producing and Exporting Countries (OPEC). The technique he helped develop at Shell is called scenario planning and at its heart involved changing the mindset of managers who previously made decisions based on typical linear thinking. Up until that time (the early 1970s), most of the managers at major oil companies worldwide had experienced enormous long-term stability in the pricing and supply of oil. Even for older employees, very little had changed in oil pricing, supply, and production. By shifting these managers' mindsets to understand the system of oil supply, including who was providing the oil and how world events at the time were likely to impact those suppliers, Wack and his group developed several scenarios of possible futures that were radically different from those being offered by the average product and marketing managers throughout the industry, not just at Royal Dutch/Shell. Through systems thinking and scenario planning, Wack and his team accurately forecasted a major disruption in both supply and pricing in the mid-1970s. The reader is referred to the articles for details and additional information on the scenario-planning process.

Conclusion

Because it is impossible for any one individual to examine more than a small part of one's environment, why understand or practice systems thinking? First, if one understands that systems thinking is a skill that can be developed, then one can work at it if so desired. Improving managers' abilities to look for the underlying systems structure of a particular problem will help them arrive at more lasting solutions and become better at creating learning environments within their groups or departments. Scenario planning, although a technique different from systems thinking, requires a systems thinking mindset to be successful. Being able to include far-ranging perspectives about problems or situations makes managers far more valuable to employees and companies as it helps them anticipate problems and develop better-fitting strategies and solutions. These skills are hallmarks of great managers, who are open to new thoughts, strategies, methods of problem solving, and ways of seeing old problems.

It is clear from research (see Senge, 1990; Bolman and Deal, 1992; Drucker, 1972) that the most successful managers think in complex ways, meaning that they flexibly adapt their management styles or their mental models to varied circumstances. Being a complex thinker is therefore usually a necessary, though probably not sufficient, characteristic of a good manager as well as employee. To foster a learning environment and to set an example as one who is constantly learning is a positive attribute. Systems thinking is a complex way of organizing our worldview and developing our problem solving style. It is a concept that we understand intuitively, yet is difficult to grasp in a way that allows us to put it into practice. In some ways, systems thinking is both intuitive and counterintuitive — intuitive because it is archetypal in nature and counterintuitive because we are not used to looking at things as wholes, particularly when popular magazines, TV programs, and news shows show us things in soundbite proportions. Nevertheless, the ability to see the system behind the problem will allow us to grasp larger perspectives and greater, more meaningful connections between events and things.

Bibliography

Birnbaum, R., *How Colleges Work: The Cybernetics of Academic Organizations and Leadership*, Jossey-Bass, San Francisco, 1988.

Bolman, L.G. and Deal, T.E., *Reframing Organizations: Artistry, Choice, and Leadership*, Jossey-Bass, San Francisco, 2003.

Burke, J., *The Pinball Effect*, Little, Brown, Boston, 1997.

Drucker, P., *Management: Tasks, Responsibilities, and Practices*, Harper & Row, New York, 1972.

Hammer, M. and Champy, J., *Reengineering the Corporation*, HarperBusiness, New York, 1993.

Kotter, J., *The General Managers*, The Free Press, New York, 1986.

Leape, L.L. et al., Systems analysis of adverse drug events, *JAMA*, 274(1), 1995, 35–43.

Liebler, G.J. and McConnell, C.R., *Management Principles for Health Professionals*, 3rd ed., Aspen Publishers, Gaithersburg, MD, 1999.

Schoderbek, P., Schoderbek, C., and Kefalas, A., *Management Systems: Conceptual Considerations*, 3rd ed., Business Publications, Plano, TX, 1985.

Senge, P., *The Fifth Discipline*, Doubleday/Currency, New York, 1990.

Wack, P., Scenarios: uncharted waters ahead, *Harv. Bus. Rev.*, September/October 1985a, pp. 73–89.

Wack, P., Scenarios: shooting the rapids, *Harv. Bus. Rev.*, November/December 1985b, pp. 139–150.

chapter three

Organizational structures

Andrew M. Peterson and David A. Ehlert

Contents

Introduction

Organizations come in a variety of shapes and sizes. Many are organized according to specialty, others by matter of convenience. The manner in which organizations are put together clearly affects how they function. There are several theories on which companies are organized, and this chapter reviews some of these theories and focuses on applications of them in professional pharmacy practice.

An organization is a group of individuals structured in such a way to work together to achieve common goals. The organizing function is designed to make the best use, in terms of efficiency and effectiveness, of the organization's resources to achieve these common goals. The organizational structure is the framework in which people are assigned jobs and responsibilities. The formal organizational structure is usually depicted by an organizational chart (Figure 3.1), which displays the job titles and

0-8493-1446-1/04/$0.00+$1.50
© 2004 by CRC Press LLC

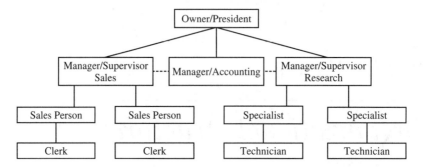

Figure 3.1 A typical organizational chart.

corresponding departments of the people within the organization. Through this graphical depiction, one can readily see the relationships and lines of authority among people and departments.

The classical organizational theory

The classical organization, the bureaucracy, was first analyzed by Max Weber in the early 1900s. Several concepts underlying the bureaucracy are specialization of labor, departmentalization, unity of command, and chain of command. These concepts, originally developed by Weber and further expanded by Henri Fayol, are based on the scientific method of analyzing processes and procedures to provide the most efficient and effective means of organizing individuals for maximum productivity. Accordingly, there are 14 points of organization and management outlined (Table 3.1). We review only a few of these points here.

Specialization of labor and departmentalization

Specialization of labor, the placement of individuals into categories based on job functions, leads to increased productivity. This increased productivity is seen by (1) an improvement in a worker's ability to do a task, resulting from a worker's concentration on one or a few tasks; (2) time saving due to minimized need for physical relocation or from adapting, or orienting, a worker to the new task; and (3) concentration on one or a few tasks increasing the likelihood of discovering easier and better methods.

Within pharmacy, there is often a specialization of labor. Specialization works not only with employees but departments as well. In pharmacy, this is seen on a large scale because there are pharmacists specializing in hospital pharmacy work and those specializing in community practice, with the subspecialization of independent vs. chain stores, and even long-term-care or managed-care pharmacy. Further, even within a given setting, pharmacists are divided based on their specialties. In hospitals, there are unit-dose phar-

Table 3.1 Fayol's Principles of Management

Authority. The right to direct and control actions of employees.

Centralization. A single, central source for decision making. Decisions are made from the top.

Discipline. Actions are governed by a strict set of rules and compliance is mandatory.

Equity. Fairness to all; does not imply equal treatment, only fair treatment.

Esprit de corps. Comradery; enthusiasm for a common goal.

Initiative. Taking on work without prompting.

Order. Each person has responsibilities and proceeds in a usual and customary manner to carry out work activities.

Personnel tenure. Dedication to the job and workers; mutual desire to stay and work at the company; longevity.

Remuneration. Fair pay for work completed.

Scalar chain (line of authority). Formal chain of command.

Specialization of labor. Workers are organized according to specialty in work function to improve productivity.

Subordination of individual interests. Workers are to focus on work.

Unity of command. Each employee has one and only one boss.

Unity of direction. Relates to centralization — orders come from the top and subordinates are to follow.

Source: Adapted from http://www.analytictech.com/mb021/fayol.htm.

macists and IV pharmacists. The IV pharmacists can be further divided into chemotherapeutic and nonchemotherapeutic.

To coordinate all these specialities, managers aid in coordinating the efforts of each division or department to produce a comprehensive work product. Weber's model suggests that such specialization is necessary and that the specific boundaries separating one department or division from another must be guided by rules, regulations, and procedures.

Unity and chain of command

In this model, it is evident that coordinating the departments of large organizations requires clear lines of authority arranged in a hierarchy. This means that all employees in the organization must know who their boss is, and all persons should always respect their boss, i.e., a chain of command. Further, there should be only one boss, i.e., unity of command. This means that only one person should be able to give subordinates orders, and people should receive orders only through their own immediate supervisors. In this way, everyone knows where the responsibilities lie, and there is assurance that orders are carried out by the best person possible.

Power and authority

Before considering specific relationships presented by an organizational design, a basis is required on which to discuss power and authority.

Sources and types of power

The literature is replete with definitions of power. Max Weber defined power as "the possibility of imposing one's will upon the behavior of others" (as cited in Fuqua et al., 2003). Others have suggested that "power is the ability to obtain compliance [or cooperation] by means of coercion, to have one's own will carried out despite resistance" (Liebler and McConnell, 1999).

Within the context of organizations, Cangemi asserted that "power is the individual's capacity to move others, to entice others, to persuade and encourage others to attain specific goals or to engage in specific behavior; it is the capacity to influence and motivate others" (as cited in Fuqua et al., 2003). Cangemi believed that successful leaders move and influence people through their power toward greater accomplishments for themselves and their organizations. Power allows organizations to function efficiently and effectively.

French and Raven classified five types of power: reward, coercive, legitimate, expert, and referent (as cited in Fuqua et al., 2003). Reward power is based on a willingness and ability to reward. Those having the ability to deliver jobs, money, or anything else that people seek will derive power. Coercive power, on the other hand, depends on the ability to administer punishment or give negative reinforcements. Legitimate power depends on a position that results in the automatic endorsement of people within that group. Expert power is based on expertise, information, and special knowledge in a given area. Part of the power of pharmacists originates in society's dependence on them for their knowledge and competency as medication use experts. Referent or charismatic power occurs when people try to emulate an individual or when they show great admiration for that person.

Legitimate, reward, and coercive powers are powers of position, or formal power. Expert and charismatic powers are considered informal or personal powers, derived from personal interactions and not by virtue of position.

Formal powers.   Legitimate power is power based on one's position. It is a formal power, bestowed on a person through appointment, selection, or election. Legitimate power allows superiors to hire or fire a person, dictate job responsibilities, and control the work of an individual by virtue of their position. In an organization, the boss has legitimate power.

Reward and coercive power are related. Reward power is based on the distribution of rewards. It involves compensating the recipient with something of value in return for work or favorable stance on an issue. For example, a manager of a pharmacy may reward a worker with a bonus for good performance. The person giving the reward holds the power, provided that the reward is of value to the recipient. Typically, managers give rewards to employees in the form of bonuses, raises, increased vacation times, and special recognitions. If the reward is of no, or little, value in relationship to the job requested, there might be no power. Conversely, coercive power involves withholding something of value, or by distributing punishments, until an action or a behavior is displayed. For example, an employee repri-manded for persistent tardiness would be experiencing a form of coercive power.

Informal powers. Expert power is power derived from a person's knowledge or expertise in a given area. Pharmacists have expert power related to drugs, particularly drug–drug interactions and adverse events. Pharmacists exercise this type of power when they call a physician to request a change in drug therapy because of a life-threatening drug–drug interaction. The pharmacist, however, must use good interpersonal skills, or charismatic power, to get the message across effectively.

Influence and authority

As noted by Liebler and McConnell (1999), "Influence is the capacity to produce effects on others or to obtain compliance, but it differs from power in the manner in which compliance is evoked. Influence differs from power in that the former is voluntary, and the latter is coercive. Authority ... is the right to issue orders, to direct action, and to command or exact compliance. It is the right given to a manager to employ resources, make commitments, and exercise control."

Max Weber discussed three forms of authority: charismatic, traditional, and rational legal. Charisma, as defined by Weber, is a "certain quality of an individual personality by virtue of which he is set apart from ordinary men and treated as endowed with supernatural, superhuman, or at least specif-ically exceptional qualities" (as cited in Lieber and McConnell, 1999). Tradi-tional authority involves a pattern of hereditary or kinship succession. Ratio-nal-legal authority is derived from formal organizations. Formal organizations in turn derive their legitimacy from the social and legal system.

Aversion to power

Although many recognize power as necessary, numerous individuals display an inherent ambivalence or distrust toward it. In fact, Kanter noted, "Power is America's last dirty word" (as cited in Pfeffer, 1992). Why are so many of us uncomfortable with power?

One reason is that all of us can identify situations and scenarios in which unchecked power was used to create undesirable effects. Power, like water, has the potential to result in both positive and negative outcomes. Water is a sustaining component of life; however, ingesting too much water can also be life threatening. The current educational system in the U.S. also helps create an aversion to power. Although power is critical in organizations, within schools interdependence is minimized and in some cases discouraged or prohibited (Pfeffer, 1992). In addition, school generally teaches us that we can achieve if we try hard and do our best. In school, achievement is gen-erally dependent on *individual* ability and effort. The academic process also ingrains in us the belief that there are right and wrong answers and that the right answer can be found at the back of the book. Unfortunately, though, we live in a world of nuances and shades of gray – rarely are there black and white answers.

Managing with power

Bennis and Nanus note that one of the major problems facing organizations at present is that individuals are reluctant to exercise power: "These days power is conspicuous by absence." Without power, leaders are unable to lead. After all, "power is the basic energy needed to initiate and sustain action," or, put another way, "the capacity to translate intention into reality and sustain it" (as cited in Pfeffer, 1992).

Despite the fact that more time is spent living with the consequences of decisions, many organizations spend an inordinate amount of time and energy in the decision-making process. Rather than getting unnecessarily bogged down in this process ("paralysis by analysis"), organizations must ensure that sufficient time is given to implementing decisions and dealing with their ramifications. As Pfeffer (1992) explains, "The important actions may not be the original choices, but rather what happens subsequently, and what actions are taken to make things work out."

Various strategies have been attempted to counteract this powerlessness phenomenon present in health care organizations. Health care literature is replete with efforts to empower the frontline health care practitioner. Empowerment is the sharing of power with those who actually do the work. For example, much has been written on the topic of shared governance within the nursing literature. There also has been recent discussion of shared governance within the profession of pharmacy.

To increase organizational power, successful leaders must develop their own personal power and be effective implementers. Power and influence are the tools required to get things done. The following strategies should be considered in managing with power:

- Manage through a shared vision or organizational culture. Such a practice will minimize the effects of hierarchical authority. Moreover, it will help engender a team spirit.
- Identify the various interests within the organization. Determine the points of view of the various individuals identified. According to Pfeffer (1992), "The real secret of success in organizations is the ability to get those who differ from us, and whom we don't necessarily like, to do what needs to be done."
- Enlist the cooperation and support of others outside the chain of command.
- Remember that formal authority is not an absolute requirement for a leader to wield power and influence.
- Understand where power comes from and how these sources of power can be developed and utilized within organizations.
- Recognize that politics is involved in innovation and change.

Line and staff authority

The bureaucratic model has led to the traditional use of lines and boxes in an organizational chart. Within the organizational chart, the reporting relationships are depicted by solid or dotted lines. The solid lines, referred to as line authority, indicate the direct authority a superior has over a subordinate. Persons with line authority over a subordinate have the ability to use all forms of power, i.e., legitimate, reward, and coercive power. The manager in this position has the ability to hire and fire a direct report, give raises to the person, or reprimand the person. In contrast, staff authority is advisory to line authority. For example, an accountant who prepares reports for the district manager has staff authority over the pharmacists within that district, but can only make recommendations to the district manager regarding actions. The accountant cannot hire or fire a pharmacist because of poor financial performance. Staff authority is usually depicted on an organizational chart as a dotted line (see Figure 3.1).

Focus of much of the classical organizational theory is on output and productivity — refining the process to be the most efficient means of producing a product. Although this was attractive to most managers, many employees felt disenfranchised with the process. Often, considerations of the employee were not taken into account. From this recognition of the human factor arose some of the modern organizational theories.

Modern organizational theories

Modern organizational theories take on a more behavioral management flavor — managing people instead of processes. In this vein, Douglas McGregor developed, in *The Human Side of Enterprise,* his dual theories of management: Theory X and Theory Y. The underlying messages in these theories are that managers maintain certain beliefs about their employees, and these beliefs affect how the managers deal with employees. Consequently, employees react to managers, at times, in manners that bring about self-fulfilling prophecies; that is, employees become what managers think they are.

Theories X, Y, and Z

Theory X states that people inherently dislike work and need to be coerced into performing a duty. Further, the theory indicates that people attempt to avoid responsibility and have relatively little ambition. They wait to be told what tasks to perform and have little or no control of or direction in their work lives. Overall, employees seek money and job security only. Theory X is considered an authoritarian style of management.

MacGregor recognized that Theory X works best in some situations. Those cases include repetitive tasks in which a high volume of output is required. Further, where following orders is important to the well-being of the organization, Theory X management style is important. Often seen as the prototype, the U.S. military is a Theory X organization. The soldiers are required to follow their superiors' orders without question.

Conversely, Theory Y states that people want to exercise self-direction and control and seek to expand their spheres of influence and accept additional responsibility. People operating under the influence of this theory tend to see job commitment as a function of rewards rather than merely of job security.

If Theory Y holds, an organization can take advantage of the motivation of its employees. By delegating authority and power, decreasing the number of levels of management, each manager will have a greater span of control and be more productive. A participative management style that involves employees in the decision-making process will also tap their creativity and provide them with more control over their work environment. Through this, employees have a greater sense of job enlargement, where the broader scope of job responsibilities adds variety and opportunities to satisfy ego needs. If properly implemented, such an environment would result in a high level of motivation and enhance employee productivity and satisfaction.

In 1981, William Ouchi developed a related motivational theory labeled Theory Z (see Venn, Theory X, Y, and Z). This theory is similar to Theories X and Y, but emphasizes more the attitudes and behaviors of the worker than the manager. The theory places a large amount of trust and responsibility with the worker; that is, responsibility for success or failure is shared between employees and management, and not only management. In many Japanese companies, employees are guaranteed a position for life, which ideally increases their loyalty to the company. Further, Japanese companies tend to take a greater interest in their employees' lives outside work. Companies operating under Theory Z tend to have more stable employment, taking care of the job security issue, and managers who tend to care about their employees, satisfying Theory Y needs.

In conclusion, Theories X and Y both work, but in different ways. On the proper occasions, Theory X can produce better short-term results. However, if people are subjected to Theory X management style consistently, it could lead to disharmony and dissatisfaction, which is counterproductive in the long term. To maintain a healthy, viable organization, managers need to keep people happy and motivated.

Using these theories about human functioning in work environments and the concepts of power and authority addressed basically, we can now explore a few organizational designs that have arisen in the past century.

Organization designs

One of the first steps in designing an organization is to determine which jobs belong in which department. This process, called job classification, allows one to determine the similarities and differences and allows jobs to be organized into larger segments, such as departments. Creating these departments allows for individuals to be grouped into manageable units. There are at least four methods to group work activities.

1. *Departmentalization by function* organizes jobs by the functions to be performed. For example, in a hospital, the department of pharmacy is created to maintain all medication-related functions for the hospital. This form of departmentalization allows the organization to gain efficiencies from combining people with similar skills, knowledge, and purposes together in common units. Figure 3.2 shows a typical hospital organizational chart, grouping workers together by function.

2. *Departmentalization by product* organizes all functions needed to make and market a particular product under one person. For example, in the pharmaceutical industry, the brand manager for a product is in charge of the marketing, research, and development functions related to the product. This allows for a coordinated and directed effort in the sales and development of the brand. Further classifications also exist, in which the company may have several cardiovascular products and may have several brand managers within the cardiovascular group.

3. *Departmentalization by geographical regions* groups jobs on the basis of territory or geography. For example, a pharmaceutical company may have its sales force organized regionally, into the northeast, southeast,

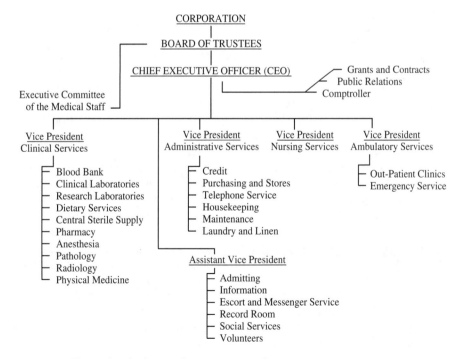

Figure 3.2 Example of a hospital organization chart.

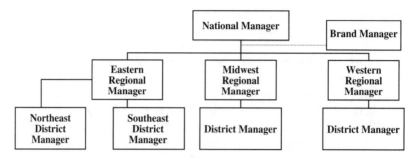

Figure 3.3 Example of a geographical organizational chart.

midwest, southwest, and northwest. This creates jobs such as regional manager for cardiovascular products (Figure 3.3).

4. *Departmentalization by customer groups* jobs on the basis of type of customer. In pharmacy, home-care or long-term-care patients represent this type of deparmentalization. Within this customer segment, the trend is to use cross-functional teams, which allow various group members chosen from different functions to work together to interdependently provide a service. Home-care organizations usually have pharmacists, nurses, pharmacy technicians, medical assistants, and others to provide the patient with the needed care.

Structure types

Organizations can be rigid, with significant structure and formality, or they can be loose, with little to no formal structure. The mechanistic organization, inherently a rigid organization, is the traditional and probably the most common structure used in medium- to large-size organizations. Mechanistic organizations have many rules and procedures, well-defined tasks, and a clear hierarchy of authority. The prototypical mechanistic organization is the bureaucracy. In mechanistic organizations, there are often multiple levels within the hierarchy, creating a "tall" organizational structure. The benefits of this type of organization are clear delineation of tasks, centralized decision making, and potential for a career ladder by which employees can progress and be promoted. Further, the specialization of labor and the functional control over the output by managers typically results in consistent productivity — up to a point. The multiple layers seen in bureaucracies, coupled with centralized decision making, make this model slow to adapt to change. This fact, coupled with the many rules and regulations associated with these organizations, creates employees who are often disillusioned by the lack of timely response and the lack of independent decision making capability. This mentality then perpetuates Theory X characteristics. In response, managers moving up the ladder continue this Theory X mentality and further perpetuate negative aspects of this style of management.

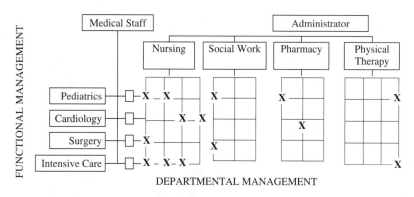

Figure 3.4 The hospital as a matrix organization.

Another form of mechanistic organization is the matrix organization. A matrix organization has a dual authority system. Employees are organized along both functional (project) and departmental lines (Figure 3.4). As such, employees report to two or more managers. Project managers have authority over activities geared toward achieving organizational goals, whereas departmental managers have authority over promotion decisions and performance reviews.

Matrix structures were developed from the aerospace industry in an effort to take advantage of employee skills when solving a difficult problem or developing a new product. This structure assigns specialists from different functional departments to work on one or more projects led by project managers. However, the matrix organization violates the unity of command principle of bureaucracies, thereby potentially creating communication and decision making conflicts as well as confusion in employee evaluation and accountability. Matrix structures may not work well as long-term strategies.

In contrast to mechanistic structures, organic structures are more flexible and more adaptable. Organic organizations use participative management as a style and are often less concerned with a clearly defined structure. Organic organizations are typically flat, with only one or two levels of management. Flat organizations emphasize a decentralized approach to decision making and encourage employee involvement in decisions. These types of organizations work well when there is a need for quick decision making and change due to the environment. In these organizations, the manager must maintain a more personal relationship, thereby adopting Theory Y characteristics, to allow for the development of trust and respect.

Professionals often work within an organic-type setting. Consider, for example, the medical team on rounds at a hospital. Typically led by a physician, multiple professions are represented on the team — medicine, nursing, pharmacy, social work, respiratory therapy, and others. In some ways, this represents a bureaucracy; that is, the physician is in charge, with staff authority over the other professionals. However, the team differs from bureaucracy in that as the team sees patients on "rounds" throughout the

hospital, decisions are made regarding the care of patients. This decentralized decision making, standardized more by the professionals themselves
than by policy and procedures, allows for more flexibility and adaptability
in the decision making when needed. In addition, even though these decisions are often costly, none of the professionals ask their bosses for permission. This professional bureaucracy is a means of allowing professionals
discriminatory decision-making power yet allowing the manager to maintain some semblance of control.

In professional bureaucracies, the patient is the central focus. All members of the organization, or team, have a primary goal in mind — for health
care professionals this is improvement in the health and well-being of the
patient. As such, health care professionals and not the managers develop the
standards by which the patient is cared for. However, one of the drawbacks
to this model is the potential for conflict among the professionals themselves,
because many of the professionals will exercise expert or charismatic power
and (most likely) the physician has primary legitimate power.

Informal organizations

Organizations come in a variety of shapes and sizes. The outward structure,
depicted by the organizational chart, can demonstrate some of the relationships that exist. However, there is also an informal organization inherent
within any formal organization. This informal organization arises within the
formal structure because of the social interaction among the organization's
members. This interaction leads to the formation of groups, both large and
small.

Small groups are the central component of the informal organization,
and membership is strongly influenced by social acceptance. Further, management has no control over the formation of these groups, but it must
recognize the negative and positive impact these groups may have on the
performance of the organization.

One of the main negative aspects of the informal organization is its
ability to thwart the efforts of the organization. It is well recognized that
what is good for the organization may not be good for the employee or a
group of employees. Increasing the prescription volume of a pharmacy without increasing staffing may seem to be a logical managerial decision, but the
pharmacist and technicians required to implement this increase might see
this as a poor decision. As such, this informal group may take steps to impede
the implementation of this objective. A good manager will take a Theory Y
approach and attempt to involve the employees in this decision-making
process, tapping the resources of the informal organization to gain support
and trust.

In contrast, the informal organization can complement and even enhance
the formal organizational structure. If there is a good relationship between
the manager and the leader of the informal group, the manager could use
this as a means to gain support for new programs, enhance communication,

and fend off rumors and misinformation. Further, the informal organization can supply the much-needed social interaction and human contact to perform work efficiently and effectively.

Conclusion

How organizations are designed and the interplay of human and other resources can provide insight into how the business operates. Organizations with strong hierarchies and mechanistic structures are good for businesses in stable environments and provide employees with orderly work environments. Businesses with organic structures will typically provide a more fluid environments in which people can work. When examining an organizational chart, one should pay attention to the line and staff authority relationships and the implied control that these relationships suggest. The structure can be organized in a variety of different fashions, along job specialty lines, geographic lines, or even product lines. However, although organizational charts may imply a formality, they may not be consistent with reality. Further, organizational charts often fail to capture the informal structure and communication that exist.

Bibliography

Anon. Bureaucracy. www.analytictech.com/bm021/bureau.htm, accessed December 16, 2002.

Anon. Classical Organization Theory. The HRM Guide Network, http://www.hrmguide.co.uk/history/classical_organization_theory.htm, accessed March 10, 2003.

Anon. Theory X and Theory Y. Net MBA Business Knowledge Center. http://www.netmba.com/mgmt/ob/motivation/mcgregor/, accessed December 29, 2003.

Fuqua HE, Payne KE, Cangemi JP. Leadership and the effective use of power. *Natl. Forum Educ. Admin. Superv. J.* 2003; 20E. http://www.nationalforum.com/12FUQUA.htm, accessed June 25, 2003.

Liebler JG, McConnell CR. Organizing. In: *Management Principles for Health Professionals*. Aspen, Gaithersburg, MD, 1999.

Longest BB. Modern health services in an organized setting. In: *Management Practices for the Health Professional*, 3rd ed. Reston Publishing, Reston, VA, 1984a, chap. 1.

Longest BB. Organizing: the framework for management. In: *Management Practices for the Health Professional*, 3rd ed. Reston Publishing, Reston, VA, 1984b, chap. 5.

McGregor D. *The Human Side of Enterprise*, Reprint edition. McGraw-Hill/Irwin, New York, 1985.

Richards B. Reflections of power. www.conncetiveintelligence.com/reflections.html, accessed March 10, 2003.

Pfeffer J. Understanding power in organizations. *Calif. Manage. Rev.* 1992; 34: 29–50.

Laschinger HK, Sabiston JA, Kutszcher L. Empowerment and staff nurse decision involvement in nursing work environments: testing Kanter's theory of structural power in organizatons. *Res. Nurs. Hlth.* 1997; 20: 341–352.

Tootelian DH, Gaedeke RM. Organizing and staffing the pharmacy. In: *Essentials of Pharmacy Management*. Mosby, St. Louis, MO, 1993.

Venn P. Theory X, Y, and Z. http://members.tripod.com/PeterVenn/brochure/complete/xyz.htm, accessed December 29, 2003.

Young D. Shared governance builds leaders, aids patient care. *Am. J. Hlth-Syst. Pharm.* 2002; 59: 2274, 2278.

chapter four

Managing professionals

David A. Ehlert

Contents

Historical context

Professions emerged in the Middle Ages when specialized practitioners began to provide nonstandardized personal services (e.g., health, religion, welfare, education) that were central to human values (Buerki and Vottero, 1996). These services required knowledge and skills that the typical client

0-8493-1446-1/04/$0.00+$1.50
© 2004 by CRC Press LLC

did not possess. In medieval times, the term *professional* was applied only to monks who professed their faith in God (Buerki and Vottero, 1996). Physicians and other modern-day health care professionals were not considered professionals in medieval times. In fact, under the Romans, medicine was considered a very low-grade occupation (Starr, 1982). It was not until late medieval times that the professionalization of medicine and pharmacy began. For instance, pharmacy can trace its professional lineage to the guild-like associations developed in the late medieval cities of Europe (Buerki and Vottero, 1996). However, the actual legal recognition and regulation of pharmacy as an occupation separate from medicine did not occur until the 13th century.

Professions and professionals

The basic contribution of health professionals is intellectual in nature in that they produce, apply, preserve, and communicate knowledge. The word *profession* literally means to "testify on behalf of" or "stand for something." Health professionals profess their commitment to serving society. Pharmacists not only profess to be experts in medication use therapy, but are also committed to helping improve a patient's quality of life through achieving optimal outcomes in medication therapy. Mrtek and Catizone describe the work of professionals as being public, special, and exclusive (as cited in Buerki and Vottero, 1996). The work of professionals is public in nature because they must demonstrate an unselfish concern for, and serve the needs of, others. The functions performed by professionals are special in nature in that they are more complex than what can be observed. For instance, there is much more to filling a prescription than what can be directly observed. Whereas an outsider could observe the acts of entering a prescription and dispensing a medication, the cognitive component of filling the prescription (e.g., screening the prescription and dose for appropriateness, checking for drug–drug, drug–disease, drug–lab, and drug–food interactions) would be indiscernible. The exclusive nature of the functions performed by professionals stems from regulations and authority granted by state and federal agencies (e.g., licensure) that determine who is permitted to practice and under what conditions.

Many individuals have identified additional characteristics and responsibilities of a professional. For instance, Abraham Flexner first identified the attributes of a profession in 1915, on which Isidor Thorner elaborated in 1942 (Buerki and Vottero, 1996). One of the attributes identified by Flexner and Thorner is that the profession provides a relatively specific function that its practitioners depend on for their livelihood and social status. Professionals perform the necessary functions for society that society cannot provide for itself. In return for this service, society grants professionals special privileges, such as internal control and autonomy in decision making within their realms of expertise. In accepting this responsibility, professionals generally rely on a code of ethics (see Appendix A for the Code of Ethics for Pharmacists) and peer review mechanisms to help maintain a standard of conduct that exceeds regulatory requirements (Buerki and Vottero, 1996).

A second attribute identified by Flexner and Thorner is that professions involve special techniques that depend on a certain set of competencies. This is closely linked with the third attribute, which states that professions are based on a specialized body of knowledge founded on general principles. Theoretical knowledge and understanding underpin the technique of every profession (Buerki and Voterro, 1996). Even though patients do not understand or use this body of knowledge directly, they do benefit from it. The fourth attribute states that the profession has ethics that put the professional's immediate interests second after attending to the needs of society. For instance, pharmacists are often required to subordinate their immediate personal needs (e.g., sleep) in the interest of patient care (e.g., being called in to prepare a stat injection after the pharmacy is closed). According to Flexner and Thorner, the fifth attribute of a profession is the existence of a formal association that fosters the ethic and improvement of performance.

Other characterizations of professionals exist. For instance, Miner refers to five characteristics of a professional (as cited in Longest, 1990):

1. *Desire to learn.* Given the explosion of medical information and estimates that knowledge and insight double in the life sciences at least every 3.5 years, it is essential for the professional to maintain a lifelong dedication to learning.
2. *Desire to work independently.* The professional maintains relationships with patients that require independent action based on an individual's best professional judgment.
3. *Desire to acquire status.* The provision of services to patients is based in part on the status granted by society, the authority granted by state and federal agencies, and the patient's recognition of the professional's expert status.
4. *Desire to help others.* The relationship between the patient and the professional is predicated on the former's expectation that the latter will help the patient as much as possible.
5. *Value-based identification within the profession.* The professional is strongly committed to the profession and upholding its conventions and ethical principles.

Professional socialization

Professional socialization is the dynamic process whereby students learn about the professional role and the expectations of performance in that role (Chalmers et al., 1995). As part of the socialization process, individuals learn formal and informal values, attitudes, beliefs, standards of practice, styles of communication, and modes of interaction as they are socialized into becoming health care professionals. "They are trained to think and act in certain ways that are consistent with the ways of their profession" (Muldary,

1983). As part of the socialization process, individuals also develop perspectives on professional identity and the ideologies that underpin the profession (Chalmers et al., 1995).

A large part of the professional socialization of pharmacists involves the training of students to provide pharmaceutical care. Although it is the subject of Chapter 15, for now readers should think of pharmaceutical care as focusing the pharmacist's abilities and responsibilities on achieving optimal outcomes in drug therapy in order improve a patient's quality of life. In addition to academic learning about drug therapy, students must learn other attributes essential to delivering pharmaceutical care, such as sensitivity and the commitment to develop caring, collaborative relationships with the patient and other care providers for the patient (Chalmers et al., 1995). To facilitate the development of these skills, professional pharmacy schools continue to emphasize the development of problem-solving skills through an emphasis on hands-on learning.

Managing health care professionals

Distinct qualities within health care

Health care is distinct from other industries in that it involves the care of human beings. Because human beings are involved, the stakes are appreciably higher, and there is an absolute necessity for a high level of quality in the work performed. Health service organizations are also unique in that a wide range of human resources is deployed in the delivery of the care, from some of the most highly trained and educated professionals and scientists to manual laborers. A high technology base and the coexistence of automated and manual work methods also help distinguish health care from other industries (Longest, 1990).

Furthermore, because of the continued growth in health care expenditures, it is no longer possible to consider only quality and ignore cost and efficiency when evaluating the delivery of health care services. National health spending is projected to reach $3.1 trillion, or approximately 18% of the gross domestic product, by 2012 (Heffler, 2003). Unstable reimbursement mechanisms and the continued erosion of reimbursement for the delivery of health care services further necessitate health care organizations to consider cost and efficiency along with quality.

Because of cost and patient care considerations, managers in health care organizations must constantly focus on maximizing quality and efficiency. Figure 4.1 depicts the dual focus required of managers in health care organizations. Managers in health care organizations must constantly strive to ensure that the provision of care falls within Quadrant I, where productivity and quality are at their highest. In the past when reimbursement for health care services was higher, efficiency was not as much of a priority, and it was easier for organizations to tolerate the provision of care that fell within Quadrant IV. Whereas the achievement of a high degree of productivity and a low to mod-

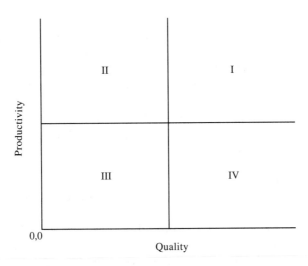

Figure 4.1 Dual focus of health care organizations.

erate level of quality may be more tolerable in other industries, the involvement of human lives in health care means that care that falls within Quadrant
II is unacceptable. The delivery of care that falls within Quadrant III is also
unacceptable in health care because both quality of care and efficiency are
compromised. Although it is commonly assumed that quality will suffer if
organizations focus to an extreme on costs, "it was found that hospitals able
to provide services in an efficient manner tend to produce services of higher
quality than those that operate less efficiently" (Longest, 1990).

Classical management theory

How does one integrate and apply an understanding of the characteristics
of professionals and the unique needs of health care into the development
of effective management techniques for health care professionals? To answer
the question, it is essential to review classical management theory. Simply
put, management is a process in which inputs, such as human and physical
resources and technology, are transformed under the influence of management into desired outputs (Longest, 1990). The five functions that comprise
the management process are planning, organizing, directing, coordinating,
and controlling. When studying the different functions of the management
process, it is helpful to think of each as an independent step. However, the
five steps are *not* a series of independent steps, but instead part of a continuous process with each step overlapping the other. The reader is referred to
Chapter 1 for a more thorough discussion of classical management theory.

Covert leadership

Although directing and controlling are frequently thought of as critical
functions in the management of human resources, the distinguishing

characteristics of professionals dictate a slightly refined management approach. For instance, because of their independence and knowledge base, professionals generally require little direction and supervision. Readers are cautioned from interpreting the preceding statement as saying that the supervision of professionals is completely unnecessary. Instead, when managing professionals, the manager must apply what is known from classical management theory and apply a sense of nuances, constraints, and limitations. Henry Mintzberg (1998) uses the term *covert leadership* to describe this concept of managing with a sense of nuances, constraints, and limitations.

Mintzberg (1998) further explains that the art of managing professionals is analogous to the work of an orchestra conductor. Mintzberg suggests that "the symphony orchestra is like many other professional organizations … in that it is structured around the work of highly trained individuals who know what they have to do and just do it." Instead of the manager providing the coordination, much of the coordination and structure comes from the profession itself. Because they are secure in what they know and how to do it, professionals, like musicians, do not need empowerment. Instead, they require an infusion of energy to help spark the inspiration necessary to complete the objectives.

Even though the profession provides some coordination and structure, management and leadership of professionals are still necessary. Without them, the system will break down. To continue the analogy of a symphony orchestra, fragmented music and even noise could result in the absence of any leadership. How then does a manager engender the support of professionals to help meet the needs of the organization?

Identifying influencers

One skill that managers of professionals need to master to be successful is the ability to identify and enlist the support of the influencers within the group. Influencers are those individuals within an organization or society to whom others turn for counsel or guidance, even though the particular individual is not identified as being in a leadership role. Bassett and Metzger (1986) describe seven strategies to identify influencers:

1. *Identify vocal people to whom others seem to listen*. The second part of this statement is critical. Vocal individuals who are frequently dismissed or ignored are not considered influencers.
2. *Identify persons who seek others out*. These individuals will often be the ones who greet and welcome new employees or comfort a distressed employee.
3. *Identify persons whom others seek out*. These individuals are the ones to whom employees turn with questions or issues.
4. *Identify the trendsetters*. People generally tend to imitate those whom they respect.

5. *Identify those who seem to reflect the consensus.* Certain individuals often stand out as representing the opinions and values of those around them.
6. *Identify those who set the work standards.* Certain individuals often set the pace for how the work is performed.
7. *Identify persons with a certain spark or charisma.* Certain individuals often emanate a certain charisma. However, it is important to note that such a spark is not always positive.

Mastering techniques to help enlist the support of influencers is as important as identifying influencers. Bassett and Metzger (1986) describe four strategies that can be used to engender the support of influencers:

1. *Ask influencers for advice or opinion.* Generally, people find it very flattering when someone in authority asks for their advice or opinion. Yet, it is important that advice should be sought from influencers only if there is a chance that the advice will be followed. In certain cases, it may be safer to seek an opinion on a potential course of action because the obligation to follow what is suggested is some-what mitigated.
2. *Give or share responsibility.* Because there are risks associated with giving or sharing responsibility, it is important not to ask for help on matters for which failure or error is unacceptable.
3. *Keep influencers in on things.* Keeping individuals in the loop about what is going on and what is being planned is critical in helping individuals respond to stress and anxiety. Moreover, when people know what is going on, they generally develop an improved outlook and favorable feelings toward those who give them the information.
4. *Match motive and reward.* One of the motivational factors for influencers is a need to be acknowledged as leaders. When influencers are recognized and respected as leaders, they will be more likely to provide additional support to meeting the overall objectives and goals.

Motivating professionals

The concept of motivation is a key determinant in influencing human behavior. At its core, motivation theory revolves around needs, actions, and goals. According to Bassett and Metzger (1986):

> *When you have a need (a wish, a desire, a want, a life requirement), it moves you into action. You stay in action, in one form or another, seeking to reach a goal that will satisfy the need. Yet action ceases when the need is satisfied, and no action takes place until the need surfaces.*

Because what another person specifically needs or wants is rarely known, applying the theory is very difficult.

Understanding what motivates people and applying that knowledge can facilitate the development and maintenance of a strong and loyal workforce. What people want from their work has changed remarkably little through the years. Surveys reveal that employees desire full appreciation for the work done, a feeling of being in on things, interesting work, and job security. Interestingly, good wages was not the highest ranked factor for employees, but instead ranked fifth (Bassett and Metzger, 1986).

A challenging job is a key motivator, especially among professionals, because it allows for a feeling of achievement, growth, responsibility, advancement, enjoyment of the work itself, and earned recognition (Longest, 1990).

Rewards and reinforcement

In 1911, Edward L. Thorndike proposed the first major theoretical treatment given to the concept of rewards and reinforcement. His law of effect states that behavior that is followed by satisfaction (reward) is more likely to recur, and behavior that is followed by discomfort (punishment) is less likely to recur. Rewards or reinforcements "are external to individuals in that they are environmental events that follow behavior." Reinforcement is therefore different from motivation in that the latter is considered an internal phenomenon (Muldary, 1983). Positive reinforcement involves the presentation of something pleasant whereas negative reinforcement involves the termination or removal of something unpleasant. Both positive and negative reinforcements serve to increase the probability that a given behavior will recur (Muldary, 1983). Managers should attempt to create situations where their employees are influenced more by positive reinforcement than by negative reinforcement.

To help satisfy employees' key needs for recognition and for feeling important, it is critical that managers acknowledge employee accomplishments. Recognition of accomplishments helps employees believe that they are accepted and approved by the institution and by their managers. It also shows them how and why they are doing useful work, and it tells them that their managers understand and appreciate their contributions (Bassett and Metzger, 1986).

In addition to recognition and praise, employees can also be rewarded through a variety of tokens including salaries, raises, promotions, bonuses, vacations, flexible scheduling, privileges, continuing education, training, equipment, and supplies. The opportunity to improve their skills through formal training and continuing education is often a powerful token for professionals (Muldary, 1983).

In granting reinforcements and rewards, managers need to be cognizant of several points. First, reinforcements and rewards need to be granted consistently and applied systematically. However, this should not be interpreted as saying that all individuals should be rewarded the same. In fact, rewarding all people the same tends to encourage mediocrity because high performers perceive that the organization does not value their extra efforts. Inaction by managers can also serve as a reinforcer. Therefore, if rewards are withheld for any reason, managers need to explain why. Continuous reinforcement is usually suboptimal because if the reinforcer is ever removed, the behavior is likely to cease quickly. As a result, the use of different schedules of reinforcement is a highly efficient way of enhancing the quality of work life and facilitating greater job satisfaction (Muldary, 1983).

The importance of communication

Even though communication is an everyday occurrence and is frequently taken for granted, it can be a key determinant in an organization's ability to achieve its objectives. Unless a manager can effectively communicate what, how, by whom, and when it is to be done, the likelihood of the objective being completed as desired is greatly diminished (Longest, 1990). The process is complicated because each communication involves at least six messages: what one means to say, what one actually says, what the other people hear, what the other people think they hear, what the other people say, and what one thinks the other people say (Bassett and Metzger, 1986). Distortion in any of the six messages can seriously impair the communication process.

Willard and Merrihue describe four principles that managers can use to ensure effective communication with their employees (as cited in Basset and Metzger, 1986). First, managers should seek to gain the confidence of their employees by being impartial and consistent, fulfilling commitments, addressing and answering any problems or concerns, representing employees' interests to others within the organization, and making it clear that the institution has a grievance process that works. Second, managers should seek to gain the respect of their employees by showing sincere interest in issues that are important to the employees, being considerate and helpful, and displaying enthusiasm about their progress. Third, there should be good upward and downward communication between managers and employees. Listening, talking, and selling skills must be developed and cultivated. Last, because half of communication is active listening, it is important to listen carefully to achieve full understanding of the information received, take action quickly based on this understanding, and communicate the results of such action. It has been said that the better the manager listens, the more the manager will inspire.

When professionals become managers

Very few people begin their careers as managers. Usually, a person is offered a management position because of past performance in some specialty or functional area. However, past success in one area does not guarantee that the person will be an effective manager. The Peter Principle states that "in a hierarchy, every person tends to rise to his [sic] level of incompetence" (McConnell, 1997). Peter recognized that good performers within a functional or specialty area tend to be singled out for promotions. He posited that "the outstanding worker at any level is likely to be promoted to the next level in the hierarchy. This process may continue until the individual reaches a level where performance is mediocre at best." Although Peter paints a rather grim picture, the situation for newly promoted managers is not as bleak as one might think. After all, management is an art, and for the most part, "the art of management is learned on the job" (Longest, 1990).

To be effective in the practice of management, new managers need to optimize their skills within three broad domains. Katz has identified the three skills as technical, human, and conceptual. Technical skill includes the ability to use the methods, techniques, and processes of a particular field. Human skill involves "the ability to get along with other people, to understand them, and to motivate and lead them in the workplace" (as cited in Longest, 1990). Conceptual skill involves the ability to visualize the factors and various interdependencies within a situation and an organization. Conceptual skill allows the manager to understand the various issues within a situation, how they fit together, and how they interact with one another. It is important to note that not all management positions utilize these three broad skills to the same degree (Figure 4.2).

Professionals and burnout

Risk factors for burnout

Health professionals experience burnout with greater frequency than people in business or industry (Muldary, 1983). Consequently, when managing professionals, it is important to understand some of the potential causes of and

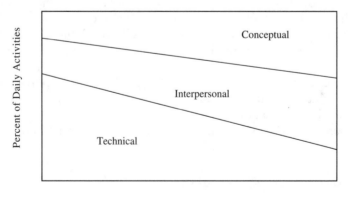

Figure 4.2 Relative application of management skills by different types of pharmacy managers.

strategies to prevent burnout in health care professionals. Although burnout in health care professionals appears to be highly individualized, Maslach and Jackson define burnout as "the loss of concern for the people with whom one is working [including] physical exhaustion [and] ... an emotional exhaustion in which the professional no longer has any positive feelings, sympathy, or respect for clients and patients" (as cited in Muldary, 1983).

Although it can be dangerous to create stereotypes or generalizations about a group, it is essential that managers of professionals understand the characteristics that predispose the professional to burnout. To reiterate, health care professionals frequently exhibit a high degree of empathy, a humanitarian orientation, a need to make an impact on the world of others, and high personal expectations about their roles and abilities to positively impact the world around them (Muldary, 1983).

The characteristics that influence individuals to become health care professionals may be the same characteristics that predispose them to burnout (Muldary, 1983). For instance, individuals with a high degree of empathy tend to be drawn to the caring professions. However, health care professionals who have a high degree of empathy tend to experience a fair amount of distress when their patients suffer. Pines and Aronson (1981) further describe that health care professionals' inherent client-centered orientation and focus predisposes them to burnout (as cited in Muldary, 1983).

Also, as described earlier in this chapter, one of the attributes of a profession is that its professionals have ethics that place their immediate interests after the needs of society. Because their individual needs and feelings are subordinated, and at times even denied, health professionals are taught to believe that it is inappropriate to satisfy their own needs while in the professional role. This results in the use of denial and repression to block the feelings and needs that are continually frustrated. In addition, health care professionals usually expect great things from themselves and often have unrealistic expectations that they will be able to function more effectively than others before them. Health care professionals frequently wind up internalizing these often unrealistic expectations that they themselves, and others, associate with their roles as health care professionals. When expectations are not met, even if through no fault of their own, health care professionals often experience anxiety and guilt, and if left unchecked, resentment and burnout may result (Muldary, 1983).

There also are certain individual personality types that if coupled with the common traits of health care professionals lend themselves to even greater risks of burnout. For instance, health care professionals who have a Type A personality or an obsessive–compulsive personality may be further predisposed to burnout. Persons with obsessive–compulsive personalities cannot accept that the world is imperfect and will strive to compensate by gaining a measure of control over anything they can. However, as the number of things that they cannot control increases, they often experience mood changes and become depressed. Individuals with obsessive–compulsive personalities also tend to be exceedingly detail-oriented and tend to focus on work and productivity at the expense of interpersonal relationships and relaxation. Moreover, they are often oriented toward achievement in order to validate their worth as human beings (Muldary, 1983).

Health care professionals plagued by self-doubt are also at higher risk for burnout. This feeling of self-doubt can be intensified whenever positive outcomes are not readily apparent in the care of patients. Another individual characteristic that can dispose an individual to burnout is a dependent personality. Dependent persons subordinate their own needs to those of others. This subordination is above and beyond that described by Flexner and Thorner as an attribute of a profession. As long as they feel needed and appreciated by the patients they serve, dependent persons will receive considerable reward from their jobs. However, if that reward is not forthcoming, the job can become more and more stressful for them. A passive–aggressive personality is another individual characteristic that can predispose an individual to burnout. Individuals demonstrating passive–aggressive behavior indirectly resist and oppose demands made on them by others (e.g., via procrastination, intentional inefficiency, or forgetfulness) to maintain or improve their current levels of performance (Muldary, 1983).

Women health care professionals may also experience unique sets of challenges and expectations within their work environments. It has been found that women "see work as a means of self-fulfillment and professional autonomy" and consequently may hold higher expectations for their careers than men (Muldary, 1983). Moreover, women health professionals who manage families in addition to their jobs have expectations to fulfill as professionals as well as wives or mothers. Expectations from each role can carry over into the other contexts and can result in little time for women to meet their personal needs. Another problem that can be experienced by women professionals is real or perceived sexism. Although beyond the scope of this chapter, real or perceived sexism can result in added frustrations and resentments that could further contribute to burnout.

Burnout and the neophyte professional

Health professionals often experience burnout within two years of beginning their jobs (Muldary, 1983). Moreover, it is frequently the neophyte professional, as opposed to the more experienced professional, who burns out during the first two years. Multiple stressors commonly experienced as part of the professional socialization process can, if left unchecked, contribute to burnout. All too often, there are discrepancies between what students learn in the somewhat idealistic environments of professional training programs and the day-to-day realities of the working world. Moreover, neophyte professionals are likely to feel stress as they encounter new situations or those for which they have not received specific training. New professionals quickly realize how much they do not know and how much they still need to learn.

If their training programs did not include stress management and conflict management techniques, new professionals can quickly become over-whelmed. Further along in the development process, health professionals can become angry and frustrated that the realities of health care are different from what they expected. They may become disillusioned when they realize that what they learned in their training programs may not occur in actual practice.

Managers of health professionals need to be aware of and watch for manifestations of these common frustrations. They need to help neophyte professionals cope with this phase of their new careers in part by helping them to realize that these feelings and experiences are not uncommon. If new professionals do not get additional guidance and support, many often begin to experience burnout. Managers need to be aware that the most enthusiastic and idealistic health professionals are often the most vulnerable to burnout (Muldary, 1983).

Managers can also help students and new professionals set realistic expectations for themselves and the work environment. Neophyte profes-sionals need to understand that it is an imperfect world and rarely are there simple solutions to problems. Moreover, outcomes of their efforts may not be immediately clear. Not all patients will get better, and in many circum-stances their efforts at helping patients may not always be appreciated. Instead of setting as an ideal that patients will always get better, it may be more realistic to set the expectation that people will not get any worse.

The manager's role

Individuals must learn how to recognize and control the stresses of their work, monitor their responses to these stressors, and adapt their behaviors accordingly (Muldary, 1983). Even though individuals are ultimately respon-sible for coping with burnout, managers must also play active roles and recognize their own influences as potential sources of stress for staff.

Availability and accessibility are critical so that staff members feel that they can approach their managers with problems. When approached with employee problems, managers need to exercise different skills. Listening is perhaps the most important strategy that a manager can use to address an employee's problems. In other cases, when a staff member's problem is related to conditions within the organization, the manager must take an advocacy role on behalf of the employee. Being an advocate demonstrates a powerful message of support and respect for staff. Confrontation is another technique that managers can use when employees need to see the role that they play in creating some of their own problems. In other situations, man-agers may need to impart information that challenges underlying assump-tions of employees. Suggestions and guidance can also be given in response to employee problems; however, advice should be doled out with caution. According to Muldary (1983), managers should answer the following ques-tions before giving advice: "What will be the consequences of providing bad advice? What will be the consequences of giving good advice? Will the individual become dependent on the [manager] for solutions? Does the [manager] know enough about the person, the problem, and the solution to give advice? Is advice giving the only recourse?"

In addition to being accessible and available, managers can help combat burnout by granting time off from work. However, managers need to be aware that this strategy can be difficult to execute at times because of the characteristic stereotypes of certain health care professionals. For instance, one of the characteristics of compulsive personalities is that "leisure does not come easily ... because it must be worked for and planned ... [Moreover,] the compulsive person does not tolerate 'doing nothing,' so even during times away from work, the person works. In many cases, the individual will often postpone vacations and leisure activities" (Muldary, 1983). Effective managers need to be vigilant about this tendency and intervene when necessary to ensure that their employees have adequate time off from work.

Conclusion

Although this chapter has discussed both theory and practical applications, there is no simple strategy for managing professionals. The management of professionals seems to follow the contingency theory of management, which states that what works best for one group in one setting may not work for another group in another setting. Part of the art of management is to use whatever methods that work to draw out the strengths of those who are managed and to direct them toward achieving objectives (Longest, 1990).

Although the following list is by no means complete or universally applicable, implementing the following steps can help facilitate the achievement of excellence in the workplace (Bassett and Metzger, 1986; Abramowitz, 2001):

- Identify how professionals' goals and efforts tie into attaining organizational objectives.
- Identify how the end results of consistent performance relate to the advancement of staff members' own careers.
- Give others credit for their ideas.
- Include professionals in developing the vision of where the organization is heading.
- Give professionals the opportunity to achieve. Achievement is a very powerful motivator.
- Help staff members create individual development plans and self-improvement goals.
- Provide frequent communication, feedback, and acknowledgment of accomplishments. Feedback in the form of annual performance evaluations is not sufficient and can cause employees to question whether

their performances are appropriate and whether they are meeting expectations.
- Express gratitude for hard work.
- Stay accessible and available.
- Recognize the human need for acceptance and approval. Demonstrate to professionals that they are accepted by their managers and the institution.
- Actively listen to staff members' problems, ideas, and concerns. Display an understanding by mirroring their ideas.
- Foster a sense of community through frequent contact with employees.
- Show interest in employees as human beings, beyond their roles as employees.

The distinguishing characteristics of professionals dictate a slightly refined management approach. As the humanist and psychoanalyst Erich Fromm once wrote, "True freedom is not the absence of structure — letting the people go off and do whatever they want — but rather a clear structure that enables people to work within established boundaries in an autonomous and creative way." Perhaps the art of leadership and managing professionals then is to facilitate true freedom.

Appendix A

Code of Ethics for Pharmacists*

Preamble

Pharmacists are health professionals who assist individuals in making the best use of medications. This Code, prepared and supported by pharmacists, is intended to state publicly the principles that form the fundamental basis of the roles and responsibilities of pharmacists. These principles, based on moral obligations and virtues, are established to guide pharmacists in relationships with patients, health professionals, and society.

I. *A pharmacist respects the covenantal relationship between the patient and pharmacist.* Considering the patient–pharmacist relationship as a covenant means that a pharmacist has moral obligations in response to the gift of trust received from society. In return for this gift, a pharmacist promises to help individuals achieve optimum benefit from their medications, to be committed to their welfare, and to maintain their trust.

II. *A pharmacist promotes the good of every patient in a caring, compassionate, and confidential manner.* A pharmacist places concern for the well-be-

---

* Copyright American Pharmaceutical Association. Adopted by the membership of the American Pharmacists Association, October 27, 1994.

ing of the patient at the center of professional practice. In doing so, a pharmacist considers needs stated by the patient as well as those defined by health science. A pharmacist is dedicated to protecting the dignity of the patient. With a caring attitude and a compassionate spirit, a pharmacist focuses on serving the patient in a private and confidential manner.

III.   *A pharmacist respects the autonomy and dignity of each patient.* A pharmacist promotes the right of self-determination and recognizes individual self-worth by encouraging patients to participate in decisions about their health. A pharmacist communicates with patients in terms that are understandable. In all cases, a pharmacist respects personal and cultural differences among patients.

IV.   *A pharmacist acts with honesty and integrity in professional relationships.* A pharmacist has a duty to tell the truth and to act with conviction of conscience. A pharmacist avoids discriminatory practices, behavior, or work conditions that impair professional judgment, and actions that compromise dedication to the best interests of patients.

V.   *A pharmacist maintains professional competence.* A pharmacist has a duty to maintain knowledge and abilities as new medications, devices, and technologies become available and as health information advances.

VI.   *A pharmacist respects the values and abilities of colleagues and other health professionals.* When appropriate, a pharmacist asks for the consultation of colleagues or other health professionals or refers the patient. A pharmacist acknowledges that colleagues and other health professionals may differ in the beliefs and values they apply to the care of the patient.

VII.   *A pharmacist serves individual, community, and societal needs.* The primary obligation of a pharmacist is to individual patients. However, the obligations of a pharmacist may at times extend beyond the individual to the community and society. In these situations, the pharmacist recognizes the responsibilities that accompany these obligations and acts accordingly.

VIII.   *A pharmacist seeks justice in the distribution of health resources.* When health resources are allocated, a pharmacist is fair and equitable, balancing the needs of patients and society.

Bibliography

Abramowitz PW. Nurturing relationships: an essential ingredient of leadership. *Am. J. Hlth.-Syst. Pharm.* 2001; 58: 479–484.

Bassett LC, Metzger N. *Achieving Excellence: A Prescription for Health Care Managers.* Aspen Publishers, Rockville, MD, 1986.

Benderev KP. The emerging leader. *Top. Hosp. Pharm. Manage.* 1986; 6: 41–45.

Buerki RA, Vottero LD. The purposes of professions in society. In: *Pharmaceutical Care.* Chapman & Hall, New York. 1996, chap.1.

Chalmers RK, Adler DS, Haddad AM, Hoffman S, Johnson JA, Woodward JMB. The essential linkage of professional socialization and pharmaceutical care. *Am. J. Pharm. Educ.* 1995; 59: 85–90.

Code of Ethics for Pharmacists. American Pharmaceutical Association. http:// www.aphanet.org/pharmcare/ethics.html, accessed June 14, 2003.

Heffler S, Smith S, Keehan S, Clemens MK, Won G, Zezza M. Health spending projections for 2002–2012. *Hlth. Aff.* 2003; 21: 207–218.

Longest BB. *Management Practices for the Health Professional,* 4th ed. Appleton-Lange, Norwalk, CT, 1990.

McConnell CR. *The Effective Health Care Supervisor,* 4th ed. Aspen Publishers, Gaithersburg, MD, 1997.

Mintzberg H. Covert leadership: notes on managing professionals. *Harv. Bus. Rev.* 1998; 76(6): 140–147.

Muldary TW. *Burnout and Health Professionals: Manifestations and Management.* Appleton-Century-Crofts, Norwalk, CT, 1983.

Starr P. *The Social Transformation of American Medicine: The Rise of a Sovereign Profession and the Making of a Vast Industry.* Basic Books, New York, 1982.

chapter five

Leadership

Andrew M. Peterson

Contents

Introduction

From the pharaohs leading Egyptians and slaves to construct the pyramids, to Jack Welch leading the United States' largest corporation into the new millennium, leadership has been the subject of considerable discussion. For centuries, theorists have attempted to determine what it takes to be a leader. All of us know a leader when we meet one, but this seemingly easy concept eludes external identification of the absolute qualities of a leader.

Leadership, the ability to influence the actions of others, is based on the interaction of three elements: the leader, the person or persons being led, and the situation in which both coexist. All three elements change, almost on a daily basis. A good leader understands each of the changes and develops strategies to work with and through others to accomplish goals.

Leaders are not always managers, and managers are not always leaders. Those who display characteristics of both are typically best for organizations. According to Bennis and Nanus (1985), "Managers are people who do things right and leaders are people who do the right thing." Managers typically focus on performing the job on behalf of the organization, routinely invoking the five functions of planning, organizing, directing, coordinating, and controlling. In contrast, leaders consider the needs of the organization as well as the needs of the people they are leading.

The purpose of leadership is to help individuals, groups, and organizations grow and develop. Individuals need leadership to aid in their personal and professional growth whereas groups need leadership to promote teamwork, cohesion, and attainment of mutually desired goals. Corporations and organizations, including professions, need leadership to assure that activities are continually aligned with collective visions and expectations.

The need for leadership in pharmacy is growing as the profession expands its horizons and takes on more patient-focused responsibilities. The rapid changes within and outside the profession require visionary leaders to help followers cope with and adjust to these changes so as to maintain and grow its professional role within society.

This chapter considers some of the theories of leadership. It is not a comprehensive analysis of the leadership literature, but instead reviews basic leadership theories and describes one model of leadership for the practicing professional.

Selected theories of leadership

Early leadership theories

Leadership studies have varied over time. Research in the early 20th century attempted to identify the traits that separate leaders from followers. The inherent traits studied include, among others, intelligence, birth order, and socioeconomic status. The learned traits, such as ambition, energy, honesty and integrity, and self-confidence, were also studied. Although many were considered quality attributes of leaders, no single trait or combination of traits fully characterized leaders. This incomplete characterization led to the investigation of other theories attempting to differentiate leaders from followers. Such theories were typically based on the task-relationship approach; that is, they looked at the situation in which the leader and the follower co-existed and then examined the interaction between the two. From this approach, theorists delineated a series of learnable behaviors that leaders exhibit in different situations.

Two of these situational theories are the situational leadership theory and the contingency theory, in which the organizational environment is considered a major factor in leader effectiveness. The path–goal theory adds another extension to these situational theories — the concept of the leader as a coach and mentor. The concepts of mentoring and coaching are more fully discussed in Chapter 7. The concept of situational leadership as developed by Paul Hersey and Kenneth Blanchard helps participants identify their own leadership styles, understand the four preferred styles available to them, and matches leadership styles to the needs of their followers (see Bennis and Nanus, 1985).

The situational leadership theory suggests that leaders assume a variety of different roles depending on the situations with which they are faced. Situational leadership is based on the premise that followers are at different readiness levels for different tasks they perform. Readiness is defined as the willingness, confidence, and ability to do a particular task. The situational leadership theory espouses four major styles that a leader assumes, depending on the readiness of the followers, both motivationally and functionally, and the resulting needed relationship. Leadership styles vary depending on the relationship the leader has with the follower as well as the complexity of the task. These styles are telling, selling, participating, and delegating. The telling style is best for inexperienced followers requiring direction and encouragement. The selling style is best used for more seasoned individuals requiring a retooling of skills, coupled with some convincing that the new way is better. The participating style is more supportive, providing a higher level of encouragement to complete a task, but the skill set of the follower is already present. Lastly, the delegating style is useful when group members are willing and able to take responsibility for completing the task.

The situational theories, both the situational leadership theory or the contingency theory, involve examining the employee's perception of the complexity of the task, which then leads to the relationship the leader must assume; that is, the relationship between the leader and the employee is contingent on the complexity of the task. (Figure 5.1). If the task is highly complex, the leader must assume a higher-level relationship with the employee; if the task has a low level of complexity, the leader should have a low-level relationship with the employee. If the task has a low level of complexity and the leader assumes a high relationship, this mismatch can lead to the employee feeling scrutinized or micromanaged. For example, an experienced pharmacist processing a routine prescription would not need her boss to check her work at each step of the process — the complexity of the task (prescription processing) is low and does not require a high-level relationship. In contrast, if an inexperienced pharmacist is given significant responsibility, without the manager around to help, this mismatch could leave the pharmacist feeling overwhelmed or swamped. The situational theories stress the complexity of the leader–follower relationship. However, these theories are unable to predict which leadership skills are necessary; they do not help identify what makes a good leader, only how a good leader should behave.

Current leadership research

Because situational theories were unable to predict which individuals would be good leaders, theorists revisited the concept of personality traits as determinants of leadership ability. These studies gave rise to the differentiation between leaders and managers and identified organizational vision as a characteristic strongly predicting leadership potential. The results indicate that good leaders have not only a vision of what the organization should be

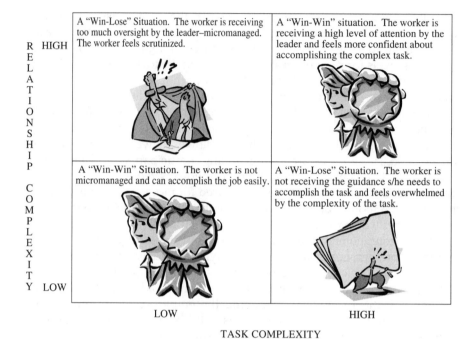

Figure 5.1 Task complexity and relationship complexity grid: outcome of matches and mismatches of complex and noncomplex situations.

doing, but also facilitate the development of a shared vision among members of the organization.

The research suggests that leaders best accomplish facilitating the shared vision when they value the human resources of their organizations. At least two contemporary theories work with this principle of valuing human resources: the transformational leadership theory and the theory of emotional intelligence.

Transformational leadership

In the 1970s, the concept of transformational leadership developed. According to this theory, researchers assert that leaders do not exhibit specific behaviors; rather there is a process by which the relationship between the leader and the follower raises both to higher levels of motivation and ethical behavior. Simply put, transformational leadership is a process through which individuals are transformed and changed. This transformation is guided by a desire to seek equality, justice, and fairness within the organization. By striving for these higher values, leaders become appealing to others and therefore develop followings. Transformational leadership goes beyond individual needs by focusing on shared visions and meeting self-actualization needs.

The transformational leadership theory focuses on the need for consensus development among followers and achievement of organizational goals.

In this model, the leader must balance the aspirations and goals of the workers with the goals of the organization. This theory of leadership concentrates on the actions and behaviors of the leader in the process of developing individuals and the organization.

Transformational leadership helps build high-quality, highly effective relationships between leaders and followers. To that end, transformational leaders display conviction to mutual goals and emphasize trust. Leaders and followers take a stand on difficult issues by presenting principles and standards relevant to both. The emphasis of the interaction is the ethical consequences of decisions. Transformational leaders become role models for followers, inculcating pride and confidence around a shared purpose. These leaders facilitate the development of a shared purpose by creating a vision of the future that is attractive to followers. Then, leaders challenge followers to perform better to achieve this shared vision. This challenge is both intellectual and emotional, often coupled with serious questioning of long-standing beliefs and traditions. By challenging these beliefs, transformational leaders encourage the development of new ideas, thus creating commitment and loyalty among workers. At the same time, these leaders treat others as individuals and consider their individual needs, abilities, and aspirations. This approach allows transformational leaders to further the employee development through purpose, directed coaching, and advising.

Emotional intelligence and leadership

Daniel Goleman (1998) introduced the concept of emotional intelligence (EI). This concept, while still controversial, merits some elucidation as it relates to leadership. Goleman and others describe EI as the "emotional needs, drives and true values of a person." EI research is akin to the trait theory of leadership, in which the core elements of successful leaders are identified. Researchers have then taken these traits and identified leadership styles in which these traits are dominant, thus allowing a person to begin using particular traits in particular situations.

Purportedly, EI largely determines the leaders' success in both their careers and relationships with others. Goleman describes EI in four separate domains: self-awareness, self-management, social awareness, and relationship management or social skill. The first two domains are personal. The last two are more externally related, characterized by an appreciation and respect for others through effective and clear communication. Each EI concept and how it relates to leadership styles is detailed in the following.

Self-awareness. Self-awareness is characterized by recognizing and understanding personal emotions and motivations and how they affect others. This understanding allows leaders to assess accurately their personal strengths and weaknesses as well as their personal value systems. This assessment allows them to know, and be comfortable with, their limitations. Armed with this knowledge, people who are self-aware become more self-confident, and therefore develop strong personal goals for self-improve-ment.

Self-management. The next step in the ladder of EI is self-management. Managing emotions, particularly disruptive emotions, is not a natural con-sequence of self-awareness. Individuals must make a conscious effort to control emotions when presented with a variety of situations. For example, a pharmacist confronted by an irate patient regarding the high cost of a medication needs to control the natural impulse to become defensive and irate as well. Self-management, not allowing disruptive emotions to interfere with professional interactions, creates an environment of trustworthiness and integrity. These are key elements to a successful leadership relationship.

Social awareness. After being able to identify and control personal emotions, a true leader also has the ability to sense the emotions of others. This skill, empathy, applies not only to the individual but the organization as well. Understanding the organizational climate is a key political skill that can be learned through proper mentoring and guidance.

Relationship management or social skill. Social skill is the culmination of the other dimensions of EI. It involves building relationships, developing teams and collaborative work relationships, and using communication as a tool for influencing and developing others to become catalysts of change. It is also key for managing conflicts. The following section applies the concepts of EI to various leadership styles.

Styles of leadership

Whereas many theories help an individual understand how to lead, there remain styles of leadership that a person can adopt to influence the actions and behaviors of others. Many of the theories discussed earlier describe some form of leadership behavior. The work of Daniel Goleman in EI provides a nice framework for describing various leadership styles.

Emotional intelligence and leadership styles

The four EIs described by Goleman can be important traits for a leader to possess, but they alone are not useful in identifying a good leader. Instead, these traits must be coupled with a repertoire of leader behaviors, or styles. Daniel Goleman has developed six styles of leadership that make use of some or all of the EIs previously described. Table 5.1 lists the leadership styles and the primary EIs associated with these styles.

Affiliative style

The affiliative style creates harmony and builds emotional bonds. This style primarily uses the external EIs of social awareness and social skill. This

Table 5.1 Styles of Leadership and Associated EIs

Affiliative
- Social awareness
- Social skill

Authoritative
- Self-awareness
- Social awareness
- Social skill

Coaching
- Self-awareness
- Social awareness
- Social skill

Coercive
- Self-management

Democratic
- Social skill

Pacesetting
- Self-management

people-come-first style works well when teams are dysfunctional or stressed (e.g., because of downsizing). The affiliative style helps create a feeling of belonging and security through feedback and reward systems. This focus on praise and belonging, though, does not help when there is poor individual performance that needs correction. The affiliative leader tends not to deliver bad news to a person, thus not allowing the employee to grow or change bad habits. The affiliative leader who lets employees arrive late to work every day without admonishing them will allow bad habits to continue and create mistrust among other employees. Therefore, the affiliative leader should, at times, employ other styles such as the authoritative or coercive style, depending on the severity of the situation.

Authoritative style

The authoritative style, although sounding "bossy," is one of the most positive styles a leader can employ. It is characterized by the self-awareness, social awareness, and social skill EIs. Individuals using the authoritative style display self-confidence, empathy, and the ability to develop cooperation and teamwork when leading the organization. A leader using this style motivates the team toward a new vision by providing a trusting environment in which individuals know their roles in achieving organizational goals. The authoritative leader develops the end vision while allowing the team to determine how to achieve the vision. This style works well in most situations, but fails when the leader is working with experts in a field who already know the vision and how to achieve it. For example, a director of pharmacy in a hospital should not typically employ an authoritative style when leading highly qualified clinical pharmacists (i.e., he or she should not tell the experts what the vision should be, but should instead use another style to help the clinical pharmacists develop their own vision of patient care).

Coaching style

Similar to the authoritative style, the coaching style uses the EIs of self-awareness, social awareness, and social skill. The focus of the coaching style is to help employees improve performance over the long term. The coach delegates responsibility to subordinates for the dual purpose of achieving outcomes and encouraging employees to develop new skills. The coach knows, though, that the task may not be accomplished quickly or, at least at first, very well. Instead, the coach uses the opportunity to provide feedback and instruction to employees. The obvious issue that exists is the leader's need to accomplish business objectives, the immediate needs vs. the employees' needs for growth and development. Balancing these two conflicting priorities takes the skill of social awareness — understanding the organization's climate and needs as well as the employees' needs. The coaching style works well when employees are ready to be coached and have identified areas for improvement. It does not work well when employees are resistant or if the business climate requires immediate results.

Coercive style

Individuals practicing the coercive style of leadership demand immediate compliance with orders and directives. This style is primarily associated with leaders displaying a strong sense of self-management, but focusing little on others. These leaders may not lack social awareness or skill; they merely do not employ these EIs routinely. When habitually used, the coercive style typically has a negative impact on employee morale and eventually productivity. The do-as-I-say attitude does not allow for employee creativity and therefore employee commitment. This creates an environment of mistrust and disrespect, which erodes the cooperation and teamwork a leader typically needs to further an organization and its people. Because of the negative impact the coercive style has on an organization, it should be employed only sparingly, such as in a crisis situation or when a poorly performing employee is not responding to education and training.

Democratic style

Democrats are participative consensus developers. They work primarily under the participative management style. Democratic leaders use social skill as the primary means for directing the activities of a group. The democratic style uses collaboration and teamwork to gain buy-in from constituents. Overall, this style has a positive impact on the climate of the organization and should be considered on par with the affiliative style in terms of effectiveness. It can be most effective when the leader is unsure of the best course of action to achieve a vision or when the leader does not have the expertise to evaluate the situation effectively. It too, though, has its drawbacks. Using a consensus-driven approach may lead to endless meetings, delayed decision making, and confusion among employees seeking a direction that the team has not developed.

Pacesetting style

In contrast to democratic leaders, pacesetters are more autocratic in their leadership style. Pacesetters set high standards of performance for themselves and expect others to have the same high standards. In this case, the pacesetting leader predominantly uses the self-management skill. The pacesetting style works well with highly motivated *and* competent teams in which there is a strong commitment to the work at hand. This style should be employed sparingly because constant pressure to keep up the pace can drive down morale. When productivity lacks because of depressed morale, pacesetters often step in and micromanage the work, indicating to the employees that they are not capable of performing the job, further eroding morale.

Newly promoted supervisors, typically well-intentioned and capable employees, tend to adopt the pacesetting style. In a short period of time, they attempt to fix every problem they encountered before the promotion. This can be disconcerting for the staff being supervised because the perception may be that the leader has become power hungry.

In summary, the authoritative and coaching styles appear best and should be used as the primary tools for leading groups and individuals. The democratic and affiliative styles are also effective, but may present additional challenges when used. Lastly, the coercive and pacesetting styles may be effective, but should be used sparingly because they have an overall negative impact on the culture when employed routinely.

Conclusion

The literature reveals that effective leadership in an organization is critical. Early examinations of leaders reported differences between leaders and followers. The early trait theories failed to predict accurately the inherent qualities of a leader. Subsequent leadership studies differentiated effective leader behaviors from noneffective leader behaviors. As such, leadership was recognized as a complex interaction among the leader, the follower, and the surrounding situation. More recent studies assert that a shared vision and collaboration with followers are important characteristics of effective leaders.

In summary, the concept of transformation leadership and the EI theory allow one to see how the behavior of the leader affects the behavior of the follower. Valuing the human aspect of the follower, that is, identifying with and appreciating the emotional and professional needs of the follower, is a key aspect of an effective leader. The transformational theory of leadership espouses a moral and ethical balance to leadership, whereas the EI theory supports the recognition of the emotional connection between the follower and the leader. According to the EI theory, there are at least six different styles of leadership, with the authoritative style typically the most effective when consistently applied. However, the coaching and affiliative styles of leadership are also effective. The pacesetting and coercive styles are effective only when used sparingly and in specific situations.

Bibliography

Bass B, From transactional to transformational leadership: learning to share the vision, *Organ. Dynam.*, Winter 1990.

Bennis WG, Nanus B. Leaders: the strategies for taking charge. Harper & Row, New York, 1985.

Bolman L, Deal T. *Reframing Organizations*. Jossey-Bass, San Francisco, 1991.

Goleman D. Leadership that gets results. *Harv. Bus. Rev.* March/April 2000, 78–90.

Goleman D. What makes a leader? *Harv. Bus. Rev.* November/December 1998, 93–102.

Kouzes JM, Posner BZ. *The Leadership Challenge*. Jossey-Bass, San Francisco, 1987.

Mintzberg H. Covert leadership: notes on managing professionals. *Harv. Bus. Rev.* November/December 1998, 140–147.

Simmons S, Sommons JC. *Measuring Emotional Intelligence: The Groundbreaking Guide to Applying the Principles of Emotional Intelligence*. Summit Publishing, Arlington, TX, 1997.

Tannenbaum R, Schmidt WH. How to choose a leadership pattern. *Harv. Bus. Rev.* 1973; 51(3): 162–172.

chapter six

Employee recruitment, retention, and compensation

Ellen Fernberger

Contents

This chapter focuses on recruiting, retaining, and compensating top talent. Although most organizations have specific guidelines and procedures, the core features of their strategies are similar.

Before any organization can look at employee recruitment, retention, and compensation, it must first understand the economic trends in the current marketplace. These trends will have a significant impact on these three keys to an organization's success. Organizations must answer these questions: How strong is the economy? What is the unemployment rate? In what fields is unemployment the highest? In the 1950s and 1960s, there was a severe shortage of engineers. Jobs were plentiful, and qualified candidates had their pick of employment opportunities. This, in turn, drove more and more students into engineering majors, which then caused a glut in the marketplace. The same cycle occurred in the high-tech industry in the 1980s and 1990s. Now, with the demise of the dotcoms and a significant influx of graduates in the technology fields, jobs are more and more difficult to come by.

Also, important demographic trends need to be assessed. For example, as the baby-boomer generation ages and begins to retire, a corresponding gap in available talent with extensive experience is developing. Will there be a reduction in the need for experienced talent or will that need also diminish? In the 2002 Workplace Demographic Trends Survey conducted by the Society for Human Resource Management (SHRM), organizations cited four key demographic trends affecting the workplace that have significant impact on their ability to staff and retain talent and to manage that talent:

- Aging population
- Ethnically diverse population
- Increase of women in the workplace
- Changing family makeup

Coupled with these demographic trends are attitudinal trends about the workplace and loyalty to an employer. The average number of years that an individual remains with an employer continues to drop. Generational differences also have strong impacts on this statistic. Only a couple of years ago, the average duration of an employment relationship was 5 years. That has now diminished to $3\frac{1}{2}$ years. Studies show that young workers, those born after the baby boomers, will hold at least 7 different jobs by the time they turn 30. By the end of their careers, they will have had an average of 15 different jobs. In a study conducted by the SHRM in 2001, only 24% of U.S. employees planned to stay with their current employer for at least 2 years.

These statistics tell employers that developing methods to accurately evaluate potential candidates, and then retain that talent once employed, is increasingly difficult yet more important than ever before. Even during these times of growing unemployment, attracting and retaining talent can impact a company's bottom-line financial success. Recruiting to fill positions costs time and money, and vacancies affect production.

Recruitment

In today's marketplace, employers cannot leave recruitment to chance. The cost of a negligent hire to an organization can easily be one to three times the salary for that position. If litigation ensues, the cost can be hundreds of thousands.

Hiring qualified candidates requires a major investment of both time and resources. There are five primary steps to the recruiting process:

- Develop a complete, up-to-date job description.
- Determine the advertising medium you will use to recruit for the position.

- Screen job applicants and plan interviews.
- Interview job candidates.
- Conduct background checks — at minimum, check references and confirm education and certification.

Develop a comprehensive and up-to-date job description

Before beginning any recruitment process, a thorough and comprehensive outline of the position must be created. Whenever possible, a complete, up-to-date job description should be prepared. This includes three key elements:

- What are the roles and responsibilities of this position? List the most important areas first and then follow up with secondary responsibilities.
- What kind of previous work experience is necessary for the position? Is this an entry-level, an intermediate, or a senior-level position? Note the minimum level of experience necessary to effectively perform the position.
- What levels of education and certification are necessary? Can significant work experience offset education?

Be honest and realistic when assessing these elements.

Determine the advertising medium

The next step in the recruiting process involves determining the advertising medium. How will you let prospective candidates know that this position is available? Are there qualified candidates internal to your organization? Many organizations have internal posting avenues: ways in which employees can learn about open positions within the organization. Recruiting resources include the following:

- Employment or recruiting agencies. They are readily available, but can be expensive.
- Electronic postings on job boards. They are abundant, such as on Monster.com, HotJobs.com, CareerMart.com, Dice.com (specializing in IT jobs), and HigherEdJobs.com (specializing in college and university jobs). In addition, many work-affiliated associations and organizations have electronic job-posting boards. In pharmacy, this might include professional organizations such as the American Pharmaceutical Association (www.aphanet.org) or the American Society of Health-System Pharmacists (ww.ashp.org). Although online recruiting resources are abundant, this medium may or may not be appropriate for all types of positions.
- Help-wanted advertisements in print media.
- Job fairs.

Screen job applicants and plan interviews

Start with the job description

You have advertised a vacant position and received a stack of applications that seem to meet or exceed the minimum qualifications for the job. Now it is time to begin narrowing the pool down to a handful of finalist candidates to interview. How do you approach the project?

At this juncture you have a comprehensive and up-to-date job description. Use that description as the basis for your thinking. You are looking for candidates who demonstrate clear evidence that they have performed comparable work and have the skills and background to do the job for which you are hiring.

The job description defines what you consider to be the essential criteria for doing the job — and for doing it well. Use these criteria to objectively evaluate each candidate's qualifications.

Develop a criteria chart

Before looking at any application, consider developing a chart (see Appendix A). List the names of the candidates across the top. Then list down the side the following criteria, taken directly from the job description:

- Education requirements
- Years-of-experience requirements
- Five or ten most important job duties or responsibilities of the position
- Five or ten most critical technical skills or competencies required of the position
- Five or ten most critical interpersonal or interactive skills required of the position

Rank the candidates

In the resulting grid, rank each candidate on a scale of 0 to 5, based on the evidence that they possess the skills or have performed duties required of the job.

Making a grid has a number of advantages. It creates an automatic first set of notes that you can refer back to during the interview process. It also allows you to concentrate on one applicant at a time, instead of trying to juggle and compare everyone simultaneously. If an unsuccessful candidate files a discrimination complaint against you for failure to hire, a grid creates a handy document that can help establish that you used legitimate, job-related criteria (rather than illegal ones such as race, gender, or age) in making your decisions.

Before filling in the chart, however, consider the following. Take a first glance through every application without looking at names. This will give some idea of the overall skills and qualifications available in the applicant pool and help you estimate an average level among the candidates' skills and experience. The average is considered 3 on the scale. Doing this will help you avoid giving the first application you see a 5 (or a 1) and then picking up the second application and wanting to give an even higher (or lower) score. After you have a sense of the average, shuffle the applications and review and score them individually in random order.

Second, give points only when there is direct evidence that a skill, knowledge, or experience exists. Be careful not to infer a skill that may or may not be there. The applicants are responsible for telling you what they know how to do; you need not guess or assume. If there is no evidence one way or the other on the existence of a certain skill or experience, give no points or note "NE" (no evidence) in the grid. Total the points across the bottom of the grid.

Watch for red flags and note questions

While reviewing, have sheets of paper handy, one for each applicant. Make notes as you go of questions that come to mind. Watch for red flags, such as unexplained gaps in employment history or inconsistent information. Be cautious of missing or vague dates and of minimal or questionable descriptions of responsibilities. If the position requires good written or verbal communication skills, for example, watch for carelessness such as typographical errors, poor grammar, or lack of clarity. You will want to pursue these issues with the candidate if you decide to interview. Attach your notes to each set of application materials for later reference.

Prepare for the interviews

Once you have narrowed down your pool to three or four strong candidates, schedule interviews. But before you bring in your first applicant, carry out preliminary planning to ensure a successful interview process.

Write interview questions in advance

Job interviews are stressful, not just for the candidate but also for the interviewer. Interviewing is not something that most hiring supervisors do often enough to develop great comfort.

Recognize that good interview questions seldom magically pop into your head during an interview — you cannot really listen to a candidate's answer to one question if you are trying to think up the next question at the same time. So it is always a good idea to develop in advance a written set of core questions that you will ask every candidate.

By asking all candidates the same basic set of core questions in exactly the same manner, you give each candidate an equal opportunity to speak about the things you are interested in, receive comparable information on all candidates, and reduce your legal risk if your hiring decision is challenged by a candidate alleging differential treatment during an interview.

Write criteria-based questions

The questions you write should be derived directly from the criteria you articulated in the job description. The questions should evoke from the candidates revealing information about the technical skills they have, how they handle interactions with others, their previous work, and how all this compares with your needs. Develop at least 10 or more good questions that will help you evaluate how the person would perform the job.

If you are interviewing for a secretary, for example, you can ask criteria-based questions such as:

- "This position requires that you keep track of ordering supplies and equipment and make sure we stay within budget. Describe a time when you have had to do something similar in other jobs."
- "This position supports the work of eight staff members, all of whom want their work done yesterday — and ahead of everyone else's. Have you ever had a job where you have had to handle many busy professionals with competing priorities? If so, what were your strategies for maintaining successful relationships?"

Write open-ended and behavior-based questions

In addition to designing questions that reflect the essential functions of the job, design the questions in a way that will elicit genuine, thoughtful, and detailed responses rather than "canned" answers. Open-ended, behavior-based questions cannot be answered by a "yes" or "no," or by a brief statement of facts. The generals begin with words or phrases such as "why," "tell me about," "describe," or "how." Open-ended, behavior-based questions require individuals to tell you stories about how they have handled specific situations in the past, situations comparable to those they will face in the position you offer.

For example, for a position requiring strong customer-service skills, you might require candidates to describe a specific incident when they were confronted by an irate customer and specifically how they handled the situation.

Avoid hypothetical questions. Do not ask, "How *would* you handle XXX?" but rather, "How *have* you handled XXX?" You do not want candidates to give you speculative answers about how they might handle a situation in a perfect case; rather, you want to know how they have really handled such situations. Remember, the best predictor of future behavior is past behavior. See Table 6.1 for examples of behavior-based questions.

Because open-ended questions force candidates to give expansive answers, and therefore do most of the talking, they should be the predominant types of questions used.

Often, however, it is necessary to verify certain facts in a candidate's interview. In this case, close-ended questions provide an efficient means of

Table 6.1   Behavior-Based Questions

The best way to get at past behavior is to phrase your questions along the following lines:

- This job will require XXX. Talk to me about a time when you have done XXX, and describe for me how you did it successfully.
- How did you handle a situation like XXX in your last job? Give me some specific examples.
- Describe the experience you have had doing XXX.
- What types of tasks do you handle well on your own, and what things do you find more comfortable with structured supervision?
- In this job you will interact with XXX types of people in XXX types of situations. Compare that to what you have done before.
- What would your current boss describe as your real strengths, and what would he or she likely describe as areas where you would benefit from constructive coaching or mentoring?
- Here is something about your work history that I wondered about as I went through your application materials. Can you help me understand it?

doing this. Close-ended questions are typically answered by a "yes" or "no," or a brief statement of facts. Close-ended questions generally begin with words and phrases such as "did/do you," "can you," or "when" (e.g., "Do you have a Bachelors degree?").

Write job-related and nondiscriminatory questions

Avoid any questions that are not directly related to the essential functions of the position or that may be construed as discriminatory. In general, it is inappropriate to ask questions about an individual's race, color, religion, sex, or national or ethnic origin (Title VII of the Civil Rights Act of 1964), their age (Age Discrimination in Employment Act of 1967), or disability status (Rehabilitation Act of 1973 and the Americans with Disabilities Act of 1990), as well as their marital status, sexual orientation, or parenting responsibilities.

If candidates volunteer personal information about one of these topics during an interview, it is best to stop them and inform them that such information is not relevant to the position and will not be considered in the decision. Document your comments in interview notes. Courts have held that it is the employer's responsibility to control the interview, and if you allow such information to be discussed, the reasons you did so may be considered discriminatory. Table 6.2 lists appropriate and inappropriate interview questions.

Decide on phone or in-person interviews

Once you have developed your core interview questions, consider whether you want to conduct telephone interviews before inviting people to in-person

Table 6.2 Appropriate and Inappropriate Interview Questions

Topic	Examples of Appropriate Interview Questions (If Asked of All Candidates)	Examples of Inappropriate Interview Questions
Age	• Are you 18 years of age or older? • If under 18, you may need a work permit. Do you have one?	• How old are you? • Are you between the ages of 18 and 65? • How many years do you plan to work before retirement?
Birthplace	• Are you eligible to work in the U.S.?	• Where were you born? • Where is your family from?
Citizenship	• Are you eligible to work in the U.S.?	• Are you a U.S. citizen? • Do you hold citizenship in any country other than the U.S.?
Criminal history	• Have you ever been convicted of a crime? If so, is the nature of the conviction relevant to this job?	• Have you ever been arrested? • Have you ever been in jail?
Disability and health status	• Can you perform the essential requirements of this job, with or without reasonable accommodation?	• Do you have any disabilities? • Do you have any conditions that might require accommodation? • What is your medical history? • Have you ever filed a workers' compensation claim at a former employer?
Family and children	**There are no appropriate questions with regard to family.**	• Where does your spouse work? • Are you the primary wage earner for your family? • Do you have children? • What are your child care arrangements? • Would you quit a job to have children?
Financial status	• Have you had financial responsibilities with other employers that are comparable to those required for this job? If so, were there ever any documented problems concerning your handling of the organization's financial resources for which you were responsible?	• How is your credit history? • Have you ever declared bankruptcy? • Have your wages ever been garnished?
Gender	**There are no appropriate questions with regard to gender.**	• Do you ever plan to quit to be a stay-at-home mom? • How does your husband feel about your working? • Are you male or female?
Language	• What is your level of fluency in the languages required to effectively perform this position (e.g., for a foreign-language instructor)?	• What is your native language? • What languages do you speak?

Table 6.2 Appropriate and Inappropriate Interview Questions (continued)

Topic	Examples of Appropriate Interview Questions (If Asked of All Candidates)	Examples of Inappropriate Interview Questions
Marital status	**There are no appropriate questions with regard to marital status.**	• Are you married, single, divorced, separated, or widowed? • Are you living with someone? • Do you have a same-sex partner? • Are you a single parent?
Military status	• What training or experience gained in your military service is relevant to this job?	• Was your discharge honorable? • Have you ever served in a foreign military?
Name	• Are there other names under which you have worked or attended school that are needed to verify your academic credentials or prior work history?	• What is your maiden name? • Have you ever changed your name? • That is an unusual name, what is its origin?
National origin	• Are you eligible to work in the U.S.?	• What is your lineage, ancestry, national origin, nationality, or parentage?
Organizational affiliations	• Are you a member of any professional, trade, or service associations that are directly related to the requirements of this job?	• Are you a member of any social clubs, fraternities, sororities, lodges, political organizations, teams, or religious organizations?
Physical characteristics	• Can you perform the essential physical requirements of this position, with or without reasonable accommodation?	• How tall are you? • How much do you weigh? • What color are your eyes or hair?
References	• Can you give me the name of an individual familiar with your work who can provide a job reference?	• Can you give me the name of your pastor or religious leader as a reference?
Relatives	• Are you related to anyone who is an employee or board member of this organization?	• To whom are you related?
Religion	• Are you available to work on the days and shifts expected of this position? • Are you able to perform the essential functions of this position, with or without reasonable accommodation?	• What is your religious affiliation? • What holidays do you observe? • Does your religion prohibit you from doing any part of this job?
Salary level	• This position falls in a hiring range of approximately $XXX. Are you interested in the position in that range?	• What is the lowest salary you will work for?
Substance abuse	• Do you currently use any illegal substances? • Do you currently use any legal substances in an illegal way?	• Do you have a history of alcohol or drug abuse? • Do you smoke? • Do you drink? • Are you taking any medications?

interviews. Preliminary phone interviews can be especially helpful in situations where many applicants look qualified on paper, and you want to narrow down the pool to a few top candidates, or candidates who otherwise would have to come in from out of town.

Schedule candidates

Scheduling enough time to conduct interviews of substance can save time and money for both your organization and the candidate. Handle all applicants consistently: if you decide to interview some candidates by phone, then conduct only phone interviews so that all interviewed candidates are treated equitably.

Telephone interviews should be scheduled in advance, like in-person interviews, so that candidates have time to prepare. Of course, if face-to-face interactive skills are essential for the job, a phone interview may not be the best option, even as a preliminary screening process. Even if you do conduct preliminary phone interviews, you will almost certainly want to invite the finalists to visit in person.

For most positions, it is virtually impossible to conduct a thoughtful and comprehensive interview, with behavior-based questions and answers, in less than one hour. Most professional positions, especially those that require several years of experience or those that involve interviews with multiple reviewers, take considerably more time.

If a candidate lives in your local community, generally a phone call is sufficient to schedule an interview. When calling candidates, be prepared to provide the following information:

- Directions to the location of the interview, and information on where they should park if driving
- Date, time, and expected duration of the interview
- Interview format (whether it will be one-on-one, with a group, etc.)
- Any materials they should bring to complete or supplement their application (e.g., portfolio of work samples, letters of recommendation, transcripts)
- Interview itinerary (when the candidates will be involved in several interview meetings)

For information on how to conduct useful and legal job interviews, see the section "Interviewing Job Candidates."

Involve relevant others

In addition to the immediate supervisor, consider involving others in the interview process, such as peer coworkers, primary constituents or users of the position's services, or subordinates who will report to the position. Ensure that these people too know the basics of legal and effective interviewing. They should ask all candidates the same core questions and keep their notes.

One advantage of involving others is the wealth of perspectives that multiple opinions can provide. Another advantage is that people able to provide feedback on the selection may have a more vested interest in helping the new employee to succeed as a member of the team.

Give finalists a copy of the job description

We previously discussed why it is important to prepare a job description or job outline, from the employer's perspective, at the beginning of the recruiting process. It is equally important to provide the candidates with a copy of that job description or outline. You want the candidates to really understand the job for which they are applying, so that both you and they can assess whether their skills and experiences are a good match for your needs. This will help keep the interview focused on the job responsibilities and the technical skills and competencies needed to be successful; further, the job description will provide an opportunity for the candidates to ask informed questions to clarify their own understanding of the job.

If you have not previously provided a copy of the job description or outline to the candidate, give them a copy before the interview. Then give the candidates 10 to 15 minutes to review the job description and a quiet space to look at the materials and organize their thoughts. This is the time when a good job description is critical; it becomes the basis on which both you and the candidates will assess their appropriateness for the job.

Can skill tests be conducted?

When evaluating individuals' abilities to perform technical or physical skills, you may wonder whether it is wise to have them take a test of some sort. Unfortunately, tests can be legally problematic unless they have been determined to be both reliable and internally valid. Other than the standard keyboarding program tests for positions that require typing or data entry skills, grammar and spelling tests, and basic math tests, there are few validated tests available in the marketplace.

That does not unilaterally prohibit you from asking applicants to demonstrate how they would perform certain tasks. A demonstration is different from a test in that it does not have a passing or failing score or a cutoff; it just provides you with a piece of information you can use in considering the applicants. However, you should exercise caution even in asking candidates to demonstrate skills. First, if you ask one applicant, you must ask all of them. Second, you must ask individuals to demonstrate only those skills that represent essential functions of the job. Third, a request for a demonstration must be accompanied by an offer to allow candidates to demonstrate the skill with or without reasonable accommodation, which may be required by individuals with a disability, and which, once requested, you may be obliged to provide. Therefore, exercise caution before taking the path of skill demonstration.

Communicate a time frame for the interview
It is important to give applicants a reasonable expectation of how long you will need to conduct the interview. They have lives too and will need to plan and schedule a realistic amount of time. Once you say, "Plan on two hours (or two days)," stick to it.

Interviewing job candidates

The process begins
You have narrowed your applicant pool down to a few top candidates. You have planned the interview process and your desired outcomes, prepared some insightful interview questions, and are now ready to meet with the candidates who look best on paper. There is far more to people than what appears on their resumes and application forms, and the interview is your chance to really explore in depth who the persons are, how they can contribute to the organization, and whether they are a good match for your needs and your goals as a manager.

Make the candidates feel welcome
When candidates come for the interviews, break the ice by being warm and welcoming. Offer coffee, offer to take their coats, and ask whether they had any trouble finding your office. A couple minutes of pleasant general talk will set a positive tone for the interviews. But do not get off-track — the limited time together is too valuable to waste on nonjob-related small talk.

Arrange for privacy and adequate interview time
Make sure you have a private place for the interviews. Forward phone calls and make other arrangements so that you are not interrupted. Nothing is more disconcerting to a candidate than a hiring manager who cannot focus on the interview because of incoming distractions. A good interview takes at least an hour. Make sure you budget enough time to get a good sense of this person who might be joining you for the better portion of your weekly waking hours.

Give the candidates an overview of the meeting
At the start of the interview, take a couple of minutes to highlight the essential functions of the job. Explain why this position is important to the accomplishment of your organization's goals and objectives.

Then explain that you will be using a set of prepared questions as a basis for the interview and that you will be taking notes. Ask the candidates to bear with you if you need a few minutes every now and then to jot down their comments or your thoughts; explain that your notes will be helpful later as you compare all the candidates. Encourage them to ask you questions that will help them better understand and evaluate the job.

Ask all candidates the same core questions

Asking all candidates the same core questions helps ensure that you receive consistent and comparable information from which you can make a defensible hiring decision. However, it is okay, even desirable, to ask follow-up questions that will vary by individual if you are seeking clarification of the candidates' responses or their specific work backgrounds.

Ask questions that elicit detailed, real-life responses

The best kinds of questions are those that elicit descriptive, real-life responses from the candidates. These questions, prepared in advance, will help get the candidates to describe situations in vivid detail, as if they are replaying a movie in their minds while describing past work experiences to you. This can be difficult for candidates. Sometimes it is hard to come up with good examples of past performance during a pressure situation such as an interview. So do not be surprised if their first tendencies are to give generalized responses such as, "I would probably just…." Such responses are merely speculative — how they think they might ideally react or how they think you want them to react. So do not settle for nonspecific responses. Explain to the candidates that you want to hear about specific incidents and examples. Acknowledge that answering such questions takes longer, assure them that they can take their time before answering, and then wait.

Wait for a good answer and avoid overtalking

Waiting in silence can be awkward for both you and the candidates. Social environments usually encourage us to fill in silences with conversation. Resist the temptation because you will distract the individuals' concentration, and you may even inadvertently prompt the candidates with clues to the answers you want to hear rather than their own answers. Once you have posed a question, allow the candidates time to think about the response, even if they seem to struggle a bit trying to think of something. Once you break the silence or move to another question, you have excused the candidates from demonstrating that they have the skills required for the position you offer.

Some candidates are natural talkers and can fill silences without actually answering questions. If candidates talk but get off track in answering a question, simply steer them back on course by saying, "I appreciate that comment, but let me make sure I understand specifically how you…."

Ask the hard questions

Just because a question may be difficult or uncomfortable to answer does not make it inappropriate or discriminatory to ask. Supervisors are sometimes reluctant to ask candidates why they left previous positions. Candidates will sometimes list stress, personality conflict, or interest in better opportunities as a reason for leaving. You can ask them about specific aspects of previous positions that they found difficult. If those same factors exist in the position you offer, the candidates may not be a good match. Sometimes, however, the circumstances that caused problems for them in the past are not present in the job you offer or were personal and have been resolved. You need this information to make a good hiring decision.

Likewise, it may be necessary to have candidates explain criminal convictions listed on their applications. Depending on how relevant the convictions may be to your position and how recently they occurred, you may choose to factor the information into your decision. There is cause for caution, however. Your questioning may reveal information that may not be used to screen out an applicant. You may learn, for example, that an individual had an arrest that did not lead to a conviction, or that an individual had a conviction on a matter that is not apparently relevant to your position. If that is the case, do not use such information in a decision not to hire. If you have any questions, consult with your human resources (HR) department or legal counsel before making a hiring decision or communicating with the candidate.

Keep all interview notes

Take comprehensive interview notes that document the candidates' verbal and nonverbal responses. Use your notes later to help determine why you did, or did not, select a candidate. Besides refreshing your memory of each applicant at the end of the interview process, notes are important documentation that you conducted a defensible interview, asking comparable questions of each candidate and asking job-related questions only. Be careful: personal comments about an applicant's ethnicity, appearance, personal habits, or personality, for example, are both inappropriate and indefensible if there is any subsequent legal action.

Maintain detailed documentation of all interviews for at least three years. Your interview notes may be your only way of reconstructing the interview and the factors that led you to the decision of not hiring a particular candidate. Unsuccessful candidates may file complaints even two or three years after you have interviewed them. By that time, it is possible that you will not even remember them. You may keep your notes in your files, or you may send them to your HR department for the position recruitment file.

As you take notes, however, be sensitive to your applicants. For candidates, it can be disconcerting if the interviewer is constantly looking down and writing. Make frequent eye contact and acknowledge that you are listening carefully. By letting candidates know in advance that you will be asking the same core questions and taking notes for each applicant, you can limit their anxieties and create an environment that communicates that you intend to be fair and objective in your decision making.

If you involve others in the interviewing process, make sure they follow the same procedures outlined.

Deflect irrelevant information volunteered by candidates

During interviews, even if you do not ask inappropriate questions, candidates may volunteer information that would be inappropriate for you to use in making your hiring decision. For example, they may tell you that they have young children, use public transportation, are pregnant, or are over 60 years of age. You cannot assume that such factors might impair their work performance. If such information is volunteered, you can say something like, "That is not information that I would consider as part of my hiring decision. The only thing I need to know is whether you can satisfactorily perform the job as it is been described to you. Can you?" Then record in your notes the transaction and how you handled it.

Let the candidates ask questions and tell the truth

Interested, engaged candidates will wonder about the job and its specifics. Encourage them to ask the questions on their minds. Be open and honest in describing the challenges that will face them if they take the position, as well as all the advantages of working there. You want your candidates to have a realistic understanding about what life will be like if they take this job — the last thing you want is to paint an unrealistically rosy picture of the work and the workplace and then present a new employee with unexpected disappointments. It is much better to let candidates know what they are getting themselves into (both upsides and downsides), so they can make informed decisions about whether they are right for the job. The right candidate will be the one who can handle the stresses and challenges as well as the joys of the job.

Share your decision timelines

A good interview will leave both you and the candidate feeling like you have a good sense of the potential match between the person and the position. At the end of the interview, let the candidates know how things will proceed from there: whether you have other candidates yet to interview and how long you expect it will be before a hiring decision can be made. Let them know that if they are finalist candidates, you will be checking their employment references and academic backgrounds. (See the section "Background and Reference Checks on Job Candidates" for more information.)

Assure the candidates that you will let them know one way or the other about the outcome of your hiring decision. And then make sure you do so

— plan to notify all unsuccessful candidates with a phone call or a note that you have made a decision to hire another qualified candidate.

Background and reference checks on job candidates

Always check references

As the hiring supervisor, you need to check references once you have narrowed down your candidate field to a couple of finalists. Always check references. Unfortunately, people are not always exactly as they portray themselves to be, and you owe it to yourself and to your organization to know whom you are hiring.

Should you also conduct a background check?

Many organizations currently also conduct background checks. This may include a criminal background check and a credit-history check. It is important for your organization to include a statement on its employment application form advising candidates that a criminal background check will be conducted. Candidates should also sign and date the application form, stating that the information contained on the application is true and correct to the best of their knowledge.

Remember, an arrest record is not pertinent to making a hiring decision. If, however, the candidate has been convicted and the crime is relevant to the position, you may wish to take this into account. For example, suppose you are recruiting for a cashier, and you discover through a criminal background check that a candidate has been convicted of stealing and using credit card numbers from patrons at a store he or she used to work. This would be germane to the hiring decision.

If you plan to conduct a credit background check, be sure that there is a legitimate, job-related reason for this investigation. For example, you may wish to investigate the credit rating for all candidates applying for a cashier position or for positions in your finance department. Under the Fair Credit Reporting Act (FCRA), there are very strict and explicit legal guidelines about conducting a credit check. Candidates must be specifically notified in writing about the credit check, they must sign a release document permitting the investigation, and if there is any negative information uncovered they must be provided with that information and given the opportunity to either clear their record or explain the circumstances. Contact your HR department or seek legal guidance before undertaking a credit check.

Risks of negligent hiring

Failure to conduct background and reference checks may mean that you make the mistake of hiring someone without the education or experience to do the job. Or it may mean that you hire someone with a history of problem performance. At the extreme, it may even mean that you create a legal liability for your organization; increasingly, courts are finding employers legally responsible for negligent hiring if they have hired someone without diligent efforts to verify the individual's history, and the person then uses the job to commit violent or other serious acts.

Insist on checking supervisory references

Candidates sometimes say that they do not want you to contact a former or current supervisor. There are two common reasons for this reluctance. The first is that they do not want their current boss to know they are job-hunting. They do not want to burn any bridges with their current employer until they know they have a new job lined up. The second reason is that they are afraid that the supervisor will say something negative about them.

If you are seriously interested in applicants, tell them that they are finalist candidates (never say *the* finalist), but that you must have a full picture of their work histories, and therefore must check with their past supervisors. In some cases, candidates may provide names of other individuals in the organization as references for their current position. Explain that you would prefer to speak with the immediate supervisor. If that is not possible, be sure that the references you receive are from other individuals in the organization who are at least at a peer level to the immediate supervisor and have had significant work-related intersection with the candidate. If you want to make a job offer to a candidate, you might make the offer contingent on a discussion with the current supervisor. If his or her current boss does not know the candidate is looking, give the candidate some time (a day or so) to go back and talk with the supervisor, so that your reference call does not catch the boss off guard.

If candidates are reluctant to provide you with references from a supervisor in a prior position, ask them to explain their reluctance and try to work through it with them. If they are afraid the supervisor will say something bad about them, ask them to describe what they think the supervisor will say and why they think the supervisor will say it. Sometimes supervisors say discouraging things, even about good employees. If there are problems in an employment relationship, the problems are sometimes with the boss and not with the employee. And sometimes there is legitimate negative information that the candidate would rather you not hear.

If candidates think that you might get negative information from a current or former supervisor, assure them that their own explanations of the situation will also help you weigh what you hear. Encourage the applicants to give you the names and phone numbers of others in the organization who might be able to give countering or balancing information.

Do not take no (information) for an answer

Even though some employers say they only give out "name, rank, and serial number," many organizations do not expressly prohibit supervisors from providing references for employees. A recent survey by the SHRM found that 78% of more than 1300 responding companies say that they do provide references.

At the very least, an HR office will usually verify (1) that the individual did work there, (2) the dates of employment, and (3) the job title. The company may or may not release salary information or why an employment relationship ended. However, many organizations verify or refute data that you provide to them. Therefore you can ask questions such as, "This person says her final salary was $30,000. Is that consistent with your records?" or "This person indicates his employment ended due to a reduction in workforce. Is that what your records show?" The respondent can then simply answer with a yes or no.

Be persistent

If one company representative is unwilling to give useful information, try contacting other references at the same company. If you tried the supervisor, then try the HR office or the supervisor's boss. You can also ask the candidates for additional names of people familiar with their work. If company representatives balk, consider asking them whether they will speak with you if the candidates provide a verbal or written release. Or ask whether they would be willing to answer your questions if you put them in writing on your organization's letterhead.

It is fine to put the responsibility on the candidates to help you get references. Good applicants will not have any trouble getting former employers to speak with you. Have the applicants track down former supervisors and alert them to your call. Be very suspicious of any candidates who cannot come up with several contactable references; if all their former employers have "gone out of business" or every former supervisor is "no longer with the company," do not hire the person. Those are clear warning signs of problems. Also be wary of reference letters provided directly by the candidates; experts will tell you that the applicants may well have written such letters themselves.

Ask questions directly related to the job only

The questions you should ask references are virtually identical to the questions you would ask the candidate. This helps to give the references a brief overview of the basic functions of the job you are trying to fill, and makes it easier for the references to compare your job to the job the candidate held with them.

You can ask whether there were documented performance problems that might be relevant to your job. For example, if reliable attendance is an important factor for your job, you can ask about the candidate's attendance record. But like in an interview, phrase your questions carefully to make sure you do not accidentally learn of medical or disability information that could have discriminatory impact on your hiring decision. One way to ask is, "Other than for legitimate medical or family leave reasons, did the individual have any documented problems with abusing attendance or time off?" Table 6.3 shows some other useful questions. (These are also questions you can rephrase and ask applicants in an interview. Then you can compare their answers with those of their boss.)

In general, stay away from any reference questions that you would not ask the candidates themselves in an interview. Do not ask personal questions not directly related to the ability to do the job.

Evaluate negative information with caution

Even if you receive negative information during a reference check, do not immediately rule out the candidate. Attempt to understand every angle of the circumstances that caused the problem. Try to get confirming or refuting information from other sources. However, if it appears that the negative information is supported by relevant facts, and if you get similar responses from several references, you may choose not to consider the candidate further.

Evaluate even positive information carefully. Some people subscribe to the "if you cannot say something nice do not say anything at all" school of giving references. Read between the lines: do you get the feeling there is something they are not telling you? If you sense there is something the references are avoiding, probe further. But do not promise that what they tell you is off the record. If you end up basing your hiring decision on that information, it will need to be part of your records.

Table 6.3   Potential Questions to Ask References

- How did this person handle a typical, specific situation such as XXX when working for you?
- How much experience did this person have doing XXX for you, and how good was the performance?
- What is the person's level of technical expertise in the essential job functions I need?
- This person would be responsible for handling XXX duties. Is there anything in the candidate's performance history that would cause you concern about his or her ability or appropriateness to do these tasks?
- What types of tasks did this person handle well alone, and what things required structured supervision?
- What do you anticipate I will find to be this person's real strengths, and what areas would benefit from constructive coaching or mentoring?
- This position interacts with XXX types of coworkers or customers in XXX types of situations. How does that compare with what the person did for you, and how well do you think will the person handle these interactions for me?
- Here is something I noticed on the person's application (or in the interview) that raised a question in my mind. Can you help me understand it?

Get at least three work references

To make a good decision, you will need feedback from at least three references going back at least five years if possible. Even for entry-level positions that require little or no prior work experience, you should speak with school counselors, internship coordinators, major professors, or coordinators of volunteer activities who are familiar with the candidate in a professional or an academic (rather than social) environment.

Do not bother with personal references

Personal or character references are seldom useful. Such individuals usually cannot offer direct information about how a candidate would perform in a work environment. And often they are personal friends, and therefore their perspectives will not be neutral and objective.

Document all reference information

Document in writing all the references you attempted to contact, or did contact, and all relevant information you received. If you get stonewalled, document whom you contacted and that they refused to give you useful information. The forms in Appendix B and Appendix C are useful tools for keeping track of pertinent information. The following sections provide further information about these forms.

Preemployment reference check and credentials check forms

Hiring qualified employees in the current labor market requires a major investment of both time and resources. Many employers use a program of preemployment background checks in order to minimize the risk of negligent hiring claims, maintain a safe and secure workplace, and protect company assets from the cost of a poor hire.

For legal tracking purposes, you should maintain this documentation for three years, along with your interview notes and your reasons for not selecting all unsuccessful candidates. (For more information on interview notes, see the section "Interviewing Job Candidates.") You can keep these materials in your departmental files if you are willing to be responsible for them or you can send them to your HR department for safekeeping once your search is over. Why do documents have to be kept for three years? Because that is the general limit within which an unsuccessful candidate can challenge your hiring decision to a state or federal equal employment opportunity agency, and you need to be able to present contemporaneous records that prove you made your decision at the time for legitimate reasons, based on verifiable information and nondiscriminatory factors.

Check both academic and employment information

Companies that conduct professional background check services say that applicants are even more likely to falsify information about their academic backgrounds than about their work history, probably because employers are less likely to check with schools for verification or to require academic transcripts. Most college registrar offices, upon request, confirm dates of attendance and graduation as well as degrees awarded and majors.

Retention

Your people resources — human capital — are your most important assets. Rarely will other factors be as key to your long-term competitive advantage. Technology is readily available to organizations, product offerings are easily copied or adapted, and market niches quickly diminish as competitors see exploitable opportunities.

Successful organizations recognize that the true source of their long-term competitive advantage is their people. Employees are the force that can drive velocity, quality, innovation, customer service and satisfaction, and the efficient use of resources.

To fully understand the importance of retention, it is important to first understand the high cost of turnover to an organization. The U.S. Department of Labor (DOL) estimates that it costs a company one-third of a new hire's annual salary to replace an hourly employee. The cost to replace management employees can easily run from 50% of their salary to in excess of 100%.

Estimating the visible cost of turnover

There are three main categories of visible cost to employee turnover: termination costs, recruitment cost, and new hire cost. Use the format found in Table 6.4 to estimate the cost of a turnover at your organization.

In addition to the visible costs, there are significant hidden costs to turnover, such as the inefficiency of the terminated employee from the time notice is given until departure and loss of productivity due to workforce reductions. These may negatively affect the morale of the remaining employees, which may decrease productivity further. Lastly, the lower productivity from the new hire — the learning curve loss — may affect your productivity and that of your remaining staff while assisting the new hire during the learning curve period. In short, it is cost effective and time efficient to retain your staff.

Why do employees stay with their current employers? What are the key components of job satisfaction? In a joint study conducted in 2002 by the SHRM and *USA Today*, the top five overall components of job satisfaction by employees are job security, benefits, communication between employees and management, employee flexibility to balance life and work issues, and compensation or pay.

Although these components differ somewhat by age category, gender, and industry type, job security is one of the top five aspects selected by all. Benefits and compensation are also in the top five in almost all categories. These trends indicate that it is important to understand the needs of your employees, i.e., what is important to them. With that information in hand, you can build a culture that meets both your needs and theirs.

Table 6.4 Estimating the Cost of Employer Turnover

Termination Costs	
• Exit interview — typically ½ hour of time for someone in your HR department to provide information about the status of the departing employee's benefits (e.g., COBRA), etc.	$_____
• Exit interview — ½ hour of the departing employee's time	$_____
• Payout of accrued unused vacation time	$_____
• Unemployment costs	$_____
Recruitment Costs	
• Cost for advertising the position	$_____
• Cost for an external retained search consultant/recruiter	$_____
• Salary of your HR department recruiter — typically 10 to 15 hours — to prepare text for advertising the position, developing a detailed description of the position, reviewing and assessing resumes as they arrive, coordinating and scheduling interviews, conducting interviews and skills testing, conducting background and reference checks, etc.	$_____
• Salary for your time — at least 10 hours — to finalize and approve advertising copy, give a detailed description of the position, interview and assess candidates, and negotiate details of the job offer	$_____
New Hire Costs	
• Salary of new hire — 2 to 3 hours — to complete the new hire paperwork, benefit review, and new hire orientation	$_____
• Salary of HR department — 2 hours — to conduct reviews and orientations	$_____
• Salary of payroll staff — ½ hour — to set up new hire on payroll	$_____
• Startup costs (business cards, office supplies, computer, etc.)	$_____
Total costs for turnover	$_____

A peculiar thing happens to many employees after they have been with an employer for a few years. The 3- to 5-year period of tenure – just when most employers believe that employees are getting comfortable with the organization — turns out to be exactly the time employees think about leaving.

Manpower International conducted a loyalty survey in 2002 that found that the top three loyalty drivers are strong leadership, strong teamwork, and open and honest communication.

Most employers focus their attention on the recruiting, hiring, and orientation phase of an employee's career. Then it is business as usual. The key concept when building a retention program is to understand that one size does not fit all. It is important that you understand the needs of your employees, which will likely differ based on age and gender.

Conducting a "reality check" with your employees is an assessment tool that should be used on a periodic and regular basis. What is important today may change tomorrow, and your employees are your best resources. Many employers are looking at different ways to meet their employees' needs. These include flexible schedules, telecommuting, job sharing, and employee assistance plans (EAPs). In addition, adoption assistance, subsidized child care, and elder care are growing in popularity. Other benefits are educational subsidies, cultural subsidies, lunch-and-learn programs, and exercise and health facilities.

Many of these programs are not difficult to establish and are relatively inexpensive to implement. A survey of your workforce can help identify the types of programs best suited to your employees. It is important to build your employees' spirit and pride in the organization and help them feel a part of the team.

Conversely, a national workforce loyalty study conducted in 2001 by Walker International identified several warning signs and ongoing trends in today's workers. This study indicated that only about half (53%) of employees are willing to recommend their organizations to others looking for a job, and only about half (54%) believe that their organizations treat employees fairly. The primary concerns are the way policies are implemented (only 45% are positive), fairness of pay and pay practices (50% are positive), and fewer than half (only 41%) believe there is a degree of trust in employees.

In the final analysis, employees want challenging and stimulating work, fair pay, the tools and resources needed to do their jobs, recognition for work done well, and involvement in the decisions that impact their daily lives. The problem is that in today's fast-paced, high-powered work environments, simply addressing the basic needs of employees and recognizing their efforts are not enough.

Compensation

Compensation refers to both direct and indirect pay, and is typically referred to as total compensation. Total compensation can include base wages, overtime, bonuses, incentive pay, sales commission, and the cost of providing benefits. Here we focus on direct pay — cash compensation.

There are three types of direct pay: base pay, variable pay, and incentives. Base pay is the basic rate of direct compensation. For a nonexempt employee, this is the hourly rate of pay. For an exempt employee, this is the basic annualized rate of pay. In both cases, base pay excludes overtime, bonuses, commissions, or any other extra types of pay.

Variable pay is the portion of an employee's pay that is considered at risk. Typically, this depends on some level of performance. Examples include commission, discretionary bonuses, management by objectives (MBO), and target bonuses. Incentive pay includes stock options, restricted stock awards, venture participation, and phantom stock grants (stock appreciation for nonpublicly held companies). Companies are increasingly moving employees' direct pay into the at-risk categories of variable and incentive pay options.

Market pricing and internal value determinations

One of the most prevalent compensation strategies is to establish a target salary that is tied to compensation for similar positions in the appropriate competitive marketplace. Market pricing is a formal process for determining the external value of a position compared to an organization's competitive market. This is a job-based method of defining compensation structure.

However, a particular position might carry more internal value in your organization than it does in the external marketplace. Then you must define an appropriate person-based compensation level. Therefore, typically some level of internal alignment is used in conjunction with external data to benchmark a position. Benchmark positions are those positions that are easily identified in competitive market salary surveys and are consistently defined by a variety of organizations, which means that most organizations can agree on the job's scope of responsibility and organizational importance.

As a part of an organization's recruitment and retention plan, a strategic plan must be developed to determine which organizations compose the competitive market and to determine how your salaries will match against that marketplace. Do you want your pay scales to target the average in the marketplace, or to be above average or below average? Are you comparing to national salary data or regional salary data? How an organization answers these questions significantly impacts the overall compensation strategy. Defining the labor market will include the industry, geographic considerations, and job functions.

The Fair Labor Standards Act

The most important piece of federal legislation affecting compensation is the Fair Labor Standards Act (FLSA), which was adopted in 1938 as a means of economic recovery from the Great Depression. The purposes of the FLSA were to create minimum wage standards, promote fair competition in interstate commerce, generate job growth and reduce unemployment, and curtail child labor.

The major provisions of the FLSA are:

- Coverage
- Minimum wage
- Exemptions (minimum wage and overtime provisions)
- Overtime and hours of work
- Child labor restrictions
- Recordkeeping requirements

The FLSA, also sometimes referred to as the Wage and Hour Law, is enforced by the U.S. DOL. Its primary objective is to eliminate detrimental working conditions and to establish protections for employees regarding minimum wage, child labor, and overtime provisions. In addition, the regulations identify and exclude certain workers (exempt) from FLSA coverage.

In some states, there are both federal and state exemptions and requirements. Compliance with both federal and state requirements is mandatory. Where federal and state regulations vary, the regulations imposing the higher standard generally apply.

The FLSA also provides that employees cannot waive their FLSA rights; nor can employers retaliate against employees who invoke their FLSA rights. Subsequent regulations further define complicated issues such as:

- Defining the employment relations — When is a consultant actually an employee?
- Hours of work — What is included in time worked for purposes of calculating overtime?
- Exemptions — Who is exempt from the overtime provisions of the FLSA?

However, the FLSA does not require that you pay for time not worked. This includes vacations, holidays, severance, sick time, meal periods of 30 consecutive minutes or more (duty free), and rest or break periods greater than 20 consecutive minutes. Also, the FLSA does not require premium pay for weekend or holiday work, or pay raises or fringe benefits.

Since the adoption of the FLSA in 1938, there have been few modifications to the original act and regulations. Other pieces of federal legislation have been passed to safeguard against discrimination in employment and pay practices, such as the Equal Pay Act of 1963 (amended in 1972), the Civil Rights Acts of 1964 and 1991, and the Americans with Disabilities Act.

In the present environment, many organizations are faced with developing compensation practices for both individual performance and team performance. Designing a program that establishes performance goals that are aligned with organizational goals, and then rewarding employees and teams for attaining those performance targets, ensures that individuals, teams, and departments are in sync.

What does it mean for a position to be exempt or nonexempt?

Employees holding nonexempt positions are those who must be paid in accordance with the overtime provisions of the FLSA. Exempt positions, on the other hand, are excluded (exempted) from coverage and do not need to be paid overtime.

How does an employer decide whether a position's duties and
responsibilities are exempt according to FLSA regulations?

There are three types of exemptions under the FLSA: executive, administrative, and professional. The exempt test criteria differ by type and are detailed in the DOL regulations 29CFR Part 541.

FLSA regulations provide guidelines and examples to assist the employer in making exempt and nonexempt determinations. Essentially, the law guides the employer in evaluating two key criteria:

- The *importance of the work* as defined by the law's guidelines
- Within the context of its importance, the extent and magnitude of the position's *independent discretion*

It is important that the employees assigned to exempt positions perform work that meets the standards of exemption. The law's objective is to protect the employee; therefore, the FLSA assumes that all positions are nonexempt and subject to the law. It is the employer's responsibility to *prove* that a job is exempt. Table 6.5 gives examples of differences between exempt and nonexempt employees.

To be exempt, work must be of substantial importance to the management or operations of a business. For example, a position whose primary function is to participate in the development of business operations or management policies would typically be exempt. In contrast, a position whose main responsibility is to ensure that management policies are being followed will not be considered exempt.

Exempt employees make analyses and draw conclusions that are important to the determination of management policies or general business operations. Importance can be measured by the degree and impact of advising, planning, and negotiating. Further, how the employee represents the company in terms of purchasing, marketing, or business development decisions is key to determining the level of importance.

Types of positions that typically perform this kind of work are advisory specialists to management auditors, managers, and supervisors; professionals such as pharmacists, lawyers, doctors, engineers, and teachers; or employees who work on special assignments or in public-relations-type positions (e.g., development officers).

Independent discretion means comparing and evaluating possible courses of conduct and recommending or making a decision after various possibilities have been considered. These recommendations need to have strong influence and are usually adopted with minimal review from higher levels of authority.

Independent discretion must be free from immediate direction or supervision and involve matters of significance. It must be different from the use of skill or knowledge in applying techniques or procedures according to

Table 6.5 Differences between Exempt and Nonexempt Work

Activity	Nonexempt	Exempt
Research	Collects and compiles information. Reviews for completeness. Identifies missing documentation. Processes documents against an established standard by following prescribed audit lists.	Identifies root cause or problem. Investigates applicable laws, policies, and procedures. Ascertains intent of transactions/issues. Creates historic record of events and repercussions.
Example	Payroll coordinator	Payroll supervisor
Analysis	Identifies problem or issue and selects or determines appropriate action within prescribed guidelines. Analyses are based on reviewing the documentation against established standards.	Compares and evaluates possible courses of conduct; acts after considering various possibilities. Considers the cause and effect of historic activities and the impact and potential repercussions of possible actions.
Example	Secretary	Director of a department
Decision making	Applies skills and knowledge in following prescribed procedures and determines whether specified standards are being met. Uses knowledge in determining which procedures to follow.	Has the power to make an independent choice free from immediate supervision. The decisions may be in the form of a recommendation usually followed with minimal, if any, review from higher levels of authority.
Example	Pharmacy technician	Pharmacist
Judgment	Determines if documentation meets standards.	Determines how best to resolve the situation.
Example	Accounts payable coordinator	Senior accountant
Independent discretion	Discretion applies to the production processes as opposed to the organization's policies or operations. Consequences may lead to loss through the choice of wrong techniques, improper application of skills, neglect, or failure to follow instructions.	Makes decisions of consequence and of real and substantial significance regarding the policies or general operations of the organization. Is able to deviate from standard policies and procedures.
Example	Carpenter	Facilities manager

specific standards. Further, independent discretion must not deal with matters of little consequence to the overall business operation.

According to the DOL, decisions in significant matters refers "to the kind of decisions normally made by persons who formulate or participate in the formulation of policy, or who exercise authority within a wide range to commit their employer in substantial respects financially or otherwise." An exempt employee must exercise this kind of discretion and independent judgment customarily and regularly (daily).

What are the consequences if the FLSA is violated?

The FLSA can be enforced by private employee lawsuits or by actions taken by the U.S. DOL. Other agencies, such as the Internal Revenue Service and state employment agencies, can also investigate. Just one employee's complaint to an agency has the potential of initiating a federal audit of the jobs of the entire company.

The DOL also has the right to seek an injunction, which means that the secretary of labor files a restraint prohibiting future violations of FLSA laws. Damages may include back pay (statute of limitations is 2 years for unintentional violations and 3 years for willful violations), penalties, attorney fees, and court costs. In a lawsuit, as opposed to an administrative audit by the DOL, employees generally collect back pay and liquidated damages in the amount of back pay (double damages).

Appendix A

Candidate Evaluation Grid

Rank each candidate on a scale of 0 to 5,
Let 0 represent either (a) evidence that the skill or requirement is *not* present
or (b) *no* evidence that it is;
Let 5 represent the highest level of demonstrated competence that you could
hope for.
Look for direct evidence in the resume and other materials and in your
interviews (do not infer skill or experience without evidence to support your
inference).

Candidate name: _____

Position title: _____Date: _____

Education , Experience, Responsibilities, and Skills	Rank: 0 to 5
Point Totals	

Appendix B

Preemployment Reference Check Form

Candidate's name:	SS#:
Hiring dept.:	Position sought:

Organization name and location:	Candidate's dates of employment confirmed as: From: To:
Candidate's last job title confirmed as:	Candidate's last rate of pay confirmed as:
End of employment reason confirmed as:	Eligible for rehire? ☐ Yes ☐ No

Name of reference:	Phone number:
Title of reference:	Relationship to candidate:

Describe the job that the candidate is being considered for, and ask the reference to compare against duties performed in the job the candidate did for them:
Comments on level of technical skills and expertise that will be relevant to job:

Comments on professional interactive skills that will be relevant to job:

Any Documented Concerns About	Yes*	No
Attendance, punctuality or reliability, other than for legitimate medical or family leave reasons?		
Integrity or effectiveness in handling the organization's resources for which they were responsible?		
Integrity or effectiveness in the professional interactions for which they were responsible?		
The ability to accept responsibility or maintain productivity on the assignments for which they were responsible?		
The ability to exhibit maturity, composure, or professional conduct under typical job stresses or challenges?		
The ability to adapt successfully to new or changing work situations, people, ideas, or structures?		

*If yes to any, note referee's comments or concerns:

Other comments about whether you would recommend this person for this job?

Reference check by:	Date:

Appendix C

Credential Check Form

Candidate name: _____

Name on credential, if different: _____

Degree/certificate/license:	Year:
School/institute:	
Address:	
Telephone number:	
Contact name:	
Verification: ☐ Yes ☐ No	

Completed by: _____ Date: _____

Bibliography

Loyalty in the Workplace: 2001 National Employee Benchmark Study, Walker International, September 2001.

SHRM 2002 Workplace Demographic Trends Survey, SHRM, December 2002.

chapter seven

Employee coaching, evaluation, and discipline

Ellen Fernberger

Contents

0-8493-1446-1/04/$0.00+$1.50
© 2004 by CRC Press LLC

Ask managers about the most difficult and nightmare-provoking portion of their jobs and you will likely hear about coaching, performance evaluation, and discipline. Most U.S. workers, both mangers and those managed, have little knowledge or capacity concerning coaching, view performance evaluations as a once-a-year required evil, and consider discipline as the only solution to make people do what we want them to do.

However, when done right, coaching should be an ongoing everyday part of our work lives, evaluations should be summaries of these coaching sessions, and discipline the last option when all else has failed. In this chapter, we look at these three components of supervising and managing.

All managers learn the inevitability that some employees perform above expectations, some at an average level, and some at substandard levels. The first step in any evaluative process must be an assessment of an employee's current performance, strengths, and weaknesses. Once this is accomplished, the manager can determine whether the appropriate relationship format is mentoring, coaching, or counseling. It can be as difficult to establish *when* to mentor, coach, or counsel as to know *how* to mentor, coach, or counsel.

Based on the outcome of your assessment, if the employee is achieving above-standard performance, you should acquire the role of a mentor; average or standard performance requires coaching; and substandard performance needs your involvement as a counselor. However, each of these techniques may be required for any employee at some time in his or her career. Even the best employee will have moments when counseling is warranted.

Mentoring relationship

There are many similarities between the mentor and coach relationships; typically, mentors explore vision, mission, and identity, whereas coaches focus on transactional responsibilities. Let us explore more closely what mentoring means, and how it differs from coaching. Mentoring deals with the broader issues of organizational, career, or personal transitions. It is possibility-centered, focused on options and exploration. Coaching deals with raising the performance bar to help employees excel. It is task-centered, linking improved individual effectiveness to organizational performance.

The mentoring relationship, by definition, includes two people: the mentor and the protégé. Mentoring is typically saved for an organization's top talent. But before a mentor program can be established, the organization must first define what top talent means. This will enable you to define who should be the protégé. But it is equally important to select the right mentor, who must be someone who not only has proven success at the organization, but also exemplifies the qualities of a leader at your organization. These are the qualities that are most highly regarded by your organization, and the ones that you wish to have passed on to the next generation of leadership. You want someone who lives the values, attitudes, and styles held in highest regard, and who also achieves top results.

Linda Kyle Stromei (2001), defines the terms *mentor, mentoring*, and *protégé* as follows:

- *Mentor.* A person at a higher level of responsibility in the organization who agrees to act as a wise or trusted counselor, leader, and role model to a person seeking to grow and develop professionally.
- *Mentoring.* A complex, interactive process in which two individuals of differing levels of experience and expertise are paired for the agreed upon goal of having the lesser-skilled person grow and develop specific competencies. The process incorporates interpersonal or psychosocial development, career or educational development, or both, and socialization functions into the relationship. This one-to-one relationship is developmental and proceeds through stages.
- *Protégé.* The beneficiary of the mentoring relationship, learning from the experience, wisdom, and counsel of the mentor.

Further, Stromei indicates:

> *Mentorship serves two functions: career-related and psychosocial. Career-related functions include providing sponsorship, exposure, visibility, coaching, protection, and challenging assignments, which directly relate to the protégé's career development. These functions assist the protégé in learning the ropes of organizational life and prepare him or her for advancement opportunities in the organization. Psychosocial functions include providing role modeling, acceptance, confirmation, counseling, and friendship, all activities that influence the protégé's self-image and competence.*

Coaching relationship

Coaching is typically used to describe an ongoing evaluation and feedback process. It answers employee questions such as, "How am I doing?" and "Where do I go from here?" It is the day-to-day effort to review work, answer questions, discuss progress (or lack of) toward meeting standards, develop skills, and perhaps, most importantly, provide positive guidance.

The supervisor is not the only person who can coach an employee. Coworkers, other supervisors, and even customers can often be in a good position to compare the employee's performance to establish standards and then give helpful feedback. Such coaching opportunities can be part of a planned coaching or customer feedback process or can occur spontaneously as a result of the employee asking these people for input.

Employees can also be their own coaches by obtaining feedback from other sources. Reviewing their own work products, data from reports, or even videotapes (when appropriate and if available) can provide employees with opportunities for self-evaluation and improvement.

Coaching through informal evaluation and feedback

The most effective way to track and refer to all this information is to set up a memory file. This can be as simple as a file folder. It can include notes on exceptional (positive or negative) performance or behavior by an employee. It can also include copies of documents such as letters of appreciation or warning. By keeping a memory file on each employee, a supervisor can track an employee's performance progress as well as what coaching has been provided. Depending on how accessible and complete the files are, employees may want to set up their own memory files to ensure that all key aspects of their performance are recorded.

Counseling

Counseling is the end stage of a process, meant for those employees who are not performing up to organizational standards. As will be discussed later in the chapter, it is important for you as a manager to try and understand why an employee is underperforming. Might it simply be that you have not accurately defined the performance standards — the "what is expected of you" discussion? Does the employee have the capability to perform, but not know how to complete the tasks? As a supervisor, you must ask yourself these and many more questions before beginning a counseling process.

Counseling in stages

Typically, organizations have a discipline, or counseling, process. Most often, these procedures are in stages: from oral warnings to written warnings, final warnings, and dismissal. If managed correctly, problem employees will actually succeed in terminating themselves. Accurate and objective documentation of performance and discipline are essential components to protect both you, as the supervisor, and your organization from costly litigation.

Performance management

Employees are most likely to be successful performers when they clearly understand their assignments, know the level of performance considered acceptable, and receive consistent feedback. Evaluation of an employee's performance is not merely a yearly activity done *by* a supervisor *to* an employee. It is an ongoing process that should involve information from coworkers, customers, the supervisor, and even the employee. Employees are as responsible for their successful performance and evaluation as is the supervisor.

A formal appraisal is an important opportunity to summarize the informal evaluations of employee performance over a long period of time. Most organizations have a policy defining timeframes for conducting formal performance appraisals, typically once every year.

Table 7.1 Objectives of the Performance Management System

Objective	Average Rank
Provide information to employees about their performance	2.8
Clarify organizational expectations of employees	2.8
Identify developmental needs	3.7
Gather information for pay decisions	4.0
Gather information for coaching	4.2
Document performance for employee records	4.6
Gather information for promotion decisions	5.2

Scale: 1 = most important; 7 = least important.

But what are the real reasons that organizations conduct annual performance evaluations? In a survey sponsored jointly by the Society for Human Resource Management (SHRM) and Personnel Decisions International (PDI) in 2000, the number one answer by survey participants was to provide information to employees about their performance and to clarify organizational expectations of employees (Table 7.1). At the bottom of the list were documenting performance for employee records and gathering information for promotion decisions.

Linking performance management to business plans and goals

In the past, organizations assessed individual performance based on completion of a task. More recently, supervisors are being asked to tie departmental goals and objectives to broader organizational goals and objectives. In turn, supervisors are requiring that individuals in their unit also have performance goals and objectives that facilitate meeting these broader business needs. Figure 7.1 depicts earlier performance models.

The new model (Figure 7.2) begins by assessing business plans and goals and translating them to the department plans and goals, and then to the individual employee's plans and goals.

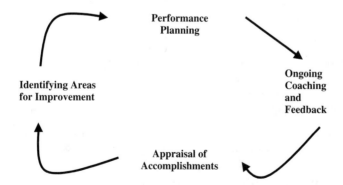

Figure 7.1 The traditional performance management system. (From SHRM/PDI 2000 Performance Management Survey.)

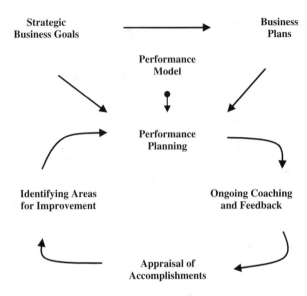

Figure 7.2 The new performance management system. (From SHRM/PDI 2000 Performance Management Survey.)

Equating performance appraisals with training and development plans

According to the SHRM/PDI survey, organizations unanimously indicate that the primary roles of a performance management system are employee-oriented — providing information about attaining performance standards, clarifying organizational expectations, and identifying developmental needs. However, the survey also showed that few organizations translate the performance appraisal into development and career planning for their employees. In fact, only 8% of survey participants provided career planning for their executives, and only 3% for their exempt and nonexempt staff. Little wonder then that employees generally regard performance appraisal simply as a way to document performance.

Supervisor and employee rights

When thinking about a performance evaluation process, it is important to be clear about your rights as a supervisor and your employees' rights. Following these simple guidelines will help you if you later become embroiled in a legal quagmire:

> *Supervisors.* They have the right of final approval on which levels of performance will be considered successful and to hold employees accountable for meeting these standards. Supervisors also have a right to evaluate employees formally on a periodic basis and provide informal feedback on a frequent basis in order to achieve the level of per-

formance required to manage a successful program, service, or department.

Employees. They have a right to be informed of performance expectations and to be evaluated as objectively as possible. Employees also have a right to periodic performance feedback and to at least one formal evaluation each year.

Assignments and job descriptions

The first step to successful performance is to ensure that employees are clear about what they have been assigned. What are the employees' roles within the organization? What are their duties and responsibilities?

Each position in a department has its own unique set of duties and responsibilities. For example, not all clerical staff perform exactly the same combination of tasks, though much of what they do is similar. An exact description of the duties and responsibilities an employee needs to perform can be provided by writing (or updating) a job description. The description should be specific to the positions in a particular department or unit. It should include the phrase "and other duties as assigned" to cover unexpected or occasional tasks and should be updated as often as is needed to keep it current.

A good job design is the basis of an employee's entire employment relationship. The job design is then articulated in the job description. A good job description is outcomes-oriented, not just a description of tasks to be completed. Therefore, it should include:

- Values to be upheld
- Technical knowledge and skills needed
- Performance levels expected
- Interactive skills required

So, for example, a better way to describe a secretarial position task such as "answers department telephone" is to include the outcome orientation, "answers telephones promptly, with warmth and courtesy, responds appropriately to callers, and routes calls or takes messages accurately and completely to ensure effective department operations." This type of description ensures that the employee understands both the task and the expected performance level, the values to be upheld, and the interactive skills required. This groundwork provides a direct link between what a job is and how it is done, linking job and performance. It makes clear that simply answering the department telephone is not good enough.

A well-designed and articulated job description is imperative to managing performance and helping employees reach positive performance outcomes. Your expectations must be set and articulated before problems arise.

It is difficult to chastise an employee for crossing the line if you have never defined where the line is.

What success looks like — establish goals

Clarifying duties and responsibilities provides a framework for the crucial activity of setting performance standards. Both the supervisor and the employee need a way of determining how well the employee is doing. It is important for the standards to be negotiated and set *before* the employee starts performing work that will be evaluated, whether the employee is new to the organization or new to the position as a result of transfer or promotion. It is also important to update the standards as the work situation changes.

Negotiation is important because many factors (e.g., staffing levels, workloads, or stressful work conditions) can affect the fairness of an expectation. The more the employee is involved in setting or updating standards and agrees they are *clear and reasonable*, the greater the chances for successful performance.

A goal refers to results that must be achieved, to ongoing performance criteria that must be met consistently, or to results that must be achieved for the employee to achieve successful performance. Goals refer to such things as the delivery of services at a specified level of quality, attendance level, accuracy rates, response times, production rates, safety thresholds, format requirements, and behavioral expectations. To write an effective goal for successful performance, it should be as *s*pecific, *m*easurable, *a*ttainable, *r*ealistic, and *t*ime-measured as possible (SMART).

Goals may be set for each duty or project assigned. They may be set for activities or behaviors that apply to many assignments or projects (e.g., computer work or cooperation). It is important that everyone who will be involved in evaluating an employee's performance is clear about which aspects of the employee's performance will be evaluated and what successful performance will look like. You should be able to match outcome-based criteria in the job description, project assignment, or both, directly to the evaluation criteria in the performance evaluation instrument.

Performance management cycle

The performance management cycle (Figure 7.3) is not a yearly procedure. It should be an ongoing circular cycle that continues throughout the year and includes planning performance and setting goals, implementing the performance plan, reviewing progress and coaching (throughout the year), and conducting annual performance reviews.

This is a team process, which needs to include both the employee and the supervisor. In some organizations, this process may also include peers and subordinates and is called a 360° review process.

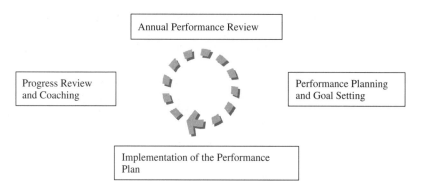

Figure 7.3 Performance management cycle.

Both the supervisor and the employee need to prepare for a performance review. The employee should prepare for the review process by:

- Reviewing the job description, responsibilities, and skills
- Assessing personal performance and identifying areas for improvement
- Preparing specific and measurable goals
- Reviewing competencies for current and desirable jobs and targeting some for developing

The supervisor should prepare for the annual review by:

- Reviewing and updating the job description, responsibilities, and skills
- Assessing employee performance and identifying areas for improvement
- Preparing specific and measurable goals
- Considering advancement or enrichment opportunities
- Scheduling uninterrupted meeting time and giving the employee advanced notice

A memory file for each employee, referred to earlier in the chapter, becomes a critical part of your assessment of a subordinate's performance. Never rely on your memory. You are likely to remember only the most recent events or some serious infraction. However, it is likely that neither of these represents the full body of your staff member's performance.

The performance appraisal meeting

The actual performance appraisal meeting can be one of the most stressful times both for you as a supervisor and your staff. Most of us have grown up learning the "golden rule" — do unto others as you would like done to you. However, you may want to employ the "platinum rule" — do unto others as they would like. This requires a clear understanding of your staff members' personalities, likes, and dislikes. What types of work or projects excite them? Each individual is different. Some employees are quiet and others social, some detail-oriented and others visionary. Understanding these differences will help you assign work and assess expectations to get the best from everyone.

When it is time for the appraisal meeting, it is important to:

- Arrange a meeting place free of interruptions, distractions, and phone calls.
- Ask for the employee's self-evaluation and review your evaluation of the employee.
- Jointly offer or suggest what would help or maintain performance.
- Agree on a developmental plan for the coming year.
- Get the employee's commitment to improve performance and schedule the first performance progress review meeting.

Performance progress reviews

The performance appraisal process does not end here. It is important that you follow up with regular, periodic performance progress review meetings. You should meet periodically with each employee to review and update goals, provide ongoing coaching and suggestions, help the employee develop relationships necessary to meet goals, run interference when necessary, and provide encouragement and reinforcement.

These meetings may be brief, depending on the employee's performance, but are crucial to continued success. They will also provide the employee with an opportunity to ask questions and clarify ongoing goals and completion timeframes.

A good supervisor exhibits these six skills:

- Sets goals and objectives
- Regularly communicates with subordinates
- Establishes values, accountability, and professionalism
- Sets expectations
- Evaluates performance
- Counsels for improvement

General tips and ideas

- *Customize.* Use the employee's first name and add your own personal touches where possible.

- *Know your employees and reward them as individuals.* For example, if the employee appreciates written praise and likes to go fishing, give the employee a recognition memo and a few hours off on a sunny afternoon.
- *Match the reward and the achievement.* Make sure that those who have completed more substantial tasks are better rewarded than those who simply had a good day.
- *Act quickly.* Recognize the employee as soon as possible following the event. Even if you are planning a more substantial reward in the future, be sure to give some verbal recognition or a quick memo right away.
- *Be as specific as possible.* Let your employees know exactly what it is that they have done right. This will help them to repeat those positive results.
- *Try not to mix recognition with advice.* This might confuse the message you are sending.
- *Convey the big picture.* Describe how the effort or result contributed to a broader goal or objective.
- *Reinforce organizational values.* When possible, point out how employees' actions support organizational values or major objectives.
- *Be genuine in your tone and wording.* Try to write in the same manner that you use when speaking.

Team evaluations

Evaluating a team is different from evaluating an individual, and it involves two levels of review. The first is to evaluate the overall team success. Then you need to look further to determine the role that each individual team member played in attaining that success. One way you can achieve the second step is to ask the team members to complete both a self-evaluation and an evaluation of each team member. This does not need to be a lengthy evaluation. See Appendix A for an example of an evaluation form that can be used for review of individual team members.

As you develop your evaluation of the team, follow these steps:

- *Praise everyone on the team.* Congratulate the entire team on its efforts.
- *Point out team players.* If someone has made a particularly strong contribution to the team effort, point it out.
- *Be specific in your team praise.* Mention a group of people who worked especially well together or point out a particular result that could not have been achieved without close cooperation.

Each individual employee is different. Therefore, you will likely have to employ different methods to motivate your staff. Are you having difficulty motivating employees? Try the tips listed in Table 7.2.

Table 7.2 Ways to Motivate Employees

- Personally thank employees for a good job both verbally and in writing. Do this in a timely manner, often, and with sincerity.
- Make the time to meet with and listen to your staff.
- Provide specific feedback about individual, departmental, and organizational progress. It is important that all staff members understand how their successes help the department to succeed, and therefore the organization to be successful.
- Strive to create an open, trusting, and fun work environment. Encourage new ideas and initiatives.
- Provide information on departmental and organizational strategies and how the individual fits in with the overall plan.
- Involve employees in decisions, especially those that affect them.
- Provide employees with a sense of ownership in their work and the work environment.
- Recognize, reward, and promote people based on their performance and deal with marginal performers.
- Give people a chance to grow and learn new skills. Create a partnership to help them meet their goals within the context of the organization's goals.
- Celebrate success — of the organization, the department, and the employees. Take time for team and morale-building meetings and activities.

Frequently asked questions

Q: What should be done about employees who become belligerent during the annual performance evaluation?

A: Holding only one evaluation session each year may cause unnecessary anxiety for both the supervisor and the employee. Consider a couple of options. First, less formal monthly or quarterly feedback sessions can provide valuable input in a less stressful manner. Another option is to ask the employee to create measurable performance standards at the beginning of the evaluation period and to provide periodic progress reports.

Q: How can an employee's cooperation skills be objectively evaluated? Isn't cooperation a highly subjective concept?

A: Cooperation is an essential component in an effective team-based environment, but it may be difficult to measure. One option to consider is asking the employee and the employee's colleagues to document examples of the employee's efforts to build and maintain relations in order to complete projects or address problems.

Q: It seems like some employees are not staying current in their field, and this may reduce the department's ability to be effective. Is there a way to mandate continuing education?

A: If staying abreast of specialized knowledge is critical to solid job performance, job knowledge should be given significant weight in the evaluation process. Demonstration of new knowledge may be evaluated by satisfactory completion of academic course work, a brief written summary of the major concepts discussed during a professional conference, or a mastery of a new product (or a new procedure) such as a computer software package or a new process for handling work assignments.

Q: Are formal evaluations pointless for truly outstanding employees?

A: Not at all. Formal evaluation for outstanding performance can be highly motivating for high achievers. Failure to acknowledge this performance may actually result in declines in future performance.

Q: What happens if an employee disputes the performance appraisal rating?

A: Typically, if the dispute cannot be resolved informally, the employee may prepare a written statement, detailing the disputed performance. This should be attached to the performance appraisal document. Employees may also choose to discuss the situation with their human resources department.

Managing performance by coaching

You have now set performance expectations by ensuring that employees know their job duties, the performance standards that will be used, and your expectations. You have monitored and evaluated employees' progress. You have identified performance problems. Any finally, you have built individual development plans. Your ongoing coaching cycle is complete.

The next step is to discover causes of problem performance (Table 7.3). Why are employees failing to succeed? Is it that they:

- *Cannot do it?* Do not have the ability or resources to do the job.
- *Will not do it?* Have the ability but do not want to do the job.
- *Do not know how to do it?* Do not understand how to do the job.

Once the causes of problem performance have been identified, then you can plan for the solutions (Table 7.3). For example, if you determine that employees are not successful because they do not know how to perform the task, providing training may be a simple solution. For instance, if you have asked your secretary to prepare a presentation for you in PowerPoint, but he or she has never used the software before, it is likely that the outcome will not be positive for either of you.

The next step is to analyze the situation to determine the performance gap — is it training or attitude? The top of this decision tree starts with the question, "Does this individual have the necessary knowledge and skill to

Table 7.3 Identifying and Solving Performance Problems

Cannot	Will Not	Does Not Know How
Causes		
• Have knowledge but lack skill after thorough instruction • Not enough time	• Believe they know it all • Poor listening skills • Unhappy with duties or responsibilities of the job	• Lack of instruction or training • Improper or lack of feedback
Solutions		
• Ensure the proper training materials are provided	• Recognize good work if appropriate • Provide a job reassignment • Disciplinary action (contact human resources)	• Provide training or retraining

perform?" How you answer that first question will take you down one of two paths (Figure 7.4).

When conducting a coaching or counseling session with an employee, it is important that you also be an effective listener. Give your undivided attention. This means that you remove all distractions, such as your telephone and e-mail, and maintain eye contact.

1. *Make sure the employee knows you understand what he or she is saying.* This builds trust with the employee by use of empathy. For example, try:
   • "What I hear you saying is …"
   • "I get the impression that …"
2. *Listen for underlying cues.* Look for the attitudes, feelings, and motives behind the employee's words. Confirm your perception by using the following examples:
   • "I can imagine that you must feel …"
   • "If it ever happened to me I would be …"
3. *Encourage the employee to elaborate.* It is important to make sure that the employee fully discusses the situation. Here are some examples of how you can probe for more information:
   • "Tell me more about …"
   • "I would like to hear your thoughts about …"
4. *Discuss implications.* You are guiding the employee to the necessary conclusion, not giving the answers. You can work toward this outcome by expanding the discussion using the following:
   • "If you did that, then would you be able to …"

- "Would that mean that …"
5. *Probe for details by using open-ended questions.* Using open-ended questions will place the employee in the position of guiding the outcomes, leading to the necessary conclusions. Some examples include:
  - "What prompted you to …?"
  - "How can I help?"
  - "Where do you think we need to focus?"

The coaching session

When conducting a coaching session, it is important that you clearly describe the problem and your expectations (see Table 7.4). Focus on what you observed:

- Speed
- Quantity
- Accuracy
- Thoroughness
- Timeliness

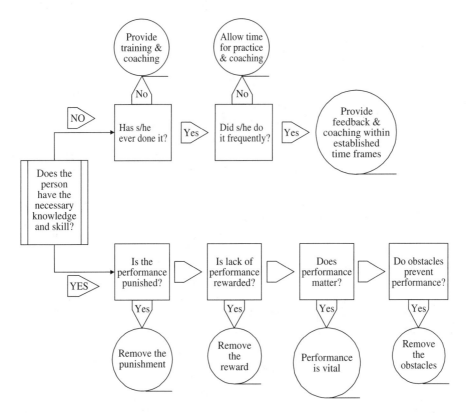

Figure 7.4 Determining the performance gap.

Table 7.4 The Four Elements of Coaching Follow-Up

1. Observe employees
   - Determine whether the objectives, goals, strategies, etc., have changed.
   - Determine ways to keep on top of performance.
   - Find opportunities for positive reinforcement and problem solving.
2. Solve problems
   - If necessary, reestablish priorities, goals, and objectives.
   - Determine ways to resolve problems in both the long term and the short term.
   - Revise work plans as needed.
3. Provide positive reinforcement
   - Reward positive performance as often as possible.
   - Use positive reinforcement to build working relationships.
   - Use positive reinforcement to encourage continuous improvement.
4. Record information and behaviors
   - Document changes in work plans.
   - Document instances to be used in formal review.
   - Record the following four facts:
     a. *When/where* — Note the time and location of the situation or circumstance.
     b. *What* did you observe? How was it different from what you expected?
     c. *Why* is it worth noting? What are the consequences?
     d. *How* is this situation going to change? Are there commitments involved?

The next step is to gain agreement on performance concerns or issues. This requires that you listen with an open mind — make every effort to approach the situation without prejudging motives. Once the employee has had the opportunity to provide full disclosure, provide more detailed feedback from your observation of performance. Then discuss the situation until you agree on the problem and the impact it has on the organization and on others.

The next step is to develop solutions together. This can be accomplished by exploring different solutions to solving the problem together. However, it is important that you let the employee take an active part in solving personal performance concerns or issues.

Then work toward developing an agreement on an action plan. Ask the employee to outline a plan for putting the solution into action. Then confirm your understanding by having the employee describe the action plan to you, thereby committing to it.

The final step in this phase of the process is to determine when you will follow up with the employee to review the progress. It is important that you establish a specific date and time for this follow-up session, so that both you and the employee understand the timeframe within which the agreed upon performance will be reached.

Prepare for the follow-up meeting

Preparing for the follow-up meeting requires you to observe whether the employee is successfully making the changes that both of you agreed upon and whether there are performance issues that could still use improvement.

Models for providing feedback

Most managers dread the process of providing feedback to employees and approach this event in one of four ways:

1. Conflict avoidance
2. The parent–child model
3. The teacher–student model
4. The adult–adult model

The parent–child model says that discipline equals punishment. The adult–adult model says that discipline equals structure. In a parent–child model, both the parent and the child react in an emotional manner. The parent says, "I set the rules" or "Because I say so." This engenders finger-wagging and a you-have-been-bad attitude. The child then responds with "I am not responsible," "Tell me exactly …," "It is not fair," or "Why do I have to?"

However, an adult–adult model is a rational interactive approach. Here you provide the facts, the organizational interests, and the consequences. In the adult–adult model it is important to:

• Focus on specific outcomes.
• Get the employees to commit to solving the problem.
• Follow up to ensure that it happens.

Ultimately, it is not your responsibility to improve your employees' behaviors — it is their responsibility. Your responsibility is to help them problem solve. Provide only the rational facts. Therefore, a discussion might be articulated in this manner, "When you do [*behavior*], the results are [*fact*], which do not meet [*desired outcome*]. In the future, I need you to do [*desired behavior*]. Failure to do so will result in [*consequence*]." (See Table 7.5.)

Typically, begin to use the process through verbal discussions of performance issues. If this fails to yield appropriate results, you may need to take the next step, using a written improvement plan process to document the discussions (Appendix B).

When making any employment-related decisions, including hiring, discharge, promotions, demotions, or discipline, you may apply, or appear to

Table 7.5 Five-Point Guide to Document Performance Issues

Describe what the *expectation* is for anyone who holds this position.
Describe how the individual's *current performance* falls short of expectations.
Describe what the individual *must do differently* in order to meet expectations, and what, if anything, you will do to help.
Describe *how long* the employee has to bring the current performance up to expectations.
Describe what will happen if the employee does not: *the consequences.*

apply, any of the following nine factors or characteristics of the employee: race, gender, religion, marital status, color, age, disability, national origin or ancestry, or veterans status. This is prohibited under federal and state law.

When you must make a decision concerning an employee's performance and potential discipline or dismissal, remember the "ouch" formula:

- *O — Objective standards.* Use standards capable of being measured. For example, "excellent typing skills" is subjective, whereas "must be able to type 50 words per minute" can be measured.
- *U — Uniformly applied standards.* Keep the nine factors listed previously in mind when making decisions. For example, ask all applicants the same questions and hold all applicants for the same position to the same requirements such as education or experience.
- *C — Consistency in effect.* Consider whether any of the requirements identified for a position effectively screen out a protected class, and, if so, determine whether that requirement is truly a bona fide job requirement. For example, requiring that a pharmacy technician be able to lift 50 lb. might effectively rule out women or individuals with disabilities. If you cannot prove that it is a primary function of the job, do not use this as a selection criterion.
- *H — Have job relatedness.* Use the job description as the starting point and make sure that all your managerial decisions are related to the job. Update the job description as needed and make sure that you provide the employees with the updated document.

It is important for managers to give due notice to employees. This includes giving employees sufficient opportunity to improve after being told that there is a problem, as well as alerting them to the seriousness with which the managers view the situation. In other words, if managers think that a particular behavior may result in termination of employment, they are responsible for telling that to the employees.

Conclusion

The evaluation and discipline processes are related through the elements of mentoring, coaching, and counseling. Managers must be able to use a variety of interpersonal skills to help employees improve their performance to achieve mutually agreed upon goals and objectives. Managers have clear responsibilities to communicate expectations and provide feedback on performance. While the formal end-of-year performance appraisal is necessary, the informal, more frequent approach to feedback and communication may help good employees perform better and the not-so-good ones become satisfactory.

Appendix A

Team Member Peer Evaluation Form

Name of team member being rated: _____

Name of evaluator: _____

Rating scale: • *Outstanding*: Team member consistently made unique and highly significant contributions • *Excels:* Team member's participation was highly effective • *Proficient:* Team member provided consistent and effective participation • *Needs improvement*: Team member was not consistent and may have also provided unacceptable participation	OUTSTANDING	EXCELS	PROFICIENT	NEEDS IMPROVEMENT
1 Knowledge of subject matter				
2 Professional demeanor and conduct				
3 Decisiveness				
4 Flexibility				
5 Initiative and creativity				
6 Team building within group				
7 Shared knowledge to identify solutions				
8 Planning and organizational skills				
9 Effective communication (written and oral)				
10 Interpersonal sensitivity				
11 Analytical skills (ability to see issues and analyze to build solutions)				

Comments: Your honesty and objectivity are very important, and will help your peers understand their strengths and weaknesses. Your evaluation will also identify areas that may need improvement. This form will not be directly shared with your team members, but will be summarized and shared.

Appendix B

Performance Improvement Plan

Identify items in which the employee has not met expectations, such as:

- Expected quality or quantity, or both, of work production
- Individual effectiveness
- Job knowledge
- Judgment and decision making
- Teamwork
- Service focus
- Project assignments
- Self-development objectives

Expectations of satisfactory completion of each item should be as specific as possible. Standards of quality, quantity, and timeliness should be stated clearly, as feasible. A meeting with the employee should then be conducted to communicate the plan. Additional follow-up meetings should be scheduled to review progress and provide additional coaching or counseling as appropriate. Use additional separate sheets as necessary.

Next scheduled progress review meeting is scheduled for: _____.

	<u>Signature</u>	<u>Date</u>
Employee's supervisor:	_____	_____
Employee:	_____	_____

Retain a copy in the department, provide a copy to the employee and forward the original to the Human Resources department.

Bibliography

Stromei L, Phillips J, eds. *In Action: Creating Mentoring and Coaching Programs.* American Society for Training and Development, Birmingham, AL, 2001.
SHRM/PDI 2000 Performance Management Survey, SHRM, December 2000.

chapter eight

Conflict management

Christy-Lee Lucas

Contents

Objective

This chapter is designed to imbue the reader with skills to manage conflict effectively. To achieve this goal, an outline of communication and listening skills is provided. A step-by-step guide is given to provide a foundation of the process involved in conflict management. Two examples of conflict models are explained to give a more specific view on types of personalities and ways to deal with them.

0-8493-1446-1/04/$0.00+$1.50
© 2004 by CRC Press LLC

Table 8.1 Health Care Professionals in Conflict

Wesley, Mrs. Montoya, and the Insurance Card

"Mrs. Montoya, do you have a new insurance card with you today?" asks Wesley, the pharmacist on duty.

Mrs. Montoya replies, "You should have my card on file. It is the same one I used last time."

Looking at the computer screen, then looking at his patient, Wesley says, "I am billing your insurance company directly on-line and they are telling me that your prescription coverage is terminated. Are you sure there isn't a new card?"

After smacking the countertop Mrs. Montoya shouts, "I've had it with you people! Every time I come to this pharmacy I have a problem. Last time you did not have my medication in stock and now this!"

The Drug Formulary Debate

Kenneth, a hospital pharmacist, receives a drug order from Dr. Decker. Mrs. Radley, one of Dr. Decker's patients, has been prescribed Prilosec®. Unfortunately for the patient, Prilosec is not on the hospital formulary. Kenneth pages the doctor to explain that the drug is not on the formulary. However, Prevacid®, a similar drug, is available. Dr. Decker refuses to change the drug and tells Kenneth to fix the problem.

The Concerta® Crisis

Andy, Brant, and Mike are assigned an important drug utilization review (DUR) of Concerta, which must be completed in 2 weeks. They meet and decide to split the project into three equal parts. Andy will determine the criteria to be studied, Brant will review charts for the pertinent data, and Mike will prepare the data into a computer presentation format. The group meets again in a week. Andy and Brant turn their information over to Mike and agree to meet in 5 days to go over the material and decide who should present what. Five days later, the trio meets again. Mike has not even started his assignment, citing vague personal problems as the culprit. He nastily adds that he thinks his partners are out to make him look bad and are heartless because he is having problems and they refuse to understand. Andy and Brant look at each other without a clue as to what they should do.

Introduction

A conflict, according to Ury et al. (1988), "begins when one person makes a claim or demand on another who rejects it." In pharmacy, conflict is part of everyday life.

Table 8.1 shows three typical scenarios in which pharmacists encounter conflict. Keep these scenarios in mind while reading through the chapter. They will be reviewed at the end to see how to help resolve conflict.

Conflict management vs. conflict resolution

Before beginning to study the nature of conflict management, it is important to understand the primary goal. Note that the title of the chapter is not "Conflict Resolution," but "Conflict Management." *Resolution*, according to the *Random House Dictionary* is a "solution, accommodation, or settling of a problem." It is not feasible to expect that all problems will be solved, accommodated, or settled. However, a person can manage, or, in other words, "control the course of affairs by one's own actions" in any conflict situation.

Good conflict management skills

Not all people are adept at conflict management. It requires skills on the part of the party handling the situation. Fortunately, these skills can be learned. Remember PILS — perception, integrity, listening skill.

Perception is the ability to read verbal as well as nonverbal behavior. Sometimes what people say is not what they mean. People with confused looks on their faces may be saying, "I understand," but do their expressions look like they mean it?

Integrity is a key factor in interactions with others, especially when emotion is involved. If people feel that someone is not trustworthy, they are less likely to reveal or identify underlying issues.

Listening is the most important and commonly used form of communication. It is also the most misused and misunderstood form.

The art of listening

According to Lucas (1994), there are several levels of listening. The listening level used can determine a person's ability to manage a conflict. The first level is called discriminative listening in which the person receiving information tries to ascertain the message through various distractions. In the following example, Tina is not using her discriminatory listening skill.

> Tina is taking a trip to the mall with her friend Gina. Gina is asking Tina's advice about an outfit she should wear for her fabulous date that night. Tina realizes that her favorite song is playing on the radio. She mentally sings the words in her head while trying to nod and listen to Gina. Tina catches snippets of what Gina is saying, but cannot physically hear all of both at the same time.

The second level is comprehensive listening. It is a deeper level of listening in which the receiver tries to assimilate the information for recall and reuse.

> Jeff is sitting in pharmacology class when his professor announces that there will be exam questions on the material he is about to cover. Hearing this, Jeff tells his friends to be quiet so he can listen to the lecture and remember the information for the exam.

Jeff wants to minimize his distractions so he can employ his comprehensive listening skill.

Therapeutic listening, the third level, involves the act of listening to information to make a plan of action. It is usually associated with an interaction that helps another person.

> "That professor is ridiculous. His test questions are so hard. Where does he pull the information from?" Amy cries to Michele after she finds that she failed the last biochemistry exam. "If I do not get an 87 on my next test, I might fail the course! What am I going to do?"

Michele will use her therapeutic listening skill as she tries to empathize with Amy's feelings of frustration.

The fourth and fifth levels of listening are combinations of the first and second levels (discriminative and comprehensive), used for different purposes. Critical listening, the fourth level, involves using these two levels of listening to assign meaning to a message in order to make a judgment on a course of action.

> Jimmy has a bad head cold and asks his pharmacist if she can recommend an over-the-counter product to make him feel better. "I feel so sick!" Jimmy complains to his pharmacist. "My head feels like it is going to explode. My nose is dripping like a faucet and I am achy all over. What can I take? Oh yeah, I have high blood pressure, too."

> Cheryl, the pharmacist, says to Jimmy, "Follow me to the cough and cold aisle and I'll help you pick something out. We do need to stay away from any products with decongestants in them because of your blood pressure."

Notice how Cheryl has discriminatively listened as well as comprehended the issue and begun to develop a course of action.

The fifth listening level is appreciative. It uses the combined effort of the first and second levels for pleasure in the case of an amusing anecdote or joke.

> Wayne says to Jen, "What kind of license does a pharmacist have?"

> Jen shakes her head and asks, "What kind?"

> Wayne replies, "A license to pill. Get it?"

How important is listening? If you are unprepared to listen to what a person is saying during a period of conflict, there is no point in addressing the conflict at that time. Listening to the other person is the only way to discover what the issues might be. Taking the time to listen also instills a feeling of trust in the aggrieved person, because you are communicating that he or she is important enough to be heard. Another bonus of listening is that it gives the speaker a chance to calm down and orally review the grievances and also gives you the time to figure out the other person's reference point.

Techniques for listening are easy to master with a little practice — and the rewards are unbelievable. First, use your discriminative listening skill to drown out all distractions. Stay focused on the person, maintaining good eye contact without staring. Nothing says you do not care like looking around at other things, fidgeting with objects, or vacantly staring. Ask for clarification of any fact that might be unclear or questionable. When doing this, use open-ended questions to draw out more information from the person. Before responding, rephrase the facts as you have heard them. Ask whether you have heard all of the information correctly and make changes as necessary.

Determination

When faced with a conflict, two major, related questions need to be answered: Is this conflict important to me? How do I know whether the situation is imperative to address? Ury et al. (1988) gauge the answers to these questions in terms of "transaction cost." The authors reason that in conflict, like in business, you want to minimize the costs. You need to consider the time cost, actual money cost, opportunity cost, and property cost and then determine the course of action that minimizes them. The answers also factor in satisfaction, long-term effects on relationships, and durability of a solution. For you, it may be helpful to analyze the person's relationship to you. Is this a significant relationship? Will you have to deal with this person in the future? Do you want things to work out? In the case of a family member, boss, subordinate, or colleague, the answer is usually "yes." With other scenarios such as a rude street vendor or casual acquaintance, the answer might be "no." If this is your decision, there is no need to continue further.

Another area of consideration is one in which you are a third party in the conflict, e.g., a fight between two siblings or two coworkers. Should you become involved? Acting as a mediator might be helpful, but make sure you are impartial. Once you have decided that management of the conflict is crucial, you are ready to move on.

Strategies for managing conflict

Getting down to it

In any conflict, a set of steps can be followed to manage the situation. The first few times you follow this algorithm, go through each step for maximum effectiveness. As you become more comfortable with your own communication and conflict resolution style, you can abbreviate or skip steps altogether.

There are seven major steps in the conflict management pathway. The first step involves identifying the correct person to speak to about the conflict. Acknowledging the feelings of the participants of the situation is the second step. The third step is finding something in common between the people in conflict. Taking the emphasis off the opposing persons and placing it on the item at hand is detailed in the fourth step. Identifying the real issue is the fifth step. The sixth step is being prepared to suggest solutions. The seventh step is how to deal with the aftermath of the conflict. Let us now discuss the conflict management steps in detail.

Step 1: Seek the right person

When you are the angry person in an incident or at the receiving end of the complaint or conflict, seek the appropriate person to speak to.

> Mr. Brody is an elderly gentleman who is taking a slew of medications for a previous myocardial infarction. Having no prescription insurance, he and his wife find it sometimes difficult to purchase his medications. This month, Mr. Brody decides to say his piece. His pharmacist, Jennifer Parker, works at a national chain pharmacy. She has a good relationship with this particular gentleman and is surprised to find him raising his voice and demanding that she lower the cost of his medications.

It does not make sense in this scenario for Mr. Brody to complain to the pharmacist at a national chain pharmacy that the costs of his drugs are too high. The pharmacist has no control over the situation and can do nothing for him. He has wasted time, emotion, and energy. Instead, he should write to the main office of the corporation or ask for the district manager's name and phone number. On the flip side, Ms. Parker is caught in a situation in which someone is making a complaint to her and she cannot meet his demands. She needs to refer Mr. Brody to the correct agency and provide him with a name or number of the agency if available (the company's district manager or corporate address and possibly the patient's physician to discuss cheaper therapy options).

Step 2: Acknowledge feelings

McClure (2000) discusses the importance of acknowledging feelings. Dealing with emotional people is not an easy task. You should not "explain away" their anger, even though your first instinct may be to explain to them why they should not be angry or upset about something.

> Pharmacist Cru: I know that you want the brand name Xanax®. We do not have it in stock right now, but the generic version is the same as the brand name.

Usually, this explanation only serves to inflame a person's anger.

Patient Luke: I do not care about that! I want my medication now!

Instead, acknowledge the emotion out loud. This will reduce people's negative emotions toward the situation. It shows that you are supportive and will aid them without being emotional yourself.

Pharmacist Cru: I understand that you are angry because we do not have your medication in stock.

Patient Luke: You're darned right I'm angry!

Step 3: Find something in common
McClure (2000), Lyles (2000), and Toropov (1997) all agree on the importance of this step. It is an excellent technique that can be used to focus a conflict on the issue instead of the emotion. People at conflict may not agree on a path to follow, but usually agree on the outcome. If you can find anything in common with the other person in the conflict, use it to bring the situation to a point where solutions can be explored.

Pharmacist Cru: Even though I do not have your medication in stock, I know we both want to find a way to get you your drug today.

Patient Luke: Yes, that is true. I do need my medication today.

The acknowledgement from the pharmacist diffuses the emotional aspect of the situation and takes the patient off the defensive. It forces the patient to look at the situation constructively so that he can reach his goal faster. (Note the finely honed listening skills exhibited by Pharmacist Cru: focusing on the patient and repeating the problem as the patient sees it.)

Step 4: Depersonalize the conflict
Arnold (1993) and McClure (2000) explore this critical step, which is a very difficult stage of conflict management. Making the conflict an impersonal "it" can be challenging in an emotional situation, especially if you feel you are the one who has been wronged. You need to take the emotional factor out of the equation in order to move forward constructively. This step is about changing your view of the situation from personal ("I cannot believe she is so lazy") to impersonal ("She has a relaxed work style"). Stewing in negative emotions will not help you accomplish a task. When you change the problem to an "it," the conflict will be easier to manage because emotional thoughts will not cloud you.

Emotions usually run high in cases of professional feedback and personal attacks. You need to learn the difference between the two, because everybody encounters each of these situations in their professional careers.

Professional feedback comes in many forms: a performance evaluation, comments after work performed, or peer reviews. This type of feedback is positive in that it can highlight your strengths and identify areas that need improvement. You learn and grow from professional feedback, assuming you can assimilate the information without being defensive. The information given is nonemotional; it is a simple statement of what the reviewer sees in your abilities. Professional feedback is given in private to prevent embarrassment of the subject. One last aspect of professional feedback is that it relates only to your work-related activities.

> "Joan, may I see you in my office for a moment?" asks Jack, the department supervisor. Joan hurries in to see Jack.
>
> "You wanted to see me?" Joan asks hesitantly.
>
> "I want to comment on your report from last week. It was insightful and well researched. I think, though, that you need to brush up on your computer skills — the graphs could have been more detailed than the way you presented them. Could you rework them for me and resubmit them? On the whole, however, it was a job well done."

On the opposite end of the feedback spectrum is a personal attack. A personal attack is negative and destructive. The only positives that may be gained from this type of feedback are to know the attacker's stance and improve your conflict management skills by diffusing the situation. The information given in a personal attack is based on emotion, personality, and communication style rather than any performance-related issue. There may or may not be facts present in the attack, which may be perpetrated in public or in private.

> "Joan!" the department supervisor, Jack, screams across the office. "I cannot believe how stupid you are! These graphs look like a two-year-old did them. I want you to stop wasting your time at the water cooler and start doing some actual work."
>
> Joan, furiously blushing, skulks back to her desk to redo the graphs.

Step 5: Get to the real issue

There is no way you can manage a conflict until you have identified the real underlying issues causing the conflict. If it is an emotionally charged situation, you may need to take some time to allow yourself and the other party to figure out what is causing the negative emotion. Once you have finished thinking about the motivations and actions leading to the conflict, you are prepared to deal with it.

Not only do you need to examine your own feelings and motivations, but you also need to examine those of the other person. Determining where a person is coming from is an invaluable asset in conflict management. Toropov (1997) suggests that Maslow's hierarchy of needs may be used to determine a person's reference point in conflict. Maslow outlines seven levels of needs:

1. Aesthetic
2. Knowledge
3. Self-actualization
4. Esteem
5. Belonging and love
6. Safety
7. Physiologic

Some sources list the aesthetic need (the need for beauty and grace) and the knowledge need as part of the self-actualization need. However, needing beauty, grace, and knowledge are not everyday aspects of pharmacy conflict. In light of this, we directly address the need for self-actualization. Self-actualization refers to the need for a person to feel fulfilled. Fulfillment issues are very common in a professional setting.

> Dominique, Alex, and Austin are given the assignment to write a review article on the diagnosis and treatment of ADHD. Francesca is asked to gather the appropriate research materials and make the information available to the three writers. Francesca thinks to herself, "Why do they never give me important assignments? Why am I never given the chance to do something challenging?"

The need for esteem can also be applied to Francesca's situation. She needs to feel good about herself. The lack of important assignments may cause her to be sullen and withdrawn around the department because she feels that she is not competent enough to be given difficult tasks.

People also have belonging and love needs. Although love is not a typical emotion involved in a professional environment, belonging and longing to be liked can be. Francesca might exhibit undesirable behaviors at work because she does not feel like an integral member of the team.

Safety issues may surface in a pharmacy, especially when dangerous chemicals are produced.

> Anthony is in the hood preparing a chemotherapy compound for a patient. He is always extremely meticulous with his safety practices. Anthony is concentrating intensely on the preparation when Melissa comes racing into the pharmacy yelling Anthony's name. Anthony explodes, "Shut up, you stupid idiot! I'm trying to make a chemo bag here without killing myself!"

The last need is physiologic. Physiologic needs are bodily needs. Conflict issues over having enough food to eat or a place to sleep are very rare in a professional atmosphere.

Maslow's hierarchy of needs may give you insight into another person's side of a conflict. The hierarchy may also help you to examine your own needs. In either case, you are more attuned to the other person's needs and motivations and are more able to accommodate them.

As you approach a person to manage a conflict (or you are approached), never resort to accusations. This will undo all the work accomplished by the first four steps. Accusations will put the other person in an immediate defensive position and will activate the "fight or flight" response inherent in us. Fighting only exacerbates a bad situation, and flight only puts the conflict on hold.

Start focusing on the real issue by stating your goal or purpose. Describe to the other person what you hope to accomplish by the end of the conflict. This will provide an outline for managing the situation.

Next, factually describe the events as you know them. This ties into the listening skills previously described. Leave no detail out. Ask whether the other party has anything to add or clarify. If the situation is serious enough, such as in a case of a medication error, take notes. You do not need to ask the person for permission to do this. Simply take out a pen and paper and write down pertinent facts. This way, you have a permanent record of the events in case they need to be specifically recalled later. It also prevents the problem of "he said/she said" that can occur in unpleasant situations.

Step 6: Be prepared to suggest solutions

If possible, do not approach a conflict without a plan to manage it. Brainstorm with the other person to gain more ideas. Write them down if necessary. Carefully inspect each idea to see whether both of you can be satisfied and reject any idea as needed.

Know beforehand what you are willing to concede. Clearly identify what you need to be satisfied in a solution. This will cut down on negotiation time and allow you to deal from a position of strength.

Step 7: Deal with the aftermath

As stated previously, although every conflict cannot be resolved, every conflict can be managed. After you have made a concerted attempt to manage a conflict, the aftermath inevitably follows. The conflict will have ended in one of two general ways: the relationship has weathered the conflict and both sides feel satisfied by the outcome; or the relationship has ended and the parties leave unsatisfied.

When the former occurs, the relationship may reach a new level because you have both faced a problem and overcome it together. This builds intimacy, which might lead to deeper fulfillment in a relationship. The parties previously in conflict can look at the conflict as a learning experience.

On the other hand, when a conflict is not resolved satisfactorily, the relationship may crumble under the strain. At this point, the lesson of letting go may help alleviate feelings of loss. Know that you did all you could to accommodate the situation in a way that could benefit both parties. If you feel that you could have done more, you might reexamine your conduct and instigate a dialogue with the other party. Again, the concept of acknowledging feelings — this time your own — comes into play. Admit to yourself that you are not happy with the way things turned out. Let yourself feel these emotions. If the relationship was a very close personal one, you may need time to grieve for the loss of it. Allowing yourself to feel will enable you to cope with the situation. Give others the space and time they need to deal with the aftermath. After a heated discussion, time apart may be the only thing that can help. Move on with your life. Do not dwell on the "what ifs." This will only undermine your healing.

Conflict models

Conflict models are helpful tools to deal with conflict in specific ways. Every author writing about conflict management has a different set of conflict models. A common model divides conflict into behavioral types and personalities. A personality is first defined by its method of operation. Once a personality is identified, a sculptured method of dealing with the personality is given.

One example of this is a personality model devised by Brinkman and Kirschner (1994). They assigned ten conflict personalities: tank, sniper, grenade, know-it-all, think-they-know-it-all, yes, maybe, nothing, no, and whiner. Each personality name indicates trademark characteristics. Tips on managing each personality are given in the following.

A *tank* is a forceful personality. Such people interrupt you and bulldoze right over you if you are in any way contrary to them. These people tend to go on tirades and do not let up. Your best bet is to hold your ground, be brief with any comments you have, and interrupt their attacks.

A *sniper* tends to make nasty personal comments in public. You know these people — in a middle of a meeting they shout out an inappropriate remark about the speaker. If you are the unfortunate speaker, you may lose your train of thought and feel embarrassed about the comment. To deal with this type, stop speaking, look the sniper directly in the eye, and ask, "What does your comment have to do with what we are talking about?"

The *grenade* is an apt title for people who never show anger until the one day they decide they cannot take any more and explode. This outburst (ranting, raving, and screaming) is so uncharacteristic that most other people are taken aback, often unaware that there was a problem. A good way to deal with grenades is to quickly get their attention and try to get to the underlying problem.

The *know-it-all*, as the name suggests, is a master in any area of expertise. These people have a propensity for being close-minded because they think that nobody can have ideas as good as theirs. When dealing with these people, you need to know your information. Any knowledge weakness and they will sniff it out. Also, present your ideas from a hypothetical angle. Ask, "What if we…."

People who *think they know it all* are tricky because they gloss over important details or exaggerate to seem like they know everything. Be sure to always ask for clarification on any items that are unclear. This way you can differentiate between what they say they know and what they truly know.

The person who says "yes" to everything is appropriately named the *yes*. Such people agree to do any task without thinking practically about how they will accomplish it. They may juggle 20 projects simultaneously, but will always take on more. Often, they are not able to fulfill certain tasks due to time constraints. Prevent being burnt by such people by making them commit to finishing your tasks and by helping them manage their time.

The *maybe* refuses to make a decision. Such people sway from side to side based on arguments presented at the time, but they avoid committing to one side. Help them come down from their fence by aiding their development of a decision-making process.

The *nothing* refuses to speak up when upset. Nothings become withdrawn. Try to guess at what is bothering them by asking them open-ended questions.

The *no* is the exact opposite of the *yes*. Such people shoot down every suggestion you have with a lot of negative reasons. Make these people useful by having them troubleshoot your ideas. They may find a potential problem where you have not. When dealing with such people, bring up negative reasons and find a way around them before they do.

The *whiner* constantly complains about everything from the weather to politics. Deal with such people by focusing on the positive aspects of the issue they are complaining about. If they continue to complain, walk away.

Table 8.2 describes each personality type and tips for dealing with each.

Toropov (1997) proposed a second conflict personality model: a four square model that includes four main personality types: the sharpshooter, the lone ranger, the professor, and the cheerleader (Table 8.3). Toropov suggests that by mirroring a personality to a specific personality type, you can more effectively manage conflicts with them. Following are scenarios that highlight characteristics of each personality type.

The sharpshooter

> Agnes, the district manager, asked Gary, the pharmacists' scheduler, to come up with a new system to schedule pharmacists. She requested that the original draft be submitted by Tuesday. It is now Friday and Gary has only a vague idea of how to frame the new system. Agnes confronts Gary, "I told you I wanted that draft 3 days ago. What is going on?"

Table 8.2 Tips for Dealing with Specific Personality Types •

Personality Type	Characteristics	Tips to Deal with the Type
Tank	• Forceful personalities • Tend to go on tirades	• Hold your ground • Be brief • Interrupt the attack
Sniper	• Interject disparaging comments in public places for maximum effect	• Stop speaking • Look directly at sniper • Ask direct questions
Grenade	• Hide anger until it reaches epic proportions • Scream	• Get their attention • Quickly get to the underlying problem
Know-it-all	• Extremely know ledgeable • Closed minded	• Know your informa-tion • Present your view hypothetically
Think-they-know-it-all	• Exaggerate • Gloss over unknown details	• Ask for clarification on specifics
Yes	• Want to please • Promise unrealistic things	• Help them manage time • Make them commit to finish things
Maybe	• Cannot or will not make a decision • Fickle	• Help them build a decision-making process
Nothing	• Refuse to speak up • Withdrawn	• Try to guess what is bothering them • Ask open-ended questions
No	• Focus on the negative	• Use them to find potential problems in a plan of action • Bring up negative items before they do
Whiner	• Constantly complain	• Focus on positives

Source: Adapted from Brinkman, R. and Kirschner, R. *Dealing with People You Can't Stand*. New York: McGraw-Hill, 1994.

Gary calmly replies, "I know how important details are to you. Instead of turning in a rough draft, I need more time to think about the scheduling system so that it runs perfectly."

Gary is mirroring Agnes' sharpshooter style by accommodating what she typically wants from him.

Table 8.3 Toropov's Four Square Model of Dealing with People

Personality Type	Description
Sharpshooter	Highly motivated; values quality over quantity
Lone ranger	Likes individual glory and undertakes massive workloads to achieve glory
Professor	Likes to find and overcome difficulties in order to maintain smooth workflow
Cheerleader	Into motivation and teamwork

Source: Adapted from Toropov, B. *The Art and Skill of Dealing with People*. Paramus, NJ: Prentice Hall, 1997.

The lone ranger

Nick and Moe cannot agree on how to market their company's new drug because Moe refuses to share any information with Nick. Nick, who is getting nervous about the situation, says to Moe, "If we are to make this deadline and turn in an outstanding marketing strategy, I need you to give me some of the information you have."

The professor

Edwin is a staff pharmacist working for Jo-Lynne at Dirt Cheap Pharmacy. Edwin is in charge of returning outdated medications to the warehouse for credit. The outdated drugs can be returned only within 2 months of their expiration or Jo-Lynne receives a drastic decrease in credit. Lately, Jo-Lynne notices that the drugs are not being pulled off the shelves in a timely fashion. When she asks Edwin why he is not performing his job, he answers, "It ruins the workflow."

Jo-Lynne returns to the pharmacy later with a checklist detailing specific days and times when the drugs should be pulled and returned, integrating this function into the workflow.

Here, Jo-Lynne is mirroring Edwin's professor style.

The cheerleader

Molly is the manager of a chain pharmacy. She notices her normally enthusiastic lead technician, Frankie, acting withdrawn and quiet. When Molly questions Frankie, she discovers that Frankie and another technician, Jane, recently argued about scheduling. Molly quietly takes Frankie aside and states, "You are an excellent technician. You are a key player on this pharmacy team and we need you at this store to make it run effectively."

Molly is the typical cheerleader, motivating Frankie.

Everyday practices to minimize conflict

Lyles (2000) discusses a major strategy to minimize the likelihood of conflict. Lyles writes that you should positively motivate those with whom you spend time. Do this by praising them, including them in important decisions, and recognizing their efforts.

Another strategy includes respecting people's personal space. There is a prescribed area that surrounds a person and should not be entered. This space decreases with your knowledge of the person. It may be disconcerting for coworkers when you stand over their shoulders, but may feel normal to close friends. People can be put on the defensive when you invade their space.

Paying close attention to your body language and that of others can help avoid conflict situations. Is someone having difficulty meeting your eye? Maybe there is a situation with them that can be taken care of before it even begins.

As in the third step of the conflict management pathway, find commonalities. Emphasize that even though there are differences among people, everyone contributes to the great whole. The teamwork mentality is more emotionally neutral than competition.

Getting the best out of yourself

To be an effective conflict manager, you must enter each situation with the same mind set. You have to be confident and project that confidence to those with whom you are in conflict. A sure way to fake confidence you do not feel is to maintain good posture and eye contact. Along with confidence, you must be enthusiastic. Apathy will get you nowhere if you are trying to resolve differences. Be a skilled listener. Practice discriminative listening at every opportunity. Make yourself understood. Use clear and concise communication. Know your influence.

Health care professionals in management

The following sections analyze the conflict scenarios in Table 8.1 using the steps of the conflict management pathway.

Wesley, Mrs. Montoya, and the insurance card

> *Step 1:* Wesley has done all he can with the insurance card Mrs. Montoya has given him. He knows that his only recourse is to go to the right "person" — the insurance company.
> *Step 2:* "Mrs. Montoya, I understand that you are upset about the insurance and feel like you have a problem every time you come to this pharmacy."
> *Step 3:* "I know we need to get this situation straightened out so we can get you your medication."

Step 4 and Step 5: Although Wesley is annoyed at Mrs. Montoya's rudeness, he tries to remember that the problem is not with Mrs. Montoya — it is an insurance problem.

Step 6: "If you do not mind waiting, I can take this up with your insurance company and find out what the problem is. If it is something that can be resolved now, then I will take care of it. Otherwise, will you be all right if I give you a few days' worth of medication to hold you until the problem can be fixed?"

Step 7: After waiting on hold, the insurance agent informs Wesley that the patient is no longer covered and that Mrs. Montoya should contact her benefits office. When Wesley relays that information to Mrs. Montoya, her face turns a mottled shade of red. Wesley offers again to give her some medication. Mrs. Montoya accepts the offer and vows to "eat her insurance company alive."

Wesley thinks that he explored every option for the patient. He can now move onto the next problem with aplomb.

The drug formulary debate

Step 1: Kenneth knows that he needs to deal with Dr. Decker in order to get a grip on the situation.

Step 2: "Dr. Decker, I can tell that you are a busy person and that your time is valuable. I can also tell that you think the hospital's formulary is restrictive."

Step 3: "You and I must work together to find a solution for Mrs. Radley. We do not want her up half the night again with stomach acid."

Step 4 and Step 5: Kenneth keeps repeating to himself that this is not about a nasty physician, but that he is working on a formulary issue.

Step 6: "If you would like, Dr. Decker, I can automatically change the order to Prevacid. If you really want the patient on Prilosec, Mrs. Radley will need you to fill out a nonformulary request sheet."

Step 7: Dr. Decker is still not happy, but grudgingly gives the okay to change the order to Prevacid. Kenneth, on the other hand, is happy that he single-handedly saved Mrs. Radley from another sleepless night.

The Concerta® Crisis

Step 1: Andy and Brant decide that they need to sit down with Mike and talk this out.

Step 2: Andy consoles Mike, "We know that you feel like we are out to make you look bad. You also feel like you are under pressure with this project considering your personal situation right now."

Step 3: Brant continues, "The three of us have to pull together to get this DUR done. The department is depending on our research of Concerta use. All of us care deeply about our jobs and the work that we do."

Step 4: On a roll, Brant says, "This is not really about personal issues. This is about time management. We have two days to finish this."

Step 5: Andy thinks that because Mike talked about some unresolved personal problems, maybe he is feeling insignificant or out of control. If Andy and Brant make Mike feel as if the work he does is crucial to the project's success (which it is), then Mike will be up to the task of doing his work.

Step 6: Andy and Brant make it clear that they will be available to Mike at any hour if he has questions or problems with the project, but they will not do his work.

Step 7: Tragedy strikes when the project is due and Mike still has not completed the project. Andy and Brant acknowledge that they tried to help Mike and did everything they could without compromising their morals. They both feel angry at Mike and embarrassed that a project that was given to them was not completed on time. The pair decides that if they are given another DUR to complete and Mike is assigned to their group, they will request to have another member take Mike's place in view of this recent development.

Conclusion

Remember that conflict does not have to be a win–lose situation. There are many layers to every problem and many ways to manage every problem. Hopefully, this chapter has provided a framework to accomplish conflict management. Good luck!

Bibliography

Arnold, J.D. *When the Sparks Fly: Resolving the Conflicts in Your Organization.* New York: McGraw-Hill, 1993.

Blanchard, K. and Johnson, S. *The One Minute Manager.* New York: William Morrow, 1982.

Blanchard, K. and O'Connor, M. *Managing by Values.* San Francisco: Berrett-Koehler Publishers, 1997.

Brinkman, R. and Kirschner, R. *Dealing with People You Can't Stand.* New York: McGraw-Hill, 1994.

Burley-Allen, M. *Managing Assertively.* New York: John Wiley & Sons, 1995.

Cloke, K. and Goldsmith, J. *Resolving Conflicts at Work.* San Francisco: Jossey-Bass, 2000.

Fujishin, R. *Discovering the Leader Within: Running Small Groups Successfully.* San Francisco: Acada Books, 1997.

Gootnick, M.M. and Gootnick, D. *Action Tools for Effective Managers.* New York: Amacom, 2000.

Hersey, P. *The Situational Leader.* New York: Warner Books, 1984.

Levey, I. *Getting the Best out of Yourself and Others.* New York: Harper & Row, 1987.

Lucas, R. *Effective Interpersonal Relationships.* New York: Mirror Press, 1994.

Lyles, D. *Winning Ways.* New York: G.P. Putnam's Sons, 2000.

McClure, L. *Anger and Conflict in the Workplace.* Manassas Park, VA: Impact Publications, 2000.

Minor, M. *Preventing Workplace Violence: Positive Management Strategies.* Menlo Park, CA: Crisp Publications, 1995.

Solomon, M. *Working with Difficult People.* Englewood Cliffs, NJ: Prentice Hall, 1990.

Toropov, B. *The Art and Skill of Dealing with People.* Paramus, NJ: Prentice Hall, 1997.

Ury, W., Brett, J.M., and Goldberg, S.B. *Getting Disputes Resolved.* San Francisco: Jossey-Bass Management and the Jossey-Bass Social and Behavioral Science Series, 1988.

Weisinger, H. *Anger at Work.* New York: William Morrow, 1995.

chapter nine

Accounting principles

Robert J. Votta

Contents

Introduction to accounting

Accounting is the essence of any business organization as it provides a useful tool for creditors, employees, investors, managers, owners, and all interested parties to make well-informed business decisions. Accounting is basically an artificial business language. Some basic accounting and financial terms include accruals, payables and receivables, yields, and evaluations. It is

0-8493-1446-1/04/$0.00+$1.50
© 2004 by CRC Press LLC

essential that this artificial language be comprehended for effective financial decision making. The more accounting knowledge a pharmaceutical professional acquires, the better armed this person will be to enter the business marketplace. The pharmaceutical professional will not only have a better understanding of accounting information, but will also know how to compile it, use it, and recognize the limitations of accounting.

The definition of accounting

Accounting is the process of analyzing, classifying, recording, summarizing, and interpreting business information into understandable financial terms to facilitate effective business decision making. The first part of the definition refers to the following:

- *Analyzing* entails examining business transactions that involve basic ongoing activities, such as investing personal cash or equipment into the business, purchasing supplies with cash or credit, and the like.
- *Classifying* refers to the activity of providing a name for each specific account analyzed in the transactions, such as assets, liabilities, and owner's equity.
- *Recording* is the process of writing the accounting transactions in journals, ledgers, and financial statements to provide a permanent record of the accounting activities.
- *Summarizing* is the totaling of the ledgers and statements in order to acquire final figures to be used in the next step.
- *Interpreting* involves the various interested parties analyzing the final totals to facilitate comprehensive and effective business decisions.

The need for accounting and the accounting entity concept

There are vital reasons for using accounting concepts. First, annually compiling and presenting the firm's financial data can provide a picture of the financial history of the organization. The financial history of a firm is not always available without accounting statements, and the financial history of a pharmacy is important in many investment decisions. Second, an immediate snapshot of a pharmacy's financial condition is provided via financial statements such as a balance sheet, income statement, or statement of owner's equity. Investors, company managers, creditors, governmental agencies, and the general public can analyze and interpret this accounting data for effective business decision making.

While there are many other advantages to accounting, one interesting use revolves around a situation referred to as the accounting or separate entity concept. An accounting entity is any organizational unit for which financial data is gathered and interpreted for decision making purposes. For example, in addition to personal items, a single entrepreneur, Amy Harris, owns a pharmacy, a restaurant, a bakery, and a delivery service. Each business owned by Harris must keep separate and distinct accounting records because all activities combined would be useless for decision making within any single unit. Therefore, she cannot pay a purchasing order for the restaurant with cash receipts from the bakery or pharmacy. A set of accounting records is developed for *each* of her individual businesses to facilitate planning and controlling decisions, and her accountants must focus on each individual business as a separate and distinct business unit. This is just one of the many accounting rules and requirements included under the generally accepted accounting principles.

Generally accepted accounting principles

Consistency is an essential aspect of accounting and because it is vital for everyone who acquires accounting reports to be able to interpret them, a set of guidelines has been developed. These guidelines describing how the accounting process should be completed are called the generally accepted accounting principles (GAAPs).

The GAAPs, developed and agreed upon by accountants, provide the rules that cover financial accounting rather than other types of accounting such as tax accounting. In relation to a pharmacy, financial accounting develops financial statements that report the pharmacy's overall performance to internal and external users.

Accounting planning and budgeting

A crucial management task is to project where the pharmacy should be in the future and consider the steps needed to achieve this goal. A vital part of this planning process is to create budgets that act as tools to facilitate these business decisions.

Budgets are usually operational (short-term) plans concerning sales and profit forecasts within the next year. In essence, they are organizational financial plans expressed in monetary terms for future periods of time. Three types of budgets are commonly used by pharmacies:

1. *Cash budget.* Is a schedule of cash receipts and disbursements reflecting a pharmacy's projected cash inflows and outflows.
2. *Operating budget.* Presents a pharmacy's anticipated revenues and expenses. In addition to the cash budget, a sales expense budget provides a vital degree of management control.
3. *Capital budget.* Shows a pharmacy's possible investment in fixed assets.

Hospitals, chain pharmacies, and long-term care pharmacy providers commonly use capital budgets more often than small local pharmacies. Because planning involves an estimate of future demand, it is an extremely difficult and inexact process. Therefore, many forecasts of demand are for the short term, usually for the next 6 to 12 months.

Users of accounting data

Compiling organized financial records guarantees that needed accounting information is available on a timely basis to internal and external users. For external purposes, these accurate accounting statements are essential for meeting the requirements of creditors, tax obligations, concerns of outside investors, and the general public. For example, the Internal Revenue Service (IRS) and regulatory agencies such as the boards of pharmacy require detailed accounting information about a pharmacy. In addition, investors and creditors may be interested in the liquidity or profitability of a specific pharmacy for their respective investment and credit-availability decisions.

Internal uses by company managers at all levels include inventory control, depreciation valuation, cash flow, and availability. Additional internal reasons for the proper use of accounting records parallel a major external concern, i.e., liquidity and profitability, which are also serious internal concerns for pharmaceutical managers.

Developing an accounting system

Numerous activities occur on a daily basis that can change assets (things that we own, e.g., a computer), liabilities (debts that we owe, e.g., notes payable), and the owner's equity (the worth of the owner, e.g., Amy Harris, capital). These changing events must be entered in accounting records. Developing a set of financial records is the responsibility of the firm's owner, and a system should be developed that is compatible with the company's owner and managers who use this information.

An entrepreneur who becomes the owner initially creates a firm with a personal investment. Then, the new firm purchases and sells assets, collects receivables, pays liabilities, and conducts many other business activities called transactions. Each transaction must be evidenced with a business document. For example, a business entity that purchases office furniture costing $500 by paying $200 in cash and the balance of $300 on credit should provide the accountant with a purchase invoice verifying the price and quantity, a check stub of the owner's checkbook or a receipt for a cash payment, and a bill that the balance of $300 is due in 30 days (an accounts payable). These documents evidence accounting information used by accountants and are available for current and future review by independent certified public accountants.

The accounting equation

Each transaction is analyzed by using the accounting equation because the financial position of a firm is affected by every transaction.

The accounting equation is as follows:

$$\text{Assets} = \text{Liabilities} + \text{Owner's equity}$$

An example of a transaction is as follows. Amy Harris invests $50,000 cash in her business as of May 1:

Assets	=	Liabilities	+	Owner's equity
+$50,000	=		+	+$50,000
$50,000	=	$50,000 = (both sides of the equation in balance)		

This example reflects the concept of double-entry accounting, in which there are offsetting entries for each transaction. In accounting terminology, for each debit entry there must be a corresponding credit entry in order to maintain a consistent balance. The possibility for error is reduced by creating the system of checks and balances.

Maintaining journals and ledgers

Many other types of transactions occur after analyzing the accounting equation and classifying different account titles, such as cash, account receivables, account payables, and capital. It is necessary to record the transactions in various journals.

Types of journals

This third part of the accounting definition outlines the process in which transactions are officially recorded. A journal provides the history of all transactions recorded by the dates of occurrence. There are many types of journals, including the general journal, the sales journal, the purchases journal, and the cash receipts journal. The following four journals reflect two main advantages for an accounting system: they strengthen managerial control and increase processing efficiency.

In a general journal, a detailed description of each transaction is provided and journalized (recorded). As it is the initial record of each transaction, this journal is referred to as the book of original entry. The general journal includes the date, type of transaction, and dollar amount involved. It is the simplest form of journal and may be the only journal used by a firm because it includes transactions that are not applicable for other types of journals. However, other journals are often used as one journal may prove too cumbersome and disorganized for a corporation. Table 9.1 presents an example of a general journal for Amy Harris's initial investment.

The previously detailed information, including the posting reference (PR) from the general journal and all other journals, is posted to the general ledger. The general ledger is outlined in the next section. A sales journal is used to record all sales of merchandise on account only and is viable for firms that survive on credit sales such as third-party prescriptions. The entries to this journal become accounts receivable. The sales journal records the sales, date, merchandise, and amount due.

Table 9.1 Example of a General Journal for Initial Investment

Date	Account Titles/Explanation Posting	Reference	Debit	Credit
2002	Cash	111	50,000	
May 1	Amy Harris, Capital	311		50,000

Note: To record the initial investment by the owner to start the firm called Harris Pharmacy.

A purchases journal is a record of all purchases made on account only and helps avoid repetition in the general journal. A purchases journal reflects the supplier, type of merchandise purchased, amount owed, and the due date for payment. The total of this journal can be completed at any time to compute the total dollar amount owed to all suppliers and the due dates for each payment.

A cash payments journal is used to record all transactions (usually by check) in which cash is paid or decreases. It also outlines disbursements to suppliers on a cash basis and credit payments previously entered in the purchases journal. The transactions are recorded by indicating to whom the payment was made, amount owed, date, any discounts included, and actual amount paid. The importance of a cash payments journal is that all outflows of money from the business are reflected here. An individual entry in the cash payments journal is usually not necessary for petty cash, which is kept in the cash register for very small transactions. These are accounted for only in the cash payments journal's total.

A cash receipts journal includes all cash receipts and cash increases. It also includes sales and payments from credit customers previously entered in the sales journal. Cash register totals, cash receipts from credit sales, and from whom the cash was received are included here. The advantage is that all transactions involving increases in cash are recorded in one place. Cash sales payable by credit customers are outlined here, and by comparing this journal with the sales journal, one can determine who pays their bills punctually and who is perennially late. In addition, by comparing this journal with the cash receipts journal, cash inflow and outflow can be determined.

Posting to the ledgers

In the sequential order of the accounting cycle, after all business transactions are analyzed, they are journalized in the general journal and then posted to the general ledger. Posting is the transfer of amounts from the general journal to the specific individual accounts in the book of final entry, the general ledger. Because it is virtually impossible to readily determine the balance of any specific account, such as cash, from the journal entries, the general ledger is maintained to provide a complete record of the individual accounts recorded initially as entries in the general journal and also reflected on the financial statements. It is essentially a book containing all the organization's accounts.

Ledgers effectively total the amounts of specific financial activities and prepare them to be used in the various statements, e.g., the balance sheet and income statement. Additional ledgers include the accounts receivable and accounts payable ledgers, and these provide a handy way to account for payments due and owed. Receivables and payables are included in the general ledger, and many companies, including pharmaceutical firms, have many suppliers and innumerable customers who need these specialized ledgers. The accounts receivable and accounts payable ledgers are used not only to facilitate convenience but also as controlling tools. In addition, credit limits established for customers and by suppliers are included in the ledgers and management is alerted when any account approaches the predetermined credit limits.

Chart of accounts

This is the arrangement of all general ledger accounts in a sequential order: assets are listed first, liabilities second, owner's equity third, revenue fourth, and expenses fifth. Table 9.2 presents a sample ledger of accounts for Harris Pharmacy. In the table, the order of accounts consists of the balance sheet accounts followed by the income statement accounts, with the account numbers preceding the account titles. In the posting process, placing the account

Table 9.2 Sample Chart of Accounts

Assets (100–199)

111	Cash
112	Accounts receivable
113	Supplies
114	Prepaid insurance
121	Equipment

Liabilities (200–299)

211	Accounts payable
212	Notes payable
213	Wages payable

Owner's Equity (300–399)

311	A. Harris, capital
312	A. Harris, drawing

Revenue (400–499)

411	Sales

Expenses (500–599)

511	Wages expense
512	Rent expense
513	Advertising expense
514	Utilities expense

number in the PR column of the journal next to the journal entry and placing the journal page number in the PR column in the specific ledger account is called cross-referencing.

Financial statements

A financial statement is a report developed by the accounting department for both internal and external users. Numerous statements are developed by way of journal and ledger entries. However, a firm uses four major financial statements to report its financial condition:

1. Income statement
2. Statement of owner's equity
3. Balance sheet
4. Statement of cash flows

These statements provide a snapshot of the business in relation to profit and losses increases and decreases in capital, status of assets and debts, and the efficient or inefficient use of cash by the firm.

Income statement

The most popular statement is the income statement, also referred to as the profit and loss statement. This statement reflects the results of all business transactions over a period of time and is a summary of all the firm's earned revenue, i.e., income from sales and services less all expenses incurred, i.e., costs associated with the earning process. The income statement usually covers a specific period of time selected by the firm, generally called a fiscal period. The fiscal period basically describes a business year, e.g., beginning on May 1, 2002, and ending on April 30, 2003. Many firms use a calendar year extending from January 1 to December 31 of the same year as their fiscal year.

Income statements are generally completed on a monthly basis, especially in a pharmacy, because it is essential to keep track of the company's profitability in a timely manner in order to institute corrective actions when necessary. When total revenue exceeds total expenses over the period selected, the remaining positive amount reflects a net income (profit).When the opposite occurs and total expenses exceed total revenue, the result is a net loss. Table 9.3 presents a brief sample of an income statement.

Many firms, such as KYW Radio in Philadelphia, sustain a loss for a number of years before the year they realize their initial profit. This station changed from a country-western format in the 1960s to all-news radio and did not realize its first year of complete profit until about 1983. Since that time, KYW has consistently been at the top of the radio market.

Table 9.3 Sample of an Income Statement

Harris Pharmacy
Income Statement
For the month ended May 31, 20–

Revenues		
Net sales[a]		$15,500
Expenses		
Salaries and wages expense	$8,200	
Rent expense	$750	
Advertising expense	$125	
Utilities expense	$230	
Miscellaneous expense	$45	
Total expenses		$9,350
Net income		$6,150

[a] Net sales represents the dollar amount of annual sales less sales tax and any sales returns and allowances.

Statement of owner's equity

This statement reflects the changes that occurred in owner's equity during the period included on the income statement. The accountant uses the net income or net loss compiled on the income statement, including withdrawals, to show how owner's equity (capital account) has changed over time, resulting in a (new) beginning capital balance for the next accounting period. This statement is also referred to as the statement in changes in stockholders' equity for a corporation since the owners are shareholders in the company. This corporate form includes retained earnings, which is the total of all net income amounts less all dividends (declared earnings distributed to stockholders on a periodic basis) paid during the life of the firm. This amount reflects the part of the shareholders' claims that the firm has earned but not contributed. Retained earnings are not the same as cash. Table 9.4 presents a brief sample of this statement.

Table 9.4 Statement of Owner's Equity

Harris Pharmacy
Statement of Owner's Equity
For the month ended May 31, 20–

A. Harris, capital, May 1, 20–		$50,000
Add: Net income for May[a]	$6,150	
Less: Withdrawals by the owner	$4,000	
Increase in capital		$2,150
A. Harris, capital, May 31, 20–		$52,150

[a] The net income amount is from the May 31 income statement.

Balance sheet

This statement is a picture of a firm's financial position as of one day in time. The balance sheet includes the distinct balances:

- Assets, e.g., cash, furniture, or land
- Liabilities, e.g., notes or wages payable
- Owner's equity, e.g., capital or retained earnings

The balance sheet changes with every transaction based on the accounting equation:

$$\text{Assets} = \text{Liabilities} + \text{Owner's equity}$$

Assets are things of value that the business owns. Liabilities are amounts that the firm owes to others such as suppliers. For example, the amount owed on the purchase of a computer is a liability. Finally, owner's equity represents claims of the owner, wherein claims can increase by personal investments from outside the business and by earning revenue as the result of conducting business. Equity that is accumulated from a successful business and kept by the firm is included in the retained earnings account. Table 9.5 shows the balance sheet for Harris Pharmacy.

Statement of cash flows

An essential consideration of financial management is liquidity: the ability to turn assets into cash quickly. Assets included on the balance sheet are

Table 9.5 Sample of a Balance Sheet

<table>
<tr><td colspan="4" align="center">Harris Pharmacy
Balance Sheet
May 31, 20–</td></tr>
<tr><td align="center">Assets</td><td></td><td align="center">Liabilities and Owner's Equity</td><td></td></tr>
<tr><td>Current Assets</td><td></td><td>Current Liabilities</td><td></td></tr>
<tr><td>Cash</td><td>$24,800</td><td>Accounts payable</td><td>$1,350</td></tr>
<tr><td>Accounts receivable</td><td>$8,425</td><td>Total current liabilities</td><td>$1,350</td></tr>
<tr><td>Merchandise inventory</td><td>$12,200</td><td>Long-Term Liabilities</td><td></td></tr>
<tr><td>Prepaid insurance</td><td>$1,460</td><td>Notes payable</td><td>$2,000</td></tr>
<tr><td>Total current assets</td><td>$46,885</td><td>(due after one year)</td><td></td></tr>
<tr><td>Fixed Assets</td><td></td><td>Total long-term liabilities</td><td>$2,000</td></tr>
<tr><td>Equipment</td><td>$5,215</td><td>Total liabilities</td><td>$3,350</td></tr>
<tr><td>Furniture and fixtures</td><td>$3,400</td><td>Owner's Equity</td><td></td></tr>
<tr><td>Total fixed assets</td><td>$8,615</td><td>A. Harris, capital[a]</td><td>$52,150</td></tr>
<tr><td></td><td></td><td>Total Liabilities and</td><td></td></tr>
<tr><td>Total Assets</td><td>$55,500</td><td>Owner's Equity</td><td>$55,500</td></tr>
</table>

[a]The new capital amount is from the May 31 statement of owner's equity.

Table 9.6 Statement of Cash Flows

Statement of Cash Flows For the period ending May 31, 20–	
Cash flow (used by) operating activities	$8,000
Cash flow from investing activities	($4,500)
Cash flow from financing activities	($1,500)
Net increase or decrease in cash	$2,000[a]

[a]The cash flows involved in operating activities concern changes in the current asset and liability accounts whereas investing relates to changes in fixed assets, except accumulated depreciation and financing activities involve changes in owner's equity accounts.

categorized as current and plant (long-term), with current assets representing assets that can be readily turned into cash within 1 year, such as cash, accounts receivable, supplies, inventory, and prepaid expenses. Plant assets, such as equipment, buildings, and land, take longer than 1 year to turn into cash and are therefore not as liquid. Note that assets are always presented in their order of liquidity. Because cash is the most liquid asset, it is vital to any organization to keep track of the inflows and outflows of this asset. The statement of cash flows outlines how cash balance and cash equivalents have changed from the beginning to the end of the fiscal year. This statement has also been referred to as the sources and uses of cash statement. In addition to determining the liquidity of the firm, this statement can aid managers in determining the company's dividend policy and evaluating potential investment opportunities and ability to borrow and make cash payments on time. To determine whether there is a positive or negative cash flow, the statement of cash flows divides cash receipts and payment into three areas: cash flows from (used by) operating activities, investing activities, and financing activities. Table 9.6 outlines a condensed example.

The accounting cycle

After becoming familiar with the accounting equation, journalizing, posting, and various financial statements, it is important to consider the remaining steps and the order of the accounting process. The accounting cycle is a process whereby accounting professionals develop a business entity's financial statements for a specific period of time, e.g., the fiscal year. This cycle is repeated for all new accounting periods, with the end product being a new set of financial statements. Table 9.7 gives an overview of the accounting cycle.

Interpretation of financial statements

Comparative financial statement analysis

Management, investors, creditors, and various other business professionals depend on accounting data to facilitate effective business decision making.

Table 9.7 Accounting Cycle

1. Begin the new period with the owner's initial investment into the business or the beginning account balances in the general ledger.
2. Analyze and classify each transaction as it occurs.
3. Journalize the transactions in the general journal.
4. Post journal entries to the ledger accounts and compute the unadjusted balance of each account at the end of the period.
5. Complete a trial balance [a listing of all ledger account balances used to check the equality of the accounting equation A = (L + OE)].
6. Complete a work sheet (includes adjusting entries that bring specific accounts up to date).
7. Journalize and post adjusting entries.
8. Journalize and post closing entries.
9. Prepare a postclosing (afterclosing) trial balance.
10. Prepare the financial statements (income statement, statement of owner's equity, balance sheet, statement of cash flows, etc.).

To evaluate accounting information, business people evaluate financial statements in three broad areas: (1) horizontal analysis, (2) vertical analysis, and (3) ratio analysis.

Analyses used by creditors, owners, and management

Horizontal analysis

Numerous business decisions depend on how the figures for sales, income, and expenses fluctuate during the period of operations. How have sales changed within the last 5 years? Are expenses increasing at a faster rate than income? Although very interesting, the answers to these questions may not be useful for decision making unless the percentage change is analyzed in any account classification, e.g., sales over time. The study of percentage changes among years in comparative statements is called horizontal analysis. The procedure to compute the percentage change in horizontal analysis requires:

- Computing the dollar amount of the change from the base (earlier) period to the latter period
- Dividing the dollar amount of change by the base period amount

Table 9.8 presents horizontal analysis.

Vertical analysis

Vertical analysis is another strategy employed by accountants to analyze financial statements. When an income statement is used for vertical analysis, each account in the statement is expressed as a percentage of net sales, i.e., dividing the total amount of any item by the total of net sales. A firm would

Table 9.8 Horizontal Analysis

	2002	2001	Increase or Decrease	Amount%
Sales	$42,430	$36,864	$5,566	15.1[a]
Net income	$17,800	$16,560	$1,240	7.5

[a] The firm has a percentage increase in sales that is approximately twice the percentage increase as net income between 2001 and 2002.

raise a red flag if it normally experiences gross profit at a rate of 40% of net sales and then suddenly records a drop in gross profit to 25%.

In a balance sheet, total assets and total liabilities should be used as denominators to determine the percentage of specific assets, liabilities, and owner's equity, respectively. All financial statement users, including shareholders, will exhibit concern because this drop in gross profit may make the firm report a net loss on the current income statement. Table 9.9 illustrates a sample of vertical analysis for a balance sheet.

Ratio analysis
In addition to using financial statements for comparative horizontal and vertical analysis, ratios are another available tool. Developing relationships among financial statement items is the crux of ratio analysis. In this type of analysis, it is extremely important for the evaluators, such as creditors or management, to select the ratio applicable to their immediate area of concern. Then, the relevant ratio can be calculated for analysis, and, finally, more research might be necessary as ratio analysis is limited.

Table 9.9 Vertical Analysis

Current Assets	December 31, 2002	Vertical Analysis%
Cash	$32,000	17.2
Accounts receivable	$14,400	7.7
Inventory	$23,720	12.7
Total current assets	$70,120	37.6
Fixed Assets		
Land	$8,000	4.3
Building	$96,000	51.5
Store equipment	$12,210	6.6
Total fixed assets	$116,210	62.4
Total Assets	$186,330	100.0

Note: (1) The vertical analysis of the balance sheet reflects any account selected as the numerator and the amount of total assets as the base or denominator (e.g., cash account $32,000/$186,330). (2) Each liability or owner equity account is divided by the total of liabilities and owner's equity.

Solvency (liquidity)

Solvency refers to an enterprise's ability to meet its long-term debt obligations on a continuing basis. All financial statement users are interested in the liquidity of a firm in addition to the obvious liquidity concerns of creditors and management. Will the firm be able to pay its short-term debts as they become due? Can the firm cover its current liabilities with its current assets? Does the firm have an efficient mix of current assets, e.g., cash and inventory? Do owners and management properly use the current assets? To effectively answer these and other financial questions, it is necessary to use the following financial tools.

Working capital

To measure a firm's ability to pay off its short-term debt with its current assets, the working capital is computed by subtracting current assets from current liabilities. Table 9.10 presents the working capital of two firms. In the example, the Blue company's working capital is as large as its current liabilities, whereas the Gold company's working capital is only one-third of its current liabilities. However, both firms have equal working capital of $100,000. Obviously, the Blue company has a stronger working capital position because its working capital is a greater percentage of current assets and current liabilities. The amount of working capital is more valuable in decision making when used as part of a financial ratio. The current ratio and the acid-test ratio make effective use of the working capital figures.

Current ratio

The most popular indicator of a firm's ability to pay off its short-term debt is the current ratio. The formula is:

$$\text{Current ratio} = \frac{\text{Current assets}}{\text{Current liabilities}}$$

Table 9.11 calculates the current ratio for the Blue and Gold companies. Although both companies have $100,000 more of current assets than current liabilities (working capital), the current ratio varies substantially. The Blue company's management has twice as many assets to pay for the current

Table 9.10 Working Capital of Two Firms

	Blue Company	Gold Company
Current assets	$200,000	$400,000
Current liabilities	$100,000	$300,000
Working capital	$100,000	$100,000

Table 9.11 Current Ratio

Blue Company	Gold Company
Current ratio = $\dfrac{\$200{,}000}{\$100{,}000}$ = 2:1	Current ratio: $\dfrac{\$400{,}000}{\$300{,}000}$ = 1.33:1

liabilities as they become due, but the Gold firm has only 1.33 of current assets for the current debt. Therefore, the current ratio reveals that the Blue company is more liquid than the Gold company. The best current ratio will vary depending on the type of industry; a ratio of 2:1 is considered ideal in most situations. A current ratio higher than 2:1 may mean that the levels of cash, accounts receivable, inventory, and so forth are too high, and it may be best to invest in some short-term securities to increase the firm's income and make effective use of available funds.

Acid-test ratio

Although the current ratio is valuable, an organization may wish to go further to evaluate liquidity. The acid-test or quick ratio is a means to consider only the most liquid of the current assets and determine whether the firm can pay its short-term debt even more quickly. The formula for the quick ratio is:

$$\text{Acid-test ratio} = \frac{\text{Cash} + \text{Accounts receivable} + \text{Short-term securities}}{\text{Current liabilities}}$$

Only the most liquid of assets are included in this ratio, and the best ratio is usually 1:1, but this varies with the industry concerned. Table 9.12 calculates the acid-test ratio. Although the Blue company has a better current ratio than the Gold company, it does not have a better acid-test ratio, and, therefore, may have to sell its inventory at discounted prices in order to raise cash for current debt that is due. The Gold company, which did not have a favorable current ratio, does have an acceptable acid-test ratio because most of its current assets are in cash, accounts receivable, and marketable securities.

Table 9.12 Quick Ratio

	Blue Company	Gold Company
Cash, A/R, and S/T securities[a]	$75,000	$300,000
Current liabilities	$100,000	$300,000
Quick ratio	0.75:1	1:1

[a]A/R = accounts receivable; S/T = short-term.

Although working capital, the current ratio, and the acid-test ratio are effective ways to analyze a firm's liquidity, they should not be the only tools employed. The statement of cash flows is as viable as these ratios for analyzing liquidity.

Profitability

The basic goal in business is the "bottom line," which is earning profit. If a firm is not as profitable as its competition, credit and new capital from stockholders may be more difficult to obtain and some companies may experience bankruptcy. In essence, the concepts of solvency and profitability are connected to planning and controlling in management. The ability to measure a firm's profit is reflected in the firm's annual report, in business journals, and by investment services; it is essential to the decision-making process of an organization. The most well-known profitability ratio is the rate of return on net sales, as follows:

$$\text{Rate of return on net sales} = \frac{\text{Net income}}{\text{Net sales}}$$

The rate of return on net sales is basically the ratio of income from continuing operations to net sales. When this ratio reflects that a company has a high rate of return, it indicates that increased net sales are providing income and fewer net sales dollars are being used for expenses. It provides data on the organization's ability to control its costs and also reflects the firm's ability to create profits from an increasing level of sales. This indicator compares a company's income from ongoing operations to net sales, but ignores the amount of investment used to generate income.

Therefore, an enterprise may have a high rate of return on net sales and still not be effective concerning creditor and stockholder interests. Financial statement users must be cognizant of the limitations of using only this ratio to evaluate an organization.

A wider method of evaluating a firm's efficiency is the rate of return on total assets. Because the accounting equation requires that total assets equal the sum of total liabilities and total stockholder's equity, this ratio provides a measure of the firm's efficiency at managing both stockholder and creditor investments:

$$\text{Rate of return on total assets} = \frac{\text{Net income} + \text{Interest expense}}{\text{Average total sales}}$$

This is the ratio of income from ongoing operations plus interest expense to the average total sales. Therefore, it is a measure of the firm's ability to effectively use its assets to earn a profit.

The rate of return on common stockholder's equity is the ratio of income from continuing operations to average stockholder equity. This ratio measures the efficiency with which a company manages its stockholder's investments. The formula is as follows:

$$\text{Rate of return on equity} = \frac{\text{Net income} - \text{Preferred dividends}}{\text{Average stockholder equity}}$$

This indicator focuses only on the rate of profit earned on the amount invested by common stockholders or the relationship between net income and the common stockholder's investment in the firm.

Another profitability indicator commonly quoted by the financial press is the price-earnings (*P/E*) ratio on common stock. It is a measure of a firm's future earning potential. Table 9.13 outlines the formula. The *P/E* ratio indicates that a share of the firm's common stock was selling for 10.7 times the amount of earnings per share (EPS) at the end of 2001; however, the common stock was selling for 12.3 times the amount of EPS at the end of 2002. This indicates favorable future earning prospects based on the relationship between market value of common stock and earnings. The optimum *P/E* ratio varies between industries; however, the Dow Jones average lists 15:1 as a favorable *P/E* ratio.

Efficiency (activity)

The efficiency ratio, also called the activity ratio, measures the speed at which a company moves its assets through operations. The efficiency and solvency ratios can be used together to effectively assess the firm's solvency position. Two of the most common activity ratios are the accounts receivable turnover and inventory turnover ratios.

Accounts receivable turnover

This ratio measures a firm's ability to collect cash from its credit customers and how the firm manages its credit. The ratio also reflects how fast the firm can expect to generate cash from the various receivables. The amount and types of the firm's receivables fluctuate continually as sales on account

Table 9.13 Price-Earnings Ratio

$$\text{P/E ratio} = \frac{\text{Market price per share of common stock}}{\text{EPS of common stock}}$$

Common Stock	2002	2001
Market price per share	$13.80	$8.80
EPS	1.12	0.82
P/E ratio	12.3	10.7

increase, whereas collections from customers lower the accounts receivables. In addition, increases and decreases in sales volume affect the accounts receivables balance. It is best to collect accounts receivables quickly to improve the firm's solvency position; the promptly collected cash can then be immediately used in operations, such as extra cash to pay off immediate debt obligations or to pay dividends and reduce to risk of losses for potential doubtful accounts. Table 9.14 presents computation of the accounts receivable turnover ratio. To acquire the average accounts receivable, the total accounts receivable for each year is divided by two. The accounts receivable turnover ratio is then computed by using the formula in Table 9.14. In the table, the increased accounts receivable turnover ratio in 2002 reflects an improvement in the collection of the firm or pharmacy's receivables or a change in their credit and collection practices, or both.

The inventory turnover ratio provides data on how quickly a firm's inventory is sold and when it must be replaced. This creates a need for immediate cash, thereby potentially making cash unavailable to meet existing current debt obligations. The ratio also indicates how many times the company sells its average level of inventory annually. The accounts receivable and merchandise inventory turnover ratios support a company's solvency by providing vital data on the timing of cash inflows and outflows from current assets. Table 9.15 shows computation of the merchandise inventory turnover ratios. Similar to the calculation for accounts receivable turnover, the total inventory for each year is divided by 2 to obtain the annual average inventory. In this example, the inventory turnover increased because of an increase in the cost of goods sold and a decrease in the average inventory. Because of the different types of firms and inventories, there is no exact number to reflect an optimal inventory turnover for every industry. However, a firm should locate and follow various inventory turnover data applicable to its specific industry and be careful to manage its inventory correctly. The cost of goods sold reflects the cost of the merchandise that a

Table 9.14 Accounts Receivable Turnover Ratio

$$\text{A/R turnover} = \frac{\text{Net sales (on account)}}{\text{Average A/R (net)}}$$

	2002	2001
Net sales on A/R (net)	$678,000	$564,000
Beginning of the year	$80,000	$100,000
End of the year	$70,000	$80,000
Total A/R	$150,000	$180,000
Average A/R	$75,000	$90,000
A/R turnover ratio	9.04 days	6.26 days

[a]A/R = accounts receivable

Table 9.15 Inventory Turnover Ratio

$$\text{Merchandise inventory turnover} = \frac{\text{Cost of goods sold}}{\text{Average inventory}}$$

	2002	**2001**
Cost of goods sold	$743,000	$522,000
Inventory		
Beginning	$140,000	$152,000
Ending	$110,000	$134,000
Total	$250,000	$286,000
Average inventory	$125,000	$143,000
Inventory turnover ratio	5.9	3.7

pharmacy has sold during the year and is a major expense for pharmacies, because there is a larger investment in merchandise inventory than most other assets. An important indicator of the liquidity of receivables and the organization's efficiency when investing in receivables is the number of days it takes to collect receivables, also called the average collection period for accounts receivables. This is calculated in Table 9.16:

$$\frac{\text{Average collection period}}{\text{Accounts receivable}} = \frac{\text{Net accounts receivable end of year}}{\text{Average daily accounts receivables}}$$

The number of days that sales are in receivables is an estimate of the length of time that accounts receivable are outstanding, i.e., the number of days between when a charge sale is completed and when payment for the sale is collected, e.g., 30- to 60-day credit terms. By comparing the average collection period (in days) with credit term data, essential information is provided on the efficiency in the calculation of receivables. As a general rule, the accounts receivable collection period should be no longer than 1.5 times the firm's credit terms. As a controlling function, this data should be compared with that of other firms in the same industry. This may reveal a deficiency in the firm's credit and collection policies and procedures, and corrective action

Table 9.16 Average Collection Period for Accounts Receivables

	2002	**2001**
(Net) A/R end of year	$75,000	$80,000
Net sales on account	$979,660	$819,700
Average days on account (net sales on acct./365)	2,684	2,246
Average collection period (A/R)	27.9 days	35.6 days

may need to be initiated. Longer collection periods indicate poor credit management and may suggest that the pharmacy's customers are not paying their bills on time.

An organization's ability to meet its long-term debt obligations is critical to the overall survival of the organization. The firm's long-term financial condition is of special interest to stockholders, bondholders, and financial institutions as regards bonds payable, long-term notes payable, and mortgages payable. Owners and long-term creditors are concerned about the firm's credit standing, the ability to borrow and pay present obligations on time. In the event of dissolution, long-term creditors have first claims on assets if the company does not pay on time and even debenture (unsecured by collateral) bondholders have prior claims on assets over stockholders' claims.

Long-term financial condition (ability to pay long-term debts)

In addition to financial statement analysis, e.g., horizontal analysis, the rate-of-debt-to-total-assets ratio and the times-interest-earned ratio can be used to evaluate the capital structure and strategic financial strengths and weaknesses of an enterprise.

Rate-of-debt-to-total-assets ratio

The rate-of-debt-to-total-assets ratio is an indicator of the percentage of assets that are financed by creditors and the extent to which financial leverage is employed. This ratio also reflects the importance of borrowed funds and the owner's investment to the creditor, and a large debt percentage is usually viewed as an unfavorable financial condition. Table 9.17 presents the calculation of this ratio.

In the example given in the table, the company is operating on a high percentage of borrowed funds and is locked into a significant amount of fixed interest charges. Therefore, the firm will need to repay a substantial amount of debt as it matures. If the firm is unable to meet this debt obligation when due, it may be forced into bankruptcy, as the limited stockholder investment provides little support or financial safety for this company. Losses of only 10% of net assets would eliminate the total owner's equity, placing the creditors in an unfavorable position.

Table 9.17 Rate-of-Debt-to-Total-Assets Ratio

$$\text{Rate of debt to total assets} = \frac{\text{Total debt}}{\text{Total assets}}$$

Total assets	$40,000
Total liabilities	$36,000
Total owner's equity	$4,000
Rate of debt to total asset ratio	$36,000/$40,000 = 90%

In another scenario, operating on high debt increases the likelihood of not being able to meet the current obligations; however, more financing might be necessary and the owners might find that the availability of new credit will be reduced due to their elevated debt situation. Most financing results from borrowing because the firm's owners rarely invest large sums of their own personal investment. If the firm fails, the owners limit their loss potential by operating on leverage.

Times-interest-earned ratio

This ratio is a measure reflecting the basic financial strength of an organization and is important to stockholders, creditors, and employees. It is also an indicator to long-term creditors of a firm's ability to meet required interest payments. To avoid the forced liquidation of a company, earnings must be sufficient to cover fixed interest costs on borrowed funds such as bond interest.

The ratio compares the incomes from continuing operations before income taxes plus the interest expense to the interest expense and measures the number of times that a firm's net income can cover its required interest payments. The formula for this ratio is as follows:

$$\text{Times-interest-earned} = \frac{\text{Net income} + \text{Interest expense}}{\text{Interest expense}}$$

The higher the ratio, the lower the risk that interest payment will not be made as earnings decrease and higher the assurance that interest payments will be continued regularly. The amount available to meet interest charges is not directly affected by income taxes, because basic interest is deductible when computing the firm's taxable income. Table 9.18 presents the computation of this ratio. In the example, the company has experienced a slight decrease in its times-interest-earned ratio. However, interest is not generally paid out of earnings as the interest obligations must be paid to creditors from the cash account. In reality, this is an indicator of earning power and

Table 9.18 Times-Interest-Earned Ratio

$$\text{Rate of debt to total assets} = \frac{\text{Total debt}}{\text{Total assets}}$$

	2002	2001
Income from operations (net income)	$600,000	$528,000
Interest expense	$200,000	$160,000
Total (numerator)	$800,000	$688,000
Times-interest-earned ratio	4	4.3

not merely a check of cash available for interest payments. In addition, when evaluating a firm's ability to meet interest payments on time, the concept of liquidity must also be considered. A favorable times-interest-earned ratio is usually 5 to 1.

Auditing (accounting accuracy)

Auditing involves the independent review of a firm's accounting records and supporting financial statements. The auditor analyzes and provides a fair opinion of the accounting records under the guidelines of the GAAPs. Many companies have their own internal auditors who also adheres to the firms' managerial policies and procedures. Usually, independent certified public accountants (CPAs) act as public auditors by preparing tax returns and occasionally designing accounting systems for these firms. The task of determining the GAAPs is a primary function performed by the Financial Accounting Standards Board (FASB), an independent group of accountants whose philosophy of accounting principles is recognized by the accounting profession, industry, and government. In addition, the FASB has been designed to be independent of the users of accounting principles.

Tax liability

Accurate tax records are essential to satisfy a firm's tax obligations because an excellent accounting system is required to document all revenues and expenses for not only the long-term success of the organization but also income tax purposes. The IRS requires proper documentation in the event of a tax audit.

Conclusion

Accounting statements and tools such as ratio analysis increase the supply of current financial information and facilitate more effective business decisions, as decision making often occurs in an uncertain and constantly changing environment.

Accounting data does not solve a problem, but it alerts the pharmaceutical professional that a problem exists in a company. The accounting process, statements, and tools help the pharmaceutical professional acquire the financial expertise to make more informed decisions, but they are not crystal balls that predict the future.

Therefore, a basic understanding of accounting concepts is essential for the operation of all pharmaceutical organizations, from neighborhood pharmacies to chain pharmacies and international pharmaceutical corporations. Accounting skills and knowledge are not only assets for pharmacy management, but also contribute to the overall success of pharmaceutical business ventures.

Bibliography

McQuaig DJ, Bille PA. *College Accounting*. 6th ed. Houghton Mifflin, Boston, 1997.
Tootelian DH, Gaedeke RM. *Essentials of Pharmacy Management*. 1st ed. Mosby-Year-book, St. Louis, MO, 1993.

chapter ten

Purchasing pharmaceuticals

James M. Hoffman

Contents

On the surface, the purchase of pharmaceuticals might appear to be one of the most mundane tasks encountered in the management of a pharmacy. Although there is little glamour associated with the purchasing process, efficient purchasing practices are essential to the operation of any pharmacy (McAllister, 1985). Pharmaceuticals represent the largest operating expense for any pharmacy, and therefore their purchase requires careful management. Depending on the pharmacy, drug purchases account for 60 to 80% of a pharmacy's expenses (Bickett and Gagnon, 1987). A sufficient quantity of pharmaceuticals must be available at all times to allow for quality patient care, but the quantity of pharmaceuticals stocked cannot be in excess so that it wastes the pharmacy's money through unnecessary inventory.

Many of the technical functions required to purchase pharmaceuticals can be delegated to nonpharmacist staff. For example, duties such as placing an order, receiving stock, and managing inventory levels can be performed by properly trained technical staff. However, the oversight and guidance of a pharmacist are required throughout the purchasing process (Vidal, 1998). Nonpharmacist personnel may not have the drug knowledge to order substitutes when a certain drug is unavailable or to determine reasonable stock quantities for drugs, especially expensive items that are not routinely used.

The management of these challenges is improved when a pharmacist takes responsibility for the purchasing process.

Purchasing pharmaceuticals is a complex process that requires the pharmacy staff to interface with a variety of other parties. This chapter reviews in detail the sources of pharmaceuticals and the purchasing process. Purchasing continues to grow in complexity, and this chapter describes the contemporary difficulties, such as restricted distribution programs and drug shortages, that face pharmacists today. Table 10.1 explains the purchasing terms used throughout the chapter.

Sources of pharmaceuticals

In general, pharmacies use two methods to obtain drugs. Pharmaceuticals are purchased directly from the product manufacturer (direct purchases) or indirectly (indirect purchases) through a pharmaceutical wholesaler (Allen, 1992). Purchasing directly from manufacturers may reduce handling fees or other additional costs charged by wholesalers. However, direct purchases require additional staff time, because multiple orders must be placed, received, and processed. Because wholesalers allow pharmacies to order multiple products from a single source, pharmaceutical wholesalers are clearly the most common source of pharmaceuticals. Consolidated ordering through a wholesaler improves purchasing efficiency by reducing personnel time spent on purchasing and improving order turnaround time. The primary disadvantage of purchasing through a wholesaler is the additional cost the wholesaler might charge for some products.

Despite the common use of wholesalers, drug manufacturers remain important sources of drugs in some situations. An example of a pharmaceutical commonly purchased directly from the manufacturer is the influenza vaccine. The vaccine must be purchased each season because its formulation changes. Each year it is adjusted to protect patients against the strains that are expected to be most prevalent during the next flu season. In early fall, pharmacies purchase a large quantity of influenza vaccine directly from the manufacturer that will be used throughout the coming months. Because organizations purchase a single large quantity of the influenza vaccine and the product changes each year, buying from the manufacturer can result in efficiencies and savings.

Other common direct purchase scenarios include orphan drugs, drug shortages, and limited distribution systems. Orphan drugs are drugs used to treat rare diseases, and they can usually only be obtained directly from the manufacturer. When a drug is in short supply, manufacturers may develop a program in which the product is available only from the manufacturer. Patients must meet criteria to obtain the drug, and the product is allocated to pharmacies based on patient need. The program may require health care practitioners to contact the manufacturer with patient-specific information (e.g., patient diagnosis or previous therapies that have failed on

Table 10.1 Key Purchasing Terms Used in the Chapter

Direct purchasing	Purchasing pharmaceuticals directly from the manufacturer.
Indirect purchasing	Purchasing pharmaceuticals from an intermediary such as a wholesaler.
Group purchasing organization (GPO)	An organization that negotiates and maintains contracts with drug manufacturers on behalf of member organizations.
Prime vendor relationship	An agreement with a wholesaler that states the pharmacy will purchase a set quantity or dollar amount of pharmaceuticals. In exchange for guaranteed sales, the wholesaler provides discounts to the pharmacy.
Wholesalers	Companies that purchase pharmaceuticals from manufacturers and resell them to pharmacies.
Restricted distribution program	A program wherein pharmaceuticals can be purchased only from the manufacturer or a designated pharmacy. These programs are usually developed for drugs that require extensive monitoring or patient education due to safety concerns.
Reverse distributor	Companies that organize and manage the return and appropriate destruction of expired pharmaceuticals.
Purchase order	A document that lists all the items to be purchased in a given order. The purchase order is used to track items that have been ordered.

the patient). The intent of these programs is to ensure that drugs in short supply are used appropriately. Limited distribution programs are systems in which manufacturers or their designees (often specialty mail order pharmacies) are the only sources for a pharmaceutical. Although these programs add complexity to the drug-purchasing process, they are usually instituted for safety reasons. Further discussion of drug shortages and limited distribution programs is provided in the sections on special situations in pharmaceutical purchasing and drug shortages.

The majority of pharmacies' drug purchases are indirect purchases through a pharmaceutical wholesaler who purchases drugs from manufacturers and sells them to pharmacies (Carroll, 1997). Wholesalers do not sell products directly to patients; instead they act as middlemen between drug manufacturers and pharmacies. Examples of the largest pharmaceutical wholesalers include McKesson Corporation, AmerisourceBergen, and Cardinal IIealth. These wholesalers provide a full range of pharmaceuticals to all types of pharmacies, but other smaller wholesalers also exist who specialize in selling specific products such as biologicals, parenterals, or oncology drugs (Allen, 1992). In recent years, pharmaceutical wholesalers have become diversified businesses that provide a variety of products and services besides drugs. Examples of these products include pharmacy automation and dispensing technology, pharmacy information systems, drug-repackaging services, and pharmacy management services.

Pharmacies often choose one pharmaceutical wholesaler and establish a prime vendor relationship. The prime vendor relationship is an agreement that stipulates that the pharmacy will purchase a set amount of drugs from the wholesaler. In return for guaranteed purchases, wholesalers provide a discount to the pharmacy. As part of the agreement, wholesalers may provide further discounts based on purchase volume. Some pharmacies might also retain a secondary wholesaler to use as an alternative source of pharmaceuticals. However, purchases from the secondary wholesaler are usually kept to a minimum so as not to jeopardize quantity discounts from the primary wholesaler.

Discounts and purchase terms from wholesalers or other suppliers may be structured several different ways. Examples of discounts include quantity, cash, and bundled discounts (Tootelian and Gaedake, 1993). Quantity or volume discounts are arranged based on the number of units or dollars of a product purchased. The discounts may be fixed and paid after a set quantity is purchased, or discounts often increase as the quantity purchased increases. Quantity discounts are usually based on multiple purchases over a set period such as a year, and a rebate is paid to the pharmacy at the end of the period. Discounts provided by manufacturers, via either direct purchases or contracts negotiated by group purchasing organizations (GPOs), are often based on purchase volume of a product or group of products. When discounts are based on purchases of a group, or a bundle of a company's products, these agreements are called bundled contracts. Quantity discounts may provide significant savings, but these contracts may encourage pharmacies to purchase more products than necessary. In the case of bundled contracts, pharmacies may purchase products they might not normally carry so that they receive the discount.

Purchase terms between pharmacies and suppliers usually provide flexibility and potential discounts. Typically, the supplier allows the pharmacy 30 or more days to pay for an order, but discounts, called cash discounts, are paid if bills are paid immediately. For example, the terms of the agreement could allow suppliers to provide a 1 to 3% discount if purchases are paid within 10 days. If pharmacies consistently take advantage of these discounts, they can result in annual savings of 15 to 30%, depending on the purchase terms. However, quick payment of drug purchases may reduce cash flow and drain the pharmacy's cash reserves.

The role of group purchasing organizations (GPOs)

The services of GPOs are used extensively in most pharmacy settings, especially in hospitals and health systems. Because they may never actually purchase drugs, the term *purchasing*, does not accurately describe the activities of most GPOs (Wetrich, 1987). Instead, GPOs negotiate contracts with drug manufacturers and other vendors on behalf of their member hospitals or pharmacies. In hospitals, GPOs establish and maintain contracts for nearly every product a hospital might need to purchase. Contracts may exist for simple and inexpensive items, such as latex gloves, or complex and expensive items, such as cardiovascular stents, pacemakers, or orthopedic implants.

Over 95% of hospitals use the services of a GPO (Young, 2002). The largest GPO in the U.S. is Novation, which resulted from the merger between the purchasing operations of VHA and the University HealthSystem Consortium (UHC). Other large purchasing groups include Premier and Ameri-Net. Community pharmacies, especially independents, also use the services of GPOs (Tootelian and Gaedeke, 1993). For example, IPC/ServAll, the largest GPO that serves independent pharmacies, contracts for over 4000 pharmacies (IPC/ServAll, 2003).

Because GPOs negotiate on behalf of hundreds or even thousands of organizations, they are able to combine the purchases of all members during contract negotiations. By pooling resources for purchases, the contracts GPOs negotiate are larger than any single pharmacy might negotiate, and they are able to demand more favorable pricing for the drugs and other products under those contracts. Drug manufacturers and other companies that enter into GPO contracts are assured significant purchases for the item under contract. Some GPOs may only contract for a limited number of drugs within a therapeutic class. These contracts are designed to help manufacturers increase market share over competing products. Although controversial (Young, 2002), these contracts allow the pharmacy to receive the best possible price for a given drug and the cost of drugs is reduced.

GPOs have evolved to provide services to pharmacies beyond contract negotiation. Purchasing organizations often provide newsletters, drug information, formulary resources, and other benefits to GPO members. Formulary resources and drug information may provide an additional benefit of converting a member hospitals' drug use to the preferred agent under the GPO's contracts.

In addition to the obvious benefit of potentially reducing drug costs, purchasing organizations may provide other advantages to member organizations (Carroll, 1997). Purchasing organizations can provide valuable information to member hospitals. For example, they often provide reports on purchasing trends and drug costs. By contracting with only a limited number of vendors, GPOs help pharmacies standardize their inventory, which can reduce costs. Because the GPO handles contract negotiation and maintenance, labor costs for this time-consuming and complex task are reduced. Drug cost savings and other advantages do not come without a cost. Pharmacies that use the services of a GPO have less control over the purchasing process. Pharmacies may also be required to institute formulary or other changes in the drug use process in order to use the product preferred by the GPO.

The pharmaceutical purchasing process

The pharmaceutical purchasing process is continuous (Figure 10.1). Drugs are ordered, received, drug inventory is managed, and the purchasing cycle is complete when pharmaceuticals are returned or destroyed.

Computer systems are the primary method for placing drug orders. A purchase order, a document with all the items to be purchased, is generated.

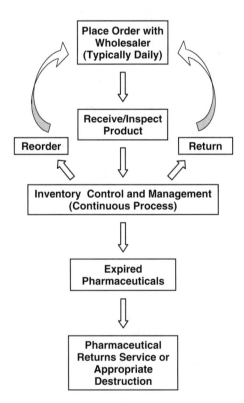

Figure 10.1 The pharmaceutical purchasing process.

The purchase order allows the pharmacy to track the items ordered. The order is then placed via a dedicated computer terminal typically provided by the wholesaler. The computer has the necessary software and connections needed to place the order with the wholesaler. As computer technology continues to expand, wholesalers are beginning to improve their systems and place ordering systems on the Internet, providing enhanced functionality and flexibility. In other cases, especially in smaller pharmacies, drug orders are placed via the phone.

Most pharmacies place an order with their wholesaler each weekday or several times each week, and the order is usually received the next day. Frequent ordering allows pharmacies to purchase drugs using a just-in-time approach. The goal of this purchasing method is to reduce inventory costs by purchasing only the minimum amount of product needed until the next order is placed. Clear procedures for receiving a drug shipment should be established and maintained (Allen, 1992). Once an order is received, care must be taken to be sure that the correct items were received (correct product, dose, quantity, and strength). The products received must be inspected for evidence of tampering or damage during shipping. Damaged products must be returned to the wholesaler, and products not received must be reordered. Before an item is added to inventory, the expiration date of the product should be verified. Items with short expiration dates (e.g., less than 12 months) should be returned to the wholesaler. To allow for double checks within the ordering system, the personnel receiving and inspecting the order should be different from the personnel who placed the order.

The drug-purchasing process does not end once drugs are ordered and received. Managing a drug inventory can be viewed as a component of the purchasing process. Because the drug inventory represents a substantial investment for any pharmacy, the goal of inventory management is to maintain the minimum amount of necessary inventory to control drug costs. Excess inventory can substantially harm the financial performance of a pharmacy. Whereas inventory should be kept to a minimum, a sufficient quantity of medications must be maintained to allow immediate access to drugs needed for patient care. The pharmacy manager should develop purchasing systems that balance product availability and cost concerns. A variety of inventory management systems can be employed and are reviewed in Chapter 11.

A systematic process should be developed and maintained to check drug expiration dates and remove expired drugs from the pharmacy inventory. For example, a system could be developed in which technical staff is assigned to perform monthly inspections in areas of the inventory for expired drugs. The types of expired drugs should be evaluated, because they might yield useful information that can be used to improve the inventory system. If the same expired product is found on a consistent basis, inventory levels of the product should be reduced.

Expired drugs are not simply discarded within the pharmacy, because they retain some value. Most manufacturers provide credit for returned expired drugs. The returns process can be complicated and multiple Drug Enforcement Administration (DEA), Environmental Protection Agency (EPA), and individual state board of pharmacy regulations must be followed. Consequently, most pharmacies outsource this function to a reverse distributor, a firm that organizes and manages the return of expired drugs to manufacturers. In exchange for these services, pharmacies pay reverse distributors a percentage of the credit value of the expired drugs. If a manufacturer does not provide credit for a certain product, reverse distributors appropriately dispose of the expired drugs.

As the final step of the purchasing cycle, proper destruction of pharmaceuticals cannot be ignored. The EPA classifies many drugs, including epinephrine, nitroglycerin, warfarin, choral hydrate, and chemotherapy agents, as hazardous waste (Smith, 2002). When discarded improperly, these and other pharmaceuticals are harmful to the environment. Although the majority of pharmaceutical waste is managed through a reverse distributor who must be registered with the EPA, pharmacies must properly manage the disposal of incidental waste such as partial containers, compounded IVs, and broken or spilled products. Hazardous, nonhazardous, and chemotherapy pharmaceutical waste should be separated. Some waste such as intravenous fluids can be disposed of through sewer systems, but all other types of pharmaceutical waste should be incinerated by a regulated medical waste disposal firm.

Special situations in pharmaceutical purchasing

Several situations increase the complexity of the purchasing process and may demand greater attention from the pharmacist managing the purchasing process. Examples of these situations include controlled substances, investigational drugs, restricted distribution programs, and drug shortages.

Different processes and additional record keeping are required to order controlled substances and investigational drugs. A DEA 222 form must be used to order and document the receipt of Schedule II controlled substances. These forms must be kept on file in the pharmacy, and a perpetual inventory of Schedule II substances must be maintained. Automated dispensing cabinets and other technology can be useful to maintain such an inventory. Investigational drugs, agents undergoing clinical trials but not yet approved by the Food and Drug Administration (FDA), can be ordered only under institutional review board approved studies or for compassionate use in individual patients. These drugs often have special handling and storage requirements, and study sponsors require strict accountability for investigational drugs. Pharmacists should develop specific procedures for handling investigational drugs and physically separate them from other pharmaceutical inventory.

Recently, restricted distribution programs have become common for drugs used in small populations or drugs with significant safety concerns.

Restricted distribution programs establish special systems for ordering and dispensing drugs, usually through a single pharmacy. Patient information, such as diagnosis, laboratory test results, or documentation of patient education, may be required to comply with the terms of the program. In many cases, these programs are developed in cooperation with the FDA as a condition of drug approval. Examples of drugs available only through restricted distribution programs include dofetilide, sodium oxybate, mifepristone, isotretinoin, bosentan, epoprostenol, and thalidomide. As these programs have become more common, pharmacists and pharmacy organizations have criticized them for their complexity, interference with the pharmacist–patient relationship, and exclusive relationship with a single pharmacy (Glaser, 2001).

An example of a restricted distribution program is the System for Thalidomide Education and Prescribing Safety (STEPS) (Young, 2002). Thalidomide, a teratogen that caused over 10,000 birth defects worldwide in the 1950s and 1960s, was recently approved for use in the U.S. Although thalidomide is indicated for the treatment of leprosy, it has become widely used for a variety of cancers, especially multiple myeloma. The program includes multiple elements to reduce the risk of birth defects in patients taking thalidomide. Prescribers are required to counsel patients on the risks of thalidomide and provide pregnancy testing to women with childbearing potential on a monthly basis. To use thalidomide, patients must use two reliable forms of contraception, and pharmacists can dispense only a single 28-day supply. The entire program is monitored by telephone surveys that prescribers, patients, and pharmacists must complete on a monthly basis.

Drug shortages

Drug shortages represent a growing challenge to the pharmacist responsible for purchasing pharmaceuticals. Within the last few years, drug shortages have become more common and severe (ASHP, 2001). Nationwide, 119 drug shortages were recorded in 2001 (Fox and Tyler, 2003). Drug shortages occur for a variety of reasons, such as raw and bulk material unavailability, manufacturing difficulties, recalls, regulatory issues, manufacturer decisions to reduce or stop production, unexpected increases in demand, and even natural disasters. One survey found that raw material shortages and regulatory issues were the most common reasons for shortage (Wellman, 2001). In another analysis, manufacturing problems and product discontinuation by the manufacturer were the most common reasons for drug shortages. Depending on the reason for shortage, they may last several weeks or continue for several years.

Besides disrupting normal purchasing operations in a pharmacy, drug shortages may have a negative impact on patient care. In some cases, no other alternative therapy is available, and patients go without optimal drug therapy. During many shortages, a similar drug is available, but health care practitioners and patients may not be familiar with the alternative therapy. During a drug shortage, pharmacists must take an active role in selecting alternative agents, determining equivalent dosages, and educating practitioners and patients on the use of the new agent.

Conclusion

Efficient pharmaceutical purchasing is a prerequisite for operating a successful pharmacy. Careful attention to the purchasing process and inventory management will result in a positive impact on the pharmacy's financial performance. The drug-purchasing process is complicated, and it will become more complex as restricted distribution programs and drug shortages become more common. Pharmacy managers must develop clear drug-purchasing systems and work proactively to eliminate inefficiencies within their system.

Bibliography

Allen SJ. Purchasing and inventory management. In: Brown TR, Ed., *Handbook of Institutional Pharmacy Practice.* Bethesda, MD: American Society of Health-System Pharmacists, 1992, pp. 73–79.

American Society of Health-System Pharmacists. ASHP guidelines on managing drug product shortages. *Am. J. Hlth.-Syst. Pharm.* 2001; 58: 1445–1450.

Bickett WJ, Gagnon JP. Purchasing and inventory control for hospital pharmacies. *Top. Hosp. Pharm. Manage.* 1987; 7: 59–74.

Carroll NV. Changes in channels of distribution: wholesalers and pharmacies in organized health-care settings. *Hosp. Pharm. Rep.* February 1997: 48–57.

Fox ER, Tyler LS. Managing drug shortages: seven years' experience at one health system. *Am. J. Hlth.-Syst. Pharm.* 2003; 60: 245–253.

Glaser M. Off limits: the growth of pharmaceuticals bearing restrictions has the profession and pharmacists worried. *Drug Top.* 2001; 5: 57.

IPC and ServAll Combine Strengths for Community Pharmacists. IPC/ServAll Web site. Available at https://www.ipcrx.com/announcements/pressrelease/final/press.htm, accessed June 11, 2003.

McAllister JC. Challenges in purchasing and inventory control. *Am. J. Hosp. Pharm.* 1985; 42: 1370–1373.

Smith CA. Managing pharmaceutical waste: what pharmacists should know. *J. Pharm. Soc. Wisc.* November/December 2002: 17–21.

Tootelian DH, Gaedeke RM. Purchasing and inventory control. In: *Essentials of Pharmacy Managment.* St. Louis, MO: Mosby, 1993, pp. 357–377.

Vidal BA. Drug procurement responsibilities [Letter], *Hosp. Pharm.* 1998; 33: 918.

Wellman GS. National supply-chain survey of drug manufacturer back orders. *Am. J. Hlth.-Syst. Pharm.* 2001; 58: 1224–1228.

Wetrich JG. Group purchasing: an overview. *Am. J. Hosp. Pharm.* 1987; 44: 1581–1592.

Young D. Investigation of GPOs yields mixed opinions. *Am. J. Hlth.-Syst. Pharm.* 2002; 1004: 10,14.

Young D. Thalidomide prescribers cannot assign survey responsibility to pharmacists. *Am. J. Hlth.-Syst. Pharm.* 2002; 1702: 4,6.

chapter eleven

Principles of inventory management

Andrew M. Peterson

Contents

Introduction

Inventory is probably the largest single investment a pharmacy can make. Regardless of whether the pharmacy is retail, hospital, or another type that serves patients, inventory investment is significant and needs to be managed well consistently. Although there is an inextricable relationship between purchasing and inventory, this chapter deals with inventory control separately.

There are a variety of reasons for managing inventory, including the need to keep costs at a minimum and to have a sufficient supply of products for good customer service. Too much inventory results in loss of profits because products remain on the shelf and do not generate cash flow. Too little inventory can result in customer dissatisfaction and employee frustration because needed products are not available.

0-8493-1446-1/04/$0.00+$1.50
© 2004 by CRC Press LLC

Costs are also associated with managing inventory. The obvious cost is the purchase price, also called the acquisition cost. It also costs money to procure and carry a product. Procurement costs, such as shipping and handling, can vary depending on the product. Similarly, carrying costs vary depending on the product and include overhead costs such as electricity and heating.

There are various ways of managing inventory, ranging from visual inspection of stocked items to computerized accounting of items entered and removed from inventory at the time of stocking and the time of purchase. Each of these strategies has advantages and disadvantages and is discussed in detail in the chapter. Lastly, because inventory comprises a significant investment, there are many ways to value it. These too are discussed further.

Inventory costs

The most obvious cost associated with an inventory is the acquisition cost. This is the cost the pharmacy pays to the supplier, be it the manufacturer, the wholesaler, or other sources. The cost associated with the acquisition cost includes the markup the wholesaler may impose, discounts offered (e.g., cash or quantity discounts), and cost of the product itself.

Procurement costs include the cost of shipping, receiving, stocking, and bookkeeping of the inventory. Shipping costs depend largely on the product itself and the quantity of product purchased. Clearly, larger, heavier products cost more money to ship. But when items are purchased in large quantities, the per-item shipping costs are typically less. The costs to receive an item include the personnel time spent receiving the item on the loading dock and checking in the inventory (i.e., to review it against the purchase order to make sure the shipment is complete). Stocking costs include the time it takes to move the items to the storeroom and then from the storeroom to the shelf. Bookkeeping costs include payment to the supplier.

Carrying costs are costs inherent in the product itself and might be difficult to quantify for individual items. The first carrying cost is the cost of storage. Also, because medications must be kept at appropriate temperatures to maintain their shelf lives, the conditions of storage must be maintained. For example, the storage cost of refrigerated items includes the purchase of a refrigerator, the electricity to run the refrigerator, and the cost of maintaining the refrigerator. Further, the pharmacist must be aware that the items have expiration dates, and if the drugs are past the expiration dates, they cannot be sold. This is also a carrying cost: if the items do not sell and expire, the money used to purchase them cannot be regained through a sale. Another hidden carrying cost is the cost of insuring the pharmacy against fire, theft, or other disasters. Typically, the higher the inventory value, the higher the insurance costs.

The opportunity cost of purchasing an item must also be considered. The opportunity cost is the cost of something in terms of something else that could be purchased and sold instead. If the pharmacy has a certain monthly budget for purchases, there is often a trade-off between purchasing large quantities of one item at a steep discount vs. purchasing a wide variety of other items. For example, if the pharmacy uses its entire monthly budget to purchase acetaminophen at a discounted price, it loses the opportunity to purchase all other medications, therefore losing the opportunity to sell other items. The cost associated with this decision is the opportunity cost.

Customer dissatisfaction is one of the hardest costs to determine, but the most easily observable. Customers expect that products typically held by a pharmacy are readily available for purchase during normal business hours. Stockouts often produce frustration and dissatisfaction among customers, but, if infrequent, may be forgiven. However, frequent stockouts can result in a loss of business. In hospitals, frequent stockouts of commonly used products can result in a decline in the quality of patient care, create frustration among the medical and nursing staffs, and promote dissension between the pharmacy and other staffs.

The mechanics of inventory control

The primary goal of inventory control is balance between having sufficient amounts of a product on hand when needed and minimizing costs associated with the inventory. Fundamentally, inventory control is assuring this balance — when to order the product and how much to order. As such, the pharmacy manager must be aware of the total cost of the inventory, which is the sum of the all the costs associated with inventory:

Total cost (TC) = Acquisition costs (AC) + Procurement costs (PC)

+ Carrying costs (CC)

How much to order

The first concern is how much the pharmacy manager should order considering all the costs. Many pharmacy managers use their intuition and decide how much to order based on prior knowledge of usage patterns and current costs. There is also a more scientific method of ordering, called the economic order quantity (EOQ). The EOQ is essentially a formula that determines the point at which the ordering and carrying costs for a product are the lowest. The EOQ should be considered whenever there is a repetitive buying pattern for a product, as it will help minimize the costs associated the inventory costs of the product.

The EOQ formula is:

$$EOQ = \sqrt{[(2 \times \text{Annual usage}) \times (\text{Ordering costs}) / (\text{Carrying costs\%} \times \text{Unit cost})]} \cdot$$

This formula considers the annual usage, per-order ordering costs, cost of the item, and carrying costs. As the order quantity increases, ordering costs decrease. However, as the order quantity increases, the carrying costs also increase. Therefore, the total cost decreases at first, until the carrying costs exceed the ordering costs. The point at which the carrying costs equal the ordering costs is the lowest total cost. This quantity, the EOQ, will produce the minimum total cost. The concept of the EOQ is best expressed graphically (Figure 11.1).

Consider the following example. A pharmacy uses 1200 bottles of aspirin annually, and each order costs $5.00. Further, a single bottle of aspirin costs $0.50, with a carrying cost of 10% of the cost. The EOQ equation would be as follows:

$$EOQ = \sqrt{[2 \times (1200) \times \$5.00 / \$0.50 \times 0.1)]}$$

$$EOQ = 490 \text{ bottles per order}$$

Therefore, the pharmacy should order 490 bottles of aspirin about 2.5 (1200/490), times per year (about every 20 weeks).

When to reorder

If, according to the EOQ model, aspirin should be ordered every 20 weeks, the idea of when to order seems inherent in the model. However, this model assumes that the usage pattern is consistent throughout the ordering period and that when the stock reaches zero, there is immediate replenishment to the EOQ. Because buying patterns vary over time and it takes time to order, receive, and stock items, the pharmacy manager needs to have an idea of the reorder point. The reorder point is that point at which the manager needs

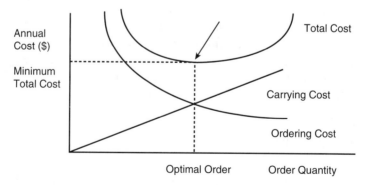

Figure 11.1 Economic order quantity cost curves.

to reorder inventory to assure adequate supply for the customer. The formula for reorder point is:

Reorder point (ROP) = Demand rate (DR) × Lead time (LT) + Safety stock (SS)

The demand rate (DR) is the amount of product used or sold within a given period of time. It is expressed as the number of units per unit of time. The lead time (LT) is the amount of time it takes to order and receive a product from a supplier. In pharmacies the LT is often 1 day, it but can be upwards of 1 to 2 weeks, depending on the product and the supplier. The safety stock (SS) is the buffer of product kept on hand to accommodate increases in demand or longer than expected LTs.

In the aspirin example, we can consider a 2-day LT, a daily usage rate of 3 bottles (1200 per year/365 days per year) and a safety stock of a 2-day supply.

Therefore, the formula would become:

$$ROP = 3 \text{ bottles} / \text{day} \times 2 \text{ days LT} + 2 \text{ days SS}$$

$$ROP = 8 \text{ bottles}$$

The pharmacy manager should reorder the EOQ of 490 bottles of aspirin when there are 8 bottles left in the pharmacy.

Controlling inventory

Inventory measurement is part and parcel of controlling inventory. One of the most common measures of inventory control is the inventory turnover rate (ITR). The ITR measures how fast inventory moves, i.e., how frequently inventory is sold and repurchased for stocking. A high ITR indicates frequent usage, which in turn indicates continued sales and profits. Therefore, typically, it is best to have a high ITR — up to a point. Recall from the EOQ model that ordering costs can influence overall costs. Ordering too frequently can increase overall inventory costs. The optimal ITR for items varies based on the total inventory costs of the product and should be individualized. Each item should have its own ITR calculated. This will allow the manager to determine specific situations in which the inventory is not turning over sufficiently. If the ITR needs to increase, purchasing a lower quantity more often should be considered. For items with a typical 20 to 30% average gross margin (GM%), the ITR is usually 5 to 6 times per year; for items with a lower average GM%, the ITR should be higher.

One can easily calculate the ITR for a product given a few pieces of information (see Chapter 9 for an example). The ITR considers the cost of goods and the average inventory investment. These factors should be taken over the same period of time, typically 1 year. How the inventory is valued must be consistent from one time period to another. The next section discusses how inventory is valued.

Valuing Inventory

There are at least three different methods for valuing inventory: (1) first-in–first-out (FIFO), (2) last-in–first-out (LIFO), and (3) weighted average cost (WAC).

The FIFO method considers that the first items brought into the pharmacy are the first ones sold. This creates an inventory of newer items. The value of the inventory is calculated by multiplying the number of units remaining in the inventory by the cost per item. If the cost of the items has risen, i.e., the items in inventory are more expensive than those already sold, the value of the inventory can be inflated using the FIFO method; conversely, if the cost of the items has declined, the value of the inventory can be underestimated.

The LIFO method assumes that the inventory on hand is the oldest inventory, and the value is calculated based on those items. In times of increasing costs, the LIFO method might underestimate the inventory value and vice versa.

The WAC method determines the weighted average of the inventory, considering the cost of the older and the newer items, thus trying to avoid the impact of increasing or decreasing prices.

See Table 11.1 and Table 11.2 for an example of each method. Table 11.2 shows the cost of goods sold (COGS) and the ending inventory value if 30 bottles remain on the shelf in April (i.e., 40 are sold).

In the FIFO method, it is assumed that the 30 remaining bottles were purchased in April (10) and March (20). Therefore, the value of the inventory is $10 \times \$65 + 20 \times \$75 = \$2150$. The LIFO method assumes that the remaining

Table 11.1 Background Information

Month	No. of Units Purchased	Cost Per Unit ($)	Total Cost ($)
January	20	60	1200
February	10	70	700
March	30	75	2250
April	10	65	650
Total	70		4800
Average			4800/70 = 68.58

Table 11.2 Valuation Methods

Method	Ending Inventory Value
FIFO	$2150 (10 × $65 + 20 × 75)
LIFO	$1900 (10 × $70 + 20 × 60)
WAC	$2057 (30 × $68.58)

bottles were purchased in February (10) and January (20) for a total value of $1900. The WAC method averages the cost of the bottles at $68.58 each for a total cost of $2057. (See Table 11.2).

To calculate the annual value of the inventory, total the value of each product in the inventory (quantity on hand times cost) at the same time each year. Use the following equation to get the company's inventory value:

Ending inventory = Beginning inventory + Net purchases – Cost of goods sold

Therefore, take what you have in the beginning, add what you have purchased, subtract what you have sold, and the result is what remains. You can also determine the annual average inventory value by calculating the monthly inventory values, adding these monthly inventory values, and dividing by 12. Regardless of the method chosen, the pharmacy manager must consistently use the same method from year to year.

Methods of inventory control

The most commonly employed method of inventory control is the visual inspection method. This method requires the pharmacist, or other designated personnel, to visually inspect the number of items remaining on a shelf. From this number, the person then determines whether there is adequate inventory or whether an order should be placed. The person may use the ROP and EOQ to help determine whether an order should be placed and the quantity of the order. This is a fixed-quantity reorder system, in which the date of reordering varies but the quantity remains the same.

Often, the manager sets up a periodic inspection schedule to aid in inventory control. In this modified visual inspection, the inventory manager routinely inspects designated inventory levels, e.g., on a daily or weekly basis, to determine whether an order should be placed. This routine examination of inventory minimizes the potential for stockouts and can potentially improve inventory control. This is a fixed-time reorder system, in which the quantity ordered might vary but the date of ordering remains the same. This is ideal for small to medium businesses for whom a prime vendor is the main supply source and the true volume of activity can be determined easily.

However, because a pharmacy contains hundreds or even thousands of items, it is difficult to use either method reliably, particularly if there are multiple vendors. In such cases, there is an added method to the periodic inspection called the ABC method of control (Figure 11.2). The ABC method of control prioritizes the items into three levels based on the theory that a small percentage of all the merchandise accounts for a large percentage of the dollar investment. A items typically comprise only 20% of the inventory items, but account for nearly 80% of the cost. Because one of the main objectives of inventory control is to minimize the inventory investment, it is

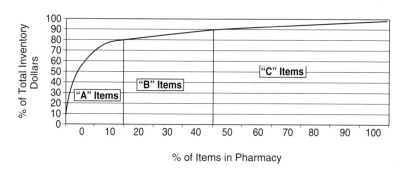

Figure 11.2 ABC method of inventory control.

only logical to focus on the items that involve the most cost. B items typically compose about 60 to 70% of the items in the inventory and about 10% of the total costs. C items account for the remaining 10 to 20% of the items and the remaining 10% of the costs.

Therefore, A items are typically inspected and reordered daily, or near daily. B items are ordered less frequently and C items even less frequently. This method allows the pharmacy to focus on those items that have a higher ITR and can be managed more efficiently.

With the advent of computers and the introduction of automated dispensing devices, the idea of a perpetual inventory is within the grasp of today's pharmacy. Further, the routine use of barcoding allows integration of point-of-care inventory management systems. In such systems, the inventory is constantly inspected and ordering and restocking takes place much faster.

Conclusion

The process of managing inventory appears mundane and routine, apparently made simple by models and strategies such as the EOQ and the ABC method. Although these models can aid the pharmacist in inventory control, they are more important in developing good purchasing and inventory control policies. These policies then must be monitored frequently and implemented daily, because inventory is the single largest investment in a pharmacy. When inventory levels change, there is a potential for loss of profits, customer dissatisfaction, or both. Therefore, the pharmacist must manage inventory continuously to assure minimized costs balanced by the maintenance of an adequate supply for customers and patients.

Bibliography

Allen SJ. Purchasing and inventory management. In *Handbook of Institutional Pharmacy Practice*, 3rd ed., Brown, T, Ed. ASHP, Bethesda, MD, 1992, chap. 9.

Carroll NV. *Financial Management for Pharmacists: A Decision-Making Approach*, 2nd ed. Lippincott Williams & Wilkins, Philadelphia, PA, 1998.

Tootelian DH, Gaedeke RM. Purchasing and inventory control. In *Essentials of Pharmacy Management*. Mosby, St. Louis, MO, 1993, chap. 19.

Huffman DC. Purchasing and inventory control. In *Effective Pharmacy Management*, 8th ed. NARD, Alexandria, VA, 1996, chap. 11.

Schreibfeder J. Why is inventory turnover important? http://www.effectiveinventory.com/article2.html, accessed August 19, 2003.

Schreibfeder J. Implementing effective inventory management. http://www.effectiveinventory.com/article3.html, accessed August 19, 2003.

chapter twelve

Pharmacy and therapeutics committee and formulary management

Andrew M. Peterson

Contents

Introduction

In the present health care market, promoting rational drug therapy is key to ensuring good clinical care. Hospitals and managed care organizations are charged with maintaining a system that promotes safe and effective drug therapy. Physicians, pharmacists, and other health care practitioners are responsible for implementing this system. These health care practitioners often use committees, such as the Pharmacy and Therapeutics (P&T) committee, as a vehicle for communicating, discussing, deciding, and monitoring which medications should be used within the organization. Further, the committees develop policies and procedures for the rational use of medications throughout the institution.

In the hospital or nursing home setting, the P&T committee is a medical staff committee reporting to the medical executive committee of the institution. The P&T committee reviews information on new and existing medications, analyzes their uses throughout the institution, and recommends the continued use or discontinuation of these medications for patients. In this capacity, the P&T committee serves as an advisory group to the medical staff, hospital administration, and the director of pharmacy with regard to drug therapy within the institution. The formulary is a list of medications developed by the P&T committee delineating the drugs approved for use within the institution or organization.

In the 1980s, managed care organizations adopted the use of P&T committees in an effort to promote rational drug use in the outpatient setting. The managed care P&T committee functions very similarly to a hospital P&T committee, but the P&T members are typically practitioners throughout the geographic region and may include academicians as well. Further, a managed care P&T committee tends to maintain a greater level of autonomy and authority for approving medications for formulary inclusion.

The P&T committee, with its role in developing medication use policies and formularies, is arguably the most important organizational committee in which a pharmacist maintains membership. In this regard, pharmacists can lead the organization in defining appropriate, cost-effective care for the patients they serve.

P&T committee

Ideally, the P&T committee oversees the development and implementation of all policies related to the use of medications within an organization. These policies can range from prescribing privileges, to determining who can order which types of medications (e.g., chemotherapy) and even to who can administer medications. Further, the P&T committee provides guidance on how medications should be used and for which diseases. The purpose of these policies is to maintain high-quality patient care, with minimial risk and reasonable cost (*Principles of a Sound Drug Formulary System*, 2000).

Structure and composition

The structure of a P&T committee varies depending on the organizational type. The committee typically has representatives from the principle users of medications, including physicians, nurses, and pharmacists, and peripheral users, such as laboratory personnel and nutritionists. Hospital administration may also be represented, because it has a vested interest in the cost of medications.

Manneback (1999) reviewed results from a survey of 187 hospitals nationwide regarding their P&T committees' structure and function. Results indicated that the average P&T committee had 19 members, 12 of whom were physicians, 3 pharmacists, 2 nurses, 1 administrator, and 1 other member.

The physician representatives of P&T committees are drawn from the medical specialty areas represented throughout the organization. Depending on the patient mix and types of services provided, physician members may be cardiologists, pediatricians, surgeons, infectious disease specialists, or internal-medicine physicians. If the organization has a center of excellence in oncology, neurology, or other specialty, physicians from those groups might also be represented. The Manneback survey (1999) showed that 99% of the chairs of P&T committees were physicians. This seems consistent because it is a medical staff committee.

Pharmacists also play key roles in P&T committees. The Manneback survey showed that in 95% of the P&T committees, the director of pharmacy served as the secretary of the committee. In this role, the secretary works with the chair to set the agenda, take and write the minutes, and communicate the recommendations of the committee to the appropriate people or departments. In this role, the primary link between the medical staff and the pharmacy staff is created and maintained.

Most P&T committees meet monthly for an average of 7 to 10 times annually (Pedersen, 2001; Manneback, 1999; Nash, 1993). The larger the institution, the more frequently the P&T committee meets (Pedersen, 2001). Most of these meetings last 60 to 90 minutes. For a P&T committee to review and act on the extraordinary workload, there often is a subcommittee structure with the P&T committee (Nash, 1993). Figure 12.1 shows the relationships among the medical executive committee, the P&T committee, and its subcommittees.

The functions of subcommittees are to expedite the review and take advantage of special skills of members. For example, there may be a gastroenterology subcommittee that consists of two or three GI physicians, one or two nurses, and one or two pharmacists. This group of specialists is in an

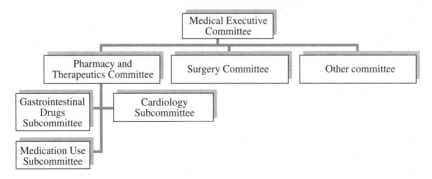

Figure 12.1 Typical organizational chart showing the relationship among the medical executive committee, the P&T committee, and the P&T subcommittees.

exceptional position to review a new GI-related drug for safety, efficacy, and cost. Further, this group's view on how the new drug should fit in the institution's current array of GI drugs is key for the larger group to make a better formulary decision. The result of the subcommittee's findings is presented to the entire P&T committee, which then reviews the merits of the drug from a system-wide perspective. At the P&T committee meeting, the impact of the drug on pediatric patients, surgical patients, cardiology patients, and others is assessed and a more informed recommendation can be made to the medical executive committee. Although this may seem a long and arduous process, the benefit of multiple reviews by experts and other users helps assure the best use of the medication within the institution.

The formulary system

The P&T committee's primary function is to maintain a drug formulary. Pedersen et al. (2001) showed that 97.5% of hospitals reported that formulary development and management was a primary function of a P&T committee. However, key elements of managing the formularies are developing and implementing policies that assure safe and effective medication therapy within institutions. These elements were also reported as primary functions by 97.1% of the hospitals surveyed. The following section reviews the formulary system and its management.

Formulary management

The formulary system is a continuous process by which an organization's P&T committee (or its equivalent) selects and evaluates those drug products considered most useful in patient care. The "Principles of a Sound Drug Formulary System" (2000), endorsed by several major pharmacy organizations, the American Medical Association, and the U.S. Pharmacopeia, defines a formulary system as "an ongoing process whereby a health care organization, through its physicians, pharmacists, and other health care professionals, establishes policies on the use of drug products and therapies, and identifies drug products and therapies that are the most medically appropriate and cost effective to best serve the health interests of a given patient population." Although some controversy exists (Horn et al. 1996; Green, 1986), the system is a powerful tool for improving the quality and controlling the cost of drug therapy (Jewesson, 2000).

The formulary

The formulary itself is a compendium of the medications and policies governing the use of medications within an organization. It is revised annually and distributed to the medical staff, heads of departments providing direct patient care, and hospital administration, and is made available on each patient care unit. Further, each pharmacist, or each pharmacy in a managed care network, receives a copy of the formulary. The "Principles" (2000) defines a formulary as a "continually updated list of medications and related information, representing the clinical judgment of physicians, pharmacists, and other experts in the diagnosis and/or treatment of disease and promotion of health." The formulary system should also have a component that enables patients to receive clinically justified medications not available on the formulary.

The formulary typically has three main parts: the policy component, the actual drug list, and the special information section. The policy component contains information on organizational policies and procedures governing the use of drugs. This includes the process for adding drugs to and deleting them from the formulary, policies and procedures for requesting nonformulary medications, and a review of the policies and procedures regarding restricted medications. This section also contains a brief description of the P&T committee, including its membership, responsibilities, and operation and organizational regulations governing the prescribing, dispensing, and administration of drugs. Table 12.1 contains a more comprehensive list of policies potentially contained in this section of a formulary.

The drug product section contains a listing of the drug products approved for use within the institution. Further, this section includes basic therapeutic information about each item, such as the generic and brand names of the drug, dosage forms, strengths, packaging, and sizes stocked by the pharmacy. The individual listing of the drug contains this basic information and may contain information regarding the relative cost of the drug or any restrictions placed on the drug.

The special information section contains information related to the use of drugs. The contents of this section vary, depending on the type of institution, and may include information on medications that should not be crushed (due to their long-acting nature), dosing conversion tables among

Table 12.1 Typical Policies Contained in a Formulary

- Approved abbreviations for prescribing drugs[a]
- Automatic stop orders
- Controlled-substances considerations
- Formulary status or tier of medication[b]
- Generic and therapeutic equivalency policies and procedures
- Investigational drug policies[a]
- Patients' use of their own medications[a]
- Rules to be followed by the drug manufacturers' representatives
- Use of drug samples
- Use of floor stock items[a]
- Verbal drug orders[a]
- Writing drug orders and prescriptions
- Quantity limit[b]

[a] Typical of a hospital or health system environment.
[b] Typical of a managed care or pharmacy benefit management (PBM) formulary.

Table 12.2 Special Information about Drugs Typically Contained in a
Formulary

- Abbreviations used for prescribing
- Analgesic equivalency tables
- Contents of emergency carts
- Dosing guidelines and nomograms
- Drugs that cannot be crushed
- List of sugar-free products
- Metric conversion tables
- Sodium content of various formulary items
- Tables of equivalent dosages of similar drugs (e.g., corticosteroids)

similar therapeutic medications, and how to administer certain medications. Table 12.2 gives a more comprehensive, but not all-inclusive, listing of information that may be contained in this section.

Types of formularies

There are at least three types of formulary systems: open, closed, and mixed. Open formularies have all medications available for use throughout the organization and have no limits placed their use. In a hospital setting, both prescription and over-the-counter medications are available for use and an individual prescriber may prescribe any medication without further approval. In a managed care setting, this may mean that all medications are paid for by the managed care organization or the pharmacy benefit manager. The implementation of open formularies in the managed care setting may take on a tiering structure to encourage cost sharing use of less expensive medications such as generics. Further, the benefit design may exclude medications available over-the-counter or cosmetic in nature. See Chapter 19 for more information.

In contrast to open formularies, closed formularies are strictly controlled. Only certain agents are available and strict therapeutic substitution with the most recognized agent within a pharmacological class is standard procedure. The purpose of this type of formulary is to assure availability of all needed products at the least cost of inventory investment. Because this mechanism of control maintains the least costly of products, it is ostensibly the most cost effective. However, significant restrictions on medication use often produce dissatisfaction and dissension among the health care practitioners and patients. Further, Horn et al. (1996) suggest that strictly controlled formularies may increase overall health care costs.

Mixed formularies attempt to take on the aspects of both open and closed formularies. There are typically two classes of drugs in a mixed formulary: drugs without limitations, which are drugs any physician can prescribe to any patient without limitations or control, and drugs with limitations. Drugs with limitations can be restricted drugs or targeted drugs. Restricted drugs can be prescribed by physicians only in certain specialties for a limited patient population. For example, chemotherapeutic agents are often restricted drugs: they can be prescribed only by oncologists to patients with cancer. There might be some exceptions to this rule, which should be noted. For example, methotrexate is an anticancer drug that may also be prescribed for rheumatoid arthritis.

Targeted drugs can be prescribed by any physician, but these drugs require approval before use and are prospectively monitored to ensure that they are used according to approved guidelines or treatment protocols. Expensive or dangerous antibiotics are often put in this classification, and approval usually comes from an infectious-disease physician or pharmacist.

Formulary product selection

For a drug to be considered for formulary inclusion, the Joint Commission on Accreditation of Healthcare Organizations (JCAHO) and other accrediting agencies look for a process in which explicit criteria are used to help judge the merits of the drug. In general, the criteria should focus on the therapeutic efficacy, safety, and cost of the medication. A brief discussion follows of how these three general areas are considered.

The process by which an institution adds a drug to formulary varies, but is typically as follows. There is an institutional policy and procedure by which the P&T committee specifies the criteria used to evaluate formulary requests. The pharmacy department submits a written new drug evaluation to the appropriate subcommittee or pharmacy and the therapeutics committee. This written new drug evaluation is called the formulary monograph, a document written by pharmacists on behalf of the subcommittee or P&T committee. It contains basic and evaluative information on the drug being considered for inclusion. This information reviews the evidence on the effectiveness, the safety, and the cost of the product. Table 12.3 lists the headings that should be included in a formulary. The purpose of the document is to educate members of the committee on the clinical use of the product. As such, the monograph contains basic information on the pharmacology, FDA-approved and non-FDA-approved uses, reviews of the clinical trials

Table 12.3 Elements Contained in a Typical Formulary Monograph

- Introduction
- Indications/Approvals
- Pharmacology
- Pharmacokinetics
- Clinical trials results/Comparative data
- Adverse effects
- Dose, how it is supplied
- Economic impact statement
- Summary and recommendation
- Bibliography

documenting the drug's efficacy and safety, and, if available, comparative information with existing drugs on the formulary. Further, the monograph contains information on how the product should be used within the institution, and cost comparisons, including an economic impact statement. The economic impact should review not only the acquisition cost of the drug, but the overall impact on laboratory, nursing, and pharmacy personnel. This should be grounded in pharmacoeconomic principles and practices in order to assure accurate information. This statement is becoming increasingly critical and needs to be a part of the final recommendation, because the acquisition cost of the drug is only part of the overall costs.

In addition, the therapeutic appropriateness of the product should be considered. This relates to the appropriateness of the drug for a specific condition. The institution should review the types of patients it cares for and develop a formulary suited to the therapeutic needs of the population it serves. When a new drug is presented for formulary consideration, the question of the population's needs should be answered before considering its inclusion. If there are few to no patients expected to need the agent, then it should not be considered for inclusion. Another characteristic of an agent is its uniqueness. There are many "me-too" products on the market. For example, as of this writing, there are 10 angiotensin-converting enzyme inhibitors (ACE inhibitors) on the market. A managed care organization or a hospital does not need to have all 11 on the formulary. Consideration should be given agents that present a unique clinical benefit to the population being served.

The availability of generic medications is also a consideration. Generic substitution is the process by which drug products that contain the same active ingredients and are chemically identical in strength, concentration, dosage form, and route of administration are used to replace the original branded product. Substitution with FDA-approved generically equivalent products is an effective means of maintaining quality care at a lower cost.

Drug use programs

Key to a successful formulary management program is the use of proven tools to assure the safe and effective use of medications. These tools include critical pathways, disease management programs, policies based on the principle of therapeutic interchange, and step-down therapy programs. All these programs can also be implemented in conjunction with the drug-use evaluation program (see Chapter 13).

Critical pathways, also known as clinical pathways or care maps, are tools of patient care management that are created by multidisciplinary teams, which are intended to lead to the most desirable patient outcome in the most desirable time frame. These programs prespecify what procedures, lab tests, medications, and dietary and exercise needs a patient should receive during a hospitalization for a specific time. There exists evidence that programs that focus on knee-replacement therapy and community-acquired pneumonia are effective at reducing the length of stay, adverse consequences, and costs associated with the treatment of these disorders (Kirk et al., 1996). Disease management programs, discussed in greater detail in Chapter 17, are also successful at improving outcomes.

Two related programs are the sequential (step-down) therapy (aka IV-to-PO switch) and the therapeutic interchange program. The sequential therapy approach consists of substituting a parenteral agent with an equivalent oral agent under specific guidelines. These guidelines are developed and reviewed at the P&T committee and approval comes from the medical executive committee. The resulting implementation occurs through the pharmacy department. Typically, pharmacists review the institution's medication records for patients on targeted IV medications (e.g., H_2-blockers or select antibiotics). Once identified, the patient's chart is reviewed and, if appropriate, an appropriate oral medication is substituted for the IV medication. The outcome typically is similar efficacy at a much lower cost. Therapeutic interchange is the automatic substitution of products within a therapeutic class that have a similar pharmacologic action and render an equivalent therapeutic effect. This occurs only under an arrangement between a pharmacist and an authorized prescriber who have previously established and jointly agreed on conditions for interchange (Chase et al., 1998). For example, a nizatidine 150-mg PO bid may be interchanged for a ranitidine 150-mg bid. These doses are, for some indications, therapeutically equivalent. The use of the less expensive nizatidine can be justified based on the equivalent efficacy and safety of the two products. However, the specific program needs to be continually monitored and updated as new efficacy and safety information becomes available.

Lastly, reporting adverse drug events and medication errors (see Chapter 16) is an important function of the P&T committee. The P&T committee is the best group of practitioners organized to identify system-wide issues regarding the appropriate use of medications. The function of the P&T committee is to analyze the systems and structures that might contribute to medication errors and implement steps to prevent these errors from being repeated. Further, the role of the P&T committee is to report medication-related adverse events to both the community in which it serves as well as the Food and Drug Administration (FDA). The FDA reporting typically is for more serious and uncommon adverse reactions. This is usually accomplished through the FDA MedWatch system, a voluntary reporting system for health care professionals. The FDA MedWatch is designed to provide the public with timely information regarding safety issues related to medications.

Conflict of interest

The organizational culture of an institution plays a significant role in the operations of the P&T committee and the subsequent development and implementation of policies related to the drug use. Effective P&T committees lead the organization through the process previously described and encourage critical thinking about the addition of expensive and potentially dangerous drugs to the formulary. Coupled with this is the issue of conflict of interest. Members of the P&T committee might have a significant financial or other interest in seeing a product attain formulary status. These interests could be stock investment in the company sponsoring the product, research support from the company, or a participant on the company's speakers bureau. Ideally, a formulary decision should be based on the benefit to the population being served and not for an individual's personal gain. To avoid supporting — or denying — a product formulary status, members of the P&T committee should refrain from voting on products in which they have a substantial interest. To help prevent conflicts of interest from entering into formulary decisions, many P&T committees require members to submit annual statements to the chair of the P&T committee, disclosing a member's financial or other interest in drug-related issues. Although these types of programs are not foolproof, they are helpful.

Coupled with this, many P&T committees have assumed the responsibility for developing policies and procedures related to pharmaceutical sales representatives. These policies are designed to ensure that the sales representatives act responsibly and provide the necessary information to the practitioners for care of patients. Further, they tend to restrict activities of sales representatives to those that provide benefit for the patient.

Conclusion

A well-organized P&T committee is essential to promoting rational, cost-effective drug therapy to a population of patients. This committee oversees the formulary development and implementation of the formulary, which, in conjunction with other drug-therapy programs and policies, promotes high-quality, cost-effective care. Pharmacists play a significant role in the functioning of the committee and the formulary system. They have the expertise necessary to lead the organization in making formulary management decisions based on sound clinical and economic judgment.

Bibliography

Chase SL, Peterson AM, Wordell CJ. Therapeutic interchange program for oral histamine H_2-receptor antagonists. *Am. J. Hlth.-Syst. Pharm.* 1998; 55: 1382–1386.

Green J. Point: the formulary system and the emperor's new clothes. *Am. J. Hosp. Pharm.* 1986; 43: 2830–2833.

Horn S, Sharkey P, Tracy ED, Horn C, James B, Goodwin F. Intended and unintended consequences of HMO cost-containment strategies: results from the managed care outcomes project. *Am. J. Manage. Care* 1996; 2: 253–264.

Jewesson PJ. Do we have evidence that formularies save money? *Can. J. Hosp. Pharm.* 2000; 53: 320–321.

Kirk JK, Michael KA, Markowsky SJ, Restino MR, Zarowitz BJ. Critical pathways: the time is here for pharmacist involvement. *Pharmacotherapy,* 1996; 16: 723–733.

Manneback MA, Ascione FJ, Gaither CA, Bagozzi RP, Cohen IA, Ryan ML. Activities, functions, and structures of pharmacy and therapeutics committees in large teaching hospitals. *Am. J. Hlth.-Syst. Pharm.* 1999; 56: 622–628.

Nash DB, Catalano ML, Wordell CJ. The formulary decision-making process in a U.S. academic medical centre. *Pharmacoeconomics* 1993; 3: 22–35.

Odendina FT, Sullivan J, Nash R, Clemmons CD. Use of pharmacoeconomic data in making hospital formulary decisions. *Am. J. Hlth.-Syst. Pharm.* 2002; 59: 1441–1444.

Pedersen CA, Schneider PJ, Santell JP. ASHP national survey of pharmacy practice in hospital settings: Prescribing and transcribing. *Am. J. Hlth-Syst. Pharm.* 2001; 58: 2251–2266.

Poirer TI. Ethical issues in pharmacy: a biblical perspective. *J. Bibl. Eth. Med.* 1993; 1: 12–14.

Principles of a sound drug formulary system, October 2000. http://www.usp.org/pdf/patientSafety/pSafetySndFormPrinc.pdf, accessed September 14, 2003.

Sullivan SD, Lyles A, Luce B, Grigar J. AMCP guidance for submission of clinical and economic evaluation data to support formulary listing in U.S. health plans and pharmacy benefits management organizations. *J. Manage. Care Pharm.* 2001; 7: 272–282.

Wade WE, Spruill WJ, Taylor AT, Longe RL, Hawkins DW. The expanding role of pharmacy and therapeutics committees: the 1990s and beyond. *Pharmacoeconomics* 1996; 10: 123–128.

chapter thirteen

Drug use evaluation

Andrew M. Peterson

Contents

Introduction

The current health care system is dependent on the appropriate use of resources. Medication use accounts for a large proportion of these resources, with the base cost of medications continually rising, at times exceeding the rate of inflation. Further, the rising salaries of the physicians, pharmacists, and nurses involved in prescribing, filling, and administering medications contributes to the increased cost of medications. Lastly, the complexity of the medication use process creates systems in which both preventable medication errors and nonpreventable adverse reactions occur, ballooning the cost of medication use. Hospitals, health care systems, managed care organizations, and pharmacy benefit management companies struggle with these costs daily. To cope with these costs, these health systems review the use of drugs within their populations to determine where improvements in the process can be made to assure high quality, cost-efficient care. The Joint Commission on Accreditation of Healthcare Organizations (JCAHO) and the National Committee for Quality Assurance (NCQA) require some form of evaluation of drug use (see Chapter

Table 13.1 Principles of Drug Use Review

1. Appropriate authority
2. Understanding the characteristics of the delivery system and population served
3. Availability of existing profiles of drug usage
4. Criteria against which drug usage can be reviewed and judged
5. A mechanism for assessing the impact of changes implemented

Source: Adapted from Brodie, DC and Smith WE. *Hospitals* 1976; 50: 143–150.

21 on accrediting organizations). This process is often referred to as drug use evaluation (DUE). Medication use evaluation (MUE), drug use review (DUR), and medication use management (MUM) are synonyms for the DUE process. The chapter describes the role of DUE as a means of improving medication use within an organization.

History of DUE/DUR

In 1972, Brodie published an important paper defining the process of reviewing and evaluating drug use as an "ongoing study of the frequency of use and cost of drugs, from which patterns of prescribing, dispensing, and patient use can be determined" (Brodie, 1972). This concept was further developed by Brodie (1976) when he published five principles of drug use review (Table 13.1). These principles remain the basic structural components of all DUR programs. As per these principles, the program must be authorized by a governing body (typically a Pharmacy and Therapeutics [P&T] committee), systematically structured to assure a continuous and consistent approach to drug use, and the use of drugs must be measured against predetermined criteria developed by professionals and experts who use the medications.

From 1981 to 1985, the JCAHO (then the Joint Commission on Accreditation of Hospitals) applied the DUE process to hospitalized patients receiving antibiotics. Adopting the terminology *antibiotic utilization review* (AUR), the JCAHO required the medical staff to review the appropriateness, safety, and efficacy of antibiotics used within an institution. Although holding the medical staff responsible, the JCAHO also insisted that this review take place with the assistance of the department of pharmacy, ostensibly through the P&T committee. In 1986, the emphasis moved from strictly antibiotics to all drugs. In 1994, the JCAHO adopted the term *medication use evaluation* (MUE). This name change was also coupled with a shifting emphasis from medical staff reviews to an interdisciplinary approach to drug use, including all users of medications (e.g., nurses and respiratory therapists).

Health policy and professional responsibilities have changed during the years since DUR was introduced into the health care system. To maintain accreditation, hospitals and health care systems are bound to conduct MUE/DUE programs. In the retail setting, the Omnibus Reconciliation Act of 1990

(OBRA 90) required that pharmacists identify and resolve drug-related problems before they reached Medicaid patients. Today, this DUR standard is applied not only to Medicaid patients but to all patients receiving health care benefits through a third-party provider (e.g., an insurance company). As such, DUR has had an enormous impact on the current health care system.

The distinction between MUE/DUE and DUR is based mainly on the origin of the terms and not on the processes. DUE is the process used to improve the use of drugs as required by the JCAHO, and DUR is that same process mandated by the OBRA 90 regulation. Recently, the NCQA promulgated new standards for utilization management, incorporating the tenets of DUE. Each organization requires that the process be an ongoing, criteria-based, systematic process designed to improve the use of drugs. Further, the responsibility does not rest only with a single practitioner; rather, the responsibility for the safe and effective use of medications is shared among all practitioners involved in the drug use process.

DUE programs are both qualitative and quantitative studies evaluating how a drug is used compared with predetermined criteria. Coupling the results of this comparison with recommendations on how to improve the use of the drug not only achieves the improved patient care objective but also provides substantial benefit to the pharmacist and prescriber.

The DUE process allows the health care organization to use the results of the evaluations to compare the quality of care delivered by practitioners. This peer evaluation is often used by managed care organizations to encourage physician compliance to use formulary drugs, generic substitution, and clinical practice guidelines.

DUE types

DUEs can be performed retrospectively, concurrently, or prospectively. Retrospective reviews are the simplest to perform but are limited in impact. In retrospective reviews, the patients have already received the drugs. Because the medications have already been administered, one can simply review the charts of patients and determine whether the drug use met predetermined criteria. Therefore, these studies are not time dependent and require limited resources. The value of these strategies is counterbalanced by the lack of impact they have on past drug use. Further, because the results of the studies are based on written records, the potential for incomplete data can lead to bias and invalid results. Retrospective reviews of drug use patterns can assist plans in developing strategies for more comprehensive and relevant prospective DURs. Retrospective DUEs are useful for identifying problems in therapeutic duplication, abuse of medications, appropriate generic use, and inappropriate durations of therapy.

In concurrent DUEs, reviews are conducted *while* patients are receiving medications. These strategies allow corrective actions to be taken during the time the patients are receiving the medications. Patients are identified as existing users of the drugs, and their profiles or charts are reviewed to determine how well the drug use meets predetermined criteria. If problems are identified, there are opportunities to effect changes in the drug use, hopefully improving the quality of care.

The benefits of concurrent reviews are balanced by the difficulties in identifying patients and reviewing problems manually. Computerized reviews can help in this arena; however, to effect timely changes, one must be able to contact prescribers and explain the situation. Often this can be difficult, and when the prescribers are reached, they may be reluctant to change therapy. Problems well suited for concurrent DUEs are drug–drug interactions, incorrect dosage, and therapeutic duplication.

Prospective DUEs occur before patients receive medications. Therefore, if problems have been identified, they can be resolved before the patients receive the medications. A major disadvantage to prospective reviews is that they require well-defined and coordinated approaches to identifying drugs targeted for review. Further, ready access to patient information and prescribers makes this difficult to implement. Problems useful for identifying and resolving before medication administration include drug–allergy and drug–disease interactions, incorrect dosage, age or disease-state contraindications, and therapeutic duplications.

Steps in conducting a DUE

Table 13.2 outlines the steps to be taken when conducting a DUE program. These steps are based on the JCAHO 10-step process for conducting DUE/ MUE programs.

Step 1 is to gain authority from the organization's stakeholders and design an appropriate reporting structure. Those with the authority typically include the organization's administration, medical staff, pharmacy staff, and nursing staff; others may be included as well. The typical source of authority is the P&T committee of the organization. The P&T committee may delegate the authority to one of its subcommittees or charge another committee with the responsibility. In any event, the clear lines of authority should be maintained and reviewed periodically.

Table 13.2 Steps in the DUE Process

1. Gain organizational authority and assign responsibility.
2. Delineate scope of drug use.
3. Identify important specific drugs to be monitored and evaluated.
4. Identify indicators.
5. Establish thresholds.
6. Collect and organize data.
7. Evaluate drug use.
8. Take actions to improve drug use.
9. Assess effectiveness of actions.
10. Communicate relevant information to appropriate individuals.

Table 13.3 Key Processes Evaluated during a DUE

1. Prescribing medications
2. Preparing medications
3. Dispensing medications
4. Administering medications
5. Monitoring efficacy and safety (outcome)

Step 2 is to delineate the scope of drug use within the organization and outline what elements of the drug use process should be reviewed. A review of peer-reviewed scientific literature, relevant clinical practice guidelines, and accrediting organization requirements should be the underpinning for this step. Table 13.3 lists the important processes evaluated in a DUE/MUE.

Step 3 is to identify the specific drugs to be reviewed. Clinicians involved in the institution's drug use process should be consulted to aid in determining which drugs should undergo the evaluation process. Information from past DUE studies, clinical judgment, and current literature help the organization decide the target drugs. Typically, drugs with high use within the organization, drugs that present a high risk to patients, or drugs with a high cost are considered for evaluation. In addition, newly introduced drugs, or drugs used for a new population of patients, may be good candidates for a DUE.

Step 4 for those involved in the process is to discuss and decide on the measures of quality pertinent to the drug being evaluated. These become the criteria for drug use. They are developed by the clinicians using the medications and are often based on both evidence from the literature as well as local experience. Often, surrogate markers of disease or outcome, or both, must be used if more clinically relevant data are not readily available in computerized records or in the patient's actual chart.

The DUE criteria should be developed in concert with the organization's programmatic goals on how medications should be used within the system. The criteria developed do not have to be comprehensive and include all five key processes for a DUE (Table 13.2); rather, the criteria can be based only on one or more of these key processes.

Step 5 is to establish thresholds for optimal use. Thresholds are the standards against which performance is measured. For example, if the criteria for dosing a medication require that all patients receive a particular dose, without variation, then the threshold will be set at 100%; that is, 100% of the patients must receive that dose. It is not necessary to set absolute standards (e.g., 0% therapeutic duplication or 100% compliance with dosage recommendations), because individual variation should be taken into account. A further example of a threshold includes the percentage of patients expected to achieve a certain outcome (e.g., goal blood pressure, 75%; adverse reaction, 12%). Clinical pharmacists and physician specialists should be involved in the development of thresholds because of their clinical experience with the drug and should help set these reasonable thresholds. See Table 13.4 for example criteria and thresholds.

Step 6 is to collect and organize the data. As noted earlier, data collection can occur retrospectively, concurrently, or prospectively. Because of the potential for misuse of information, and the old adage "garbage in – garbage out," having a clear plan of collecting the data is essential. Information specialists and clinicians must come together to determine the data to be collected and the most efficient means of doing so.

In *Step 7*, once the data are collected, comparing and evaluating the results with predetermined thresholds rests with the clinicians. Often, initial results are reviewed by an experienced clinical pharmacist and then brought back to all stakeholders for their review. All clinicians involved in the criteria and threshold development should jointly agree on conclusions from the data. Sometimes, this process also uncovers new, appropriate trends in prescribing. See Table 13.4 for an abbreviated DUE report to a P&T committee.

Step 8 is to identify solutions to the problems identified in Step 7. This step includes formulating educational programs to improve the knowledge of the users of medications, developing restrictions to drug use based on inappropriate use, or even removing the drug from the formulary because of the potential dangers it might present. See Table 13.5 for example recommendations that may come from a DUE report. Education is the most common means of corrective action and often becomes the cornerstone of all interventions to improve drug use. This is discussed in more detail later.

Steps 9 and 10 involve assessing the effectiveness of the actions taken in Step 8; a continuous quality improvement (CQI) process (see Chapter 14); and communicating the findings, actions, and follow-up to the appropriate individuals involved. These individuals may be the patients, the provider, or the managed care organization.

Educational programs

The results of a DUE program should be shared with all the health care providers involved in the medication use process. There are several strategies for communicating these results, including a one-on-one education by pharmacists to providers, workshops, seminars, and newsletters.

Typically, presenting DUE results directly to a health care professional more effectively changes how a provider uses the medication. This type of process, called academic detailing, was studied by Avorn and Soumerai (1983). In their classic study, the researchers targeted 435 physicians and assigned them randomly to one of three groups: (1) face-to-face education by clinical pharmacists, (2) mailed printed materials, or (3) control group (no material provided). The study found that the best means of affecting prescribing changes was through the one-on-one discussions, and that mailed printed materials had no significant effect over providing no material.

Table 13.4 Abbreviated DUE Report for the Example Drug Peterpenem

Criteria	Threshold (%)	Performance (n = 25 Patients) (%)	Comments
Indications Serious Gram-negative infections	100	92	• 2 patients were treated for *Mycobacterium avium intracellularae* (MAI)
Dosing 250–500 mg q6h	100	72	• 4 patients were not dose adjusted based on estimated creatinine clearance
• For CrCl b/t 20–50 ml/min, then 500 mg q8-q12h	100	88	• 2 patients received greater than 50 mg/kg/d
• No doses >50mg/kg and no single dose > 500 mg	100	92	• 1 patient received a loading dose of 1 g
Lab Studies • Scr at baseline and daily	100	100	All labs were appropriately ordered
• Cultures and sensitivity testing baseline and daily	100	100	
• Others as indicated	100	100	
Efficacy • Temperature ≤ 99°F	85	76	• The 2 MAI patients passed away
• Negative cultures	85	72	• 1 patient developed resistant *Pseudomonas aeruginosa*
• No change in blood pressure	90	88	• 1 patient died of multiple organ dysfunction 2° to a motor vehicle accident, with septic shock
Safety/Adverse Reactions • Diarrhea	4	16	• 4 patients experienced diarrhea
• Infusion reactions	1	4	• 1 patient experienced pain at injection site
• Seizures	<1	4	• 1 patient experienced a seizure — recovered (dose was not adjusted for renal function)
• Other			• 2 patients experienced allergic reactions (whole body rash, hives)

Table 13.5 Example Recommendations for the P&T Committee Based on an Example DUE Report

1. Consider adding MAI to the approved list of peterpenem use indications.

2. A letter to the medical, nursing, and pharmacy staffs requiring the following:
   - The department of pharmacy is to adjust the dosing for all patients receiving peterpenem based on the following criteria:
     For patients with $CrCl_{est}$ > 50 ml/min: 500 mg q6-8h
     For patients with $CrCl_{est}$ 20–50 ml/min: 500 mg q8-12h
     For patients with $CrCl_{est}$ < 20 ml/min: 500 mg q12h-24h
   - Doses higher than these must be approved by the infectious disease attending and clinical pharmacist.
   - An educational program for all pharmacists and physicians *must* be conducted before implementing the above recommendations.

3. All patients' allergy status *must* be verified before initiating peterpenem therapy.

Coupled with this academic detailing, data suggest that early involvement of respected peers in the design and implementation of a DUE program aid in the successful change of medication use. Further, offering clinicians short summaries of guidelines or recommendations for change, using one of the respected peers, also improves medication use.

Tips for a successful program

One of the first and most harmful mistakes in conducting a DUE program is not assuring agreement among the stakeholders regarding the scope and authority of the program. By assuring medical staff concordance (most often through the P&T committee) and administrative authority, the DUE program is more likely to effect a true and meaningful change in drug use throughout the organization. Further, not communicating results to all the individuals involved in the drug use can impede progress on improving the drug use. Lastly, all DUE results must be well documented so that when questions regarding the results arise, they can be readily answered.

Conclusion

The responsibility for assuring appropriate drug use rests with all professionals in the medication use process, but pharmacists have the opportunity to take the lead in continually improving this process. The DUE process has evolved into a core function for pharmacists and will continue to evolve as more sophisticated tools of identifying and resolving medication-related problems are developed.

Bibliography

Academy of Managed Care Pharmacy. Concepts in managed care: drug use evaluation. Alexandria, VA. 1999.

Bowman L. Drug use evaluation is DUE: healthcare utilization evaluation is over-DUE. *Hosp Pharm.* 1996; 31: 347–353.

Brodie DC. Drug utilization review-planning. *Hospitals* 1972; 46: 103–112.

Brodie DC, Smith WE. Constructing a conceptual model of drug utilization review. *Hospitals* 1976; 50: 143–150.

Enlow M. Drug-usage evaluation by disease state: developing protocols. *Pharm. Pract. Manage. Q.* 1996; 16: 18–25.

Hlynka JN, Smith Jr. WE, Brodie DC. Developing drug-use profiles from drug-charge records. *Am. J. Hosp. Pharm.* 1979; 36: 1347–1351.

Joint Commission on the Accreditation of Healthcare Organizations (JCAHO). *1995 Comprehensive Accreditation Manual for Hospitals.* JCAHO, Oakbrook Terrace, IL, 1994.

Kubacka RT. A primer on drug utilization review. *J. Am. Pharm. Assoc.* 1996; NS(4): 257–261.

Peroutka JA. Designing drug-usage evaluation to meet Joint Commission requirements. *Pharm. Pract. Manage. Q.* 1996; 16(2): 26–35.

Soumerai SB, Avorn J. Improving drug-therapy decisions through educational outreach. A randomized controlled trial of academically based "detailing." *N. Engl. J. Med.* 1983; 308: 1457–1463.

Soumerai SB, McLaughlin TJ, Avorn J. Improving drug prescribing in primary care: a critical analysis of the experimental literature. *Milbank Q.* 1989; 67: 268–317.

Stoler M. Drug use review: operational definitions. *Am. J. Hosp. Pharm.* 1978; 33: 225–230.

Todd MW. Drug use evaluation. In *Handbook of Institutional Pharmacy Practice.* American Society of Hospital Pharmacists, Bethesda, MD, 1996, chap. 24, pp. 261–271.

chapter fourteen

Continuous quality improvement

Susan Skledar

Contents

Continuous quality improvement (CQI), most simply, can be defined as a structured method for continually improving all activities involved with organizational performance. CQI is a systematic, organizational approach for continually improving all processes that deliver quality services and products.[1] Inherent in improvement of quality is the need to meet and exceed customer expectations in the most time-efficient manner while incurring the least economic burden.

To integrate CQI into organizational performance, it must be embraced as a leadership style and management philosophy. Table 14.1 lists the underlying concepts of CQI for improving organizational performance. Organizational leaders must integrate CQI into vision, mission, and value statements, and develop a way for employees at every level of the organization to understand CQI. Engaging employees in problem-solving efforts is a

Table 14.1 CQI Concepts for Improving Organizational Performance[1-3]

- Define CQI for your organization.
- Develop a strong customer and patient focus.
- Design structured processes for solving problems and identifying solutions.
- Use employee work teams to improve quality.
- Develop and conduct educational programs at every level to promote CQI methodology.
- Create an atmosphere that supports employee risk taking and support of ideas.
- Know that the person doing the job at the front line is the most knowledgeable about the work.

successful way to promote improvement. CQI in practice depends on enabling the workforce to study work processes and suggest changes in their normal course of work. The underlying premise is that employees want to do the best work possible, and that each is both an employee and a customer. As new programs are developed and implemented within an organization, CQI techniques should be instinctively applied and explained. This will allow work teams, supervisors, and administrative leadership to fully understand application of CQI principles to daily practice. In the present health care market, it is also essential to keep processes and activities current. The method of continual evaluation of organizational performance, at the most broad and most narrow levels, will keep the organization at the forefront of rapid changes in health care.

Essential components of CQI

Essential components of CQI problem solving include the project work team, a structured method to study the problem, collected data, and data analysis tools to evaluate outcomes.

CQI work teams

Employee work teams should be multidisciplinary and have clear direction on the scope of the problem and aspects they are trying to improve. Members should include those who can provide guidance (guidance team) and those who best know and will do the frontline work (project team). The guidance team provides the overall direction to the group with the project aim or mission. It can also enlist administrative support for programmatic changes and resources that may be necessary to improve performance. Team members should have defined roles, e.g., project leader, discussion group facilitator, and progress recorder. Defined roles will promote ownership of the problem and a vested interest in continual improvement and monitoring. Overall, team members should feel comfortable identifying improvement opportunities, actively analyze problem causes, brainstorm improvement strategies, educate fellow employees and customers, and help analyze outcomes of improvement.

CQI methodology

A structured process to solve problems is essential for thorough, consistent improvement programs. For continuous improvement of quality, the most widely used structural method is the *plan–do–check–act* (PDCA) cycle.[1,4,5] Designed by Walter Shewart in the 1920s, the PDCA cycle is a model in which the project is planned by evaluating baseline practices compared with desired results from internal, published, or benchmark standards; designing an improvement action; establishing criteria to measure improvement; and continually refining or expanding the project. The PDCA process is used to guide measurement of outcomes as improvement interventions are designed, evaluated, and implemented.[6] Incremental changes are implemented and evaluated over defined time periods; successes are expanded and lessons learned emerge. Figure 14.1 depicts the PDCA cycle.

Data-driven development

It is important that improvement efforts be derived from demonstrated problems and not from assumptions that problems exist. Identifying opportunities and reporting progress and outcomes should be data driven.[7] Internal baseline data can be analyzed according to best published practices or standard operating procedures for safety, e.g. health care protocols can be compared with published care plans for drug utilization or disease management. Patient safety issues can be benchmarked against local, national, and regional standards, and the most applicable improvement efforts can be selected for improving processes of care. Displaying information by using CQI tools, such as flowcharts, cause and effect diagrams, statistical process

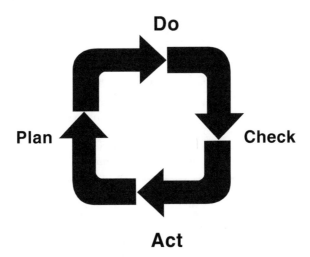

Do

Plan

Check

Act

Figure 14.1 The PDCA cycle.

control charts, and pareto charts, helps systematically identify where variations are present, focus efforts on the root cause of the problem, and measure the outcome of implemented improvement efforts.[1,7] In the 1960s, Avedis Donabedian first identified the relationship of structure, process, and outcome in evaluating the quality of health care.[9-11] Donabedian explains that the link between process and outcome must be understood clearly before CQI efforts can be initiated.[11] Focusing efforts only on the structure and process of health care delivery without evaluating the outcomes of changes made is an incomplete effort. Structure influences process, and better processes (how things happen) lead to better outcomes (what things happen).

CQI application to pharmacy practice

The CQI methodology provides the structure to evaluate services and monitor improvement. Table 14.2 lists ideas for CQI projects in pharmacy prac-

Table 14.2 Examples of CQI Application in Pharmacy Practice

CQI Project	Example
Clinical practice guidelines	*C. difficile*-associated diarrhea Community acquired pneumonia Surgical antimicrobial prophylaxis
Formulary decisions	Restricting broad spectrum antibiotics to infectious disease service Designating more expensive, equal-efficacy drug to nonformulary status Cost-effectiveness analyses
Drug use evaluation	Determine drug shortage alternative plan Evaluate use of chemical restraints
Preprinted order set design	Hypokalemia Sliding scale insulin Continuous renal replacement therapy
Promoting patient safety	Patient-controlled analgesia Automated dispensing systems Pharmacokinetic dosing service Anticoagulation service Renal dosing program Determine use of unsafe medical abbreviations Computerized medication administration records Computerized physician order entry Antibiotic management programs
Improving pharmacy services	Decentralized pharmacy services Patient education programs Cost-justifying clinical pharmacy services Missing dose evaluation

tice.[6,12-13] CQI efforts must focus on answering three questions: (1) What is the major aim of the project? (2) How will it be known that improvement has occurred? and (3) What actions can be taken to ensure improvement?[14,15] The CQI methodology should be used to plan operational improvements, expand clinical services, and determine formulary decisions. Table 14.3 lists published CQI projects and indicator measures.[16-29]

With the rapid change of health care and constant advances in science and technology in the era of cost containment, CQI is essential to providing quality care while balancing use of resources. In health care, this CQI strategy may be used to integrate published evidence with expert clinical practice to deliver optimal patient outcomes and promote cost-effective care. It has been stated that CQI is an extension of the diagnostic and treatment "scientific method" of medicine to health care (and industry) management.[30] Additionally, CQI allows the problem to be viewed as a series of structure and process connections that can be evaluated and improved collectively to change and improve practice.

A stepwise approach to applying the PDCA cycle includes defining the problem, determining baseline practices, solving for the root cause of the problem, implementing improvement efforts, and monitoring change. Table 14.4 details steps in applying the PDCA cycle to problem solving.[2] The following pharmacy CQI case example demonstrates application of the PDCA cycle.

Focused case example: using CQI to design a clinical pharmacy competency program

You are the new director of pharmacy at a community hospital. At a mock inspection by your institution's regulatory compliance team, you are asked to provide documentation of pharmacist competency assessment. You provide the information, but it is not easy for you to gather. Additionally, you find that less than half the pharmacists whose records you pulled (4/10; 40%) have their annual competency requirements completed. The staff has commented to you that they do not feel that the competency assessment program is effective or efficient. After the mock inspection is complete, you identify that the pharmacy competency program should be evaluated.

Plan phase

Step 1: Define the problem

Background. Focusing efforts to clearly define the problem is the first step to undertake. The problem statement should be specific and measurable and denote a timetable for improvement. As the work team is assembled (see Step 2 of the Plan phase), having a defined project aim will focus the group and ensure understanding of the project at hand. It is also very important to relate the CQI project to organizational performance. Data,

Table 14.3 Selected Published CQI Indicator Measurement Projects

Topic	Focus	Example Indicators
Drug related morbidity quality indicators[16]	Focused preventable drug-related morbidity projects	Use of long half-life hypnotic anxiolytics Use of carbamazepine without complete blood count measured
Diabetes care[17–20]	Diabetes	HbA1c above 8%
	Hypertension	Blood pressure readings >140/90 mmHg
	Adverse events	Thiazolidinedione patients with serum ALT measured Yearly dilated eye exam Yearly microalbumin test
Medication adherence[21]	Compliance with taking prescribed medications	Self-report of missed doses over a designated time period
Formulary management[22]	Antibiotic restrictions	Compliance with prescribing according to institution-specific guidelines
Surgical antimicrobial prophylaxis[23–24]	Timing, selection, and duration of antibiotic prophylaxis	Preoperative doses administered 60 min before surgical incision Postoperative antimicrobial duration less than 48 h
Pneumonia disease prevention[25]	Increasing use of pneumococcal vaccine	At-risk vaccination rates Elderly vaccination rates Pneumonia readmission rates
Asthma[26–27]	Short-term control	Symptom-free days Use of short-acting $beta_2$-agonists
Pain[28]	Medium- or long-term control	Asthma exacerbations
	Analgesic use	Around-the-clock analgesic use
	Pain severity assessment	Pain assessment on admission Pain reassessment after analgesic dose
Cardiovascular disease[29]	Cholesterol management	Adherence with taking cholesterol-lowering medications Patients at risk for cardiovascular disease
	Cardiac rehabilitation	Patients attending cardiac rehabilitation programs

Table 14.4 Action Steps of the PDCA Cycle

PDCA Cycle Phase	Action Step
Plan	
• Develop project	1. Define the problem
• Set timetable for improvement	2. Create multidisciplinary team to address the issue
	3. Review the literature and/or published standards
	4. Define quality indicators
	5. Analyze baseline data
	6. Review current practices
	7. Perform root cause analysis
	8. Create action plan for change
Do	
• Implement	1. Implement recommendation
• (Pilot if appropriate)	2. Multidisciplinary, multifaceted education
Check	
• Study	1. Reassess indicator progress
	2. Identify barriers to progress
	3. Identify lessons learned
Act	
• Standardize change	1. Design future plans
• Ensure ongoing monitoring	2. Establish system for continued monitoring

both from the current problem and from published literature, should drive the need for performance improvement. Directives for CQI in health care originate from sources such as the Joint Commission on Accreditation of Healthcare Organizations (JCAHO), Health Care Financing Administration (HCFA), Agency for Healthcare Research and Quality (AHRQ), American College of Surgeons (ACS), and various managed care organizations.[30] CQI efforts should not be initiated based on assumptions or anecdotal reports. It is also important that the solution is not assumed or implied in the statement of the problem.

Competency case application.   A fundamental part of the mission of your organization is to provide optimum patient care by ensuring quality services, promoting patient satisfaction, educating patients and practitioners, and continually improving care. Connecting the competency project to your organizational mission is easily achieved. Although the competency program passed the mock inspection, not only was it difficult to gather the competency information efficiently, but less than 40% of pharmacist files audited had complete information. This is the internal data that supports the need for this CQI project. A focal point of JCAHO is competency assessment, which provides further support for the need for a strong competency program.[31] The competency problem statement is defined as follows: "The aim of this project is to improve efficiency of the pharmacist clinical competency program over the next year to achieve 100% of records complete."

Step 2: Create a multidisciplinary team

Background. Involvement of the appropriate team members is essential to project success. The multidisciplinary team can be composed of members from the medical, nursing, or pharmacy staffs, the respiratory care team, support services, patient groups, and risk management, managed care, and quality assurance groups. Having a team with the correct membership will lead to better acceptance of the project and ensure that the problem is examined from many different perspectives. The group should comprise the major stakeholders in the problem, and defining all customers and their expectations helps ensure that all correct participants are part of the work team. Establishing roles for work team members is important, and having administrative and concept guidance for the team keeps the project progressing.

Competency case application. Members of the multidisciplinary team include staff pharmacists, pharmacy students, pharmacy administrators, clinical pharmacists, drug information specialists, computer specialists, secretarial support, and quality assurance specialists. Guidance is provided by the directors of pharmacy and regulatory compliance. Table 14.5 details customers and their expectations. The team is responsible for reviewing and refining the project aim statement in Step 1 of the Plan phase, gathering and reviewing literature, problem solving of root causes, developing recommendations, designing implementation strategies, and evaluating changes. The remaining CQI action steps are outlined next.

Step 3: Review the literature

Background. With the problem identified and the work team assembled, the next step is to generate specific questions and search the published

Table 14.5 Customers and Expectations

Customers	Expectations
Pharmacists	Available educational materials and understanding clinical topics
Pharmacy administrators	Demonstrating competence
Secretaries	Decreasing paperwork
JCAHO readiness group	Documenting competence
Nursing and medical staff	Knowledgeable and competent practitioners
Patients	Safe medication practices

literature.[32] Narrowing the topic scope is essential to focusing group efforts to perform a complete search. Often, particularly if your problem involves management of a disease, primary literature can be most helpful. Also, pharmacoeconomic evaluations, meta-analyses, systematic reviews, and consensus guidelines can be used. Practice guidelines for many disease states and health care topics exist from national associations and expert panels, such as the American Diabetes Association or the American Heart Association. The JCAHO, HCFA, and other regulatory agencies also have established best practice recommendations. The work team needs to thoroughly search the available external information to gather evidence. The CQI project, however, might be an internal process or operational improvement issue, and therefore other information such as internal policies and procedures can be consulted. All this information is then critically evaluated by the work team and summarized to show which approaches might be most applicable to the current problem. Benchmarking is a technique that also can be used to identify best practices. [29] Although strategies for improvement are not always published, available information should be gathered for review. The group may also engage in clinical queries of other institution practices via phone surveys, focus groups, and electronic list service message posting to gather information.

Competency case application. A wide array of information is available for competency assessment. From an internal perspective, your institution has a pharmacy department policy denoting that the department must address, maintain, and continually improve staff competency. Also, the institution has a broad policy statement indicating that providing continuing education and evaluation of practitioner competency is one of the core objectives of its overall mission. External standards for competency assessment and program strategies are available from the JCAHO.[31,33] Its accreditation manual states in the human resources standards that institutions must provide for competency staff; verify education, experience, and ability of new employees; and evaluate continued ability of staff to perform via ongoing competency assessment. [31] Institutions also have published statements on the importance of competency assessment and strategies they have used to design and implement programs.[34–36]

Step 4: Define quality indicators

Background. Creating measurement indicators is the next step in the CQI process. Measurement of current practices will denote the baseline data for the project. Indicators must be rate based, reporting percent frequency of occurrence over time. The indicator should have a defined data source (utilization records, laboratory records, billing records, etc.), and include a numerator, denominator, reporting frequency and responsibility, patient population, and threshold goal for improvement. Outcome indicators can be economic, clinical, humanistic, or process measures. Kozma and colleagues defined the ECHO (economic, clinical, and humanistic outcome) model to integrate different types of health care outcomes.[6,37] Process outcomes are important also, as processes are strongly linked to clinical, economic, and humanistic outcomes. The process of care is a sequence of linked steps that are intended to cause a defined medical outcome.[38] Horn and colleagues have also developed a sophisticated clinical practice improvement (CPI) model for improving patient care that considers three types of data — patient, process, and outcome measures — and allows adjustment for differing patient populations and severity.[38] Data on these three variables are measured and analyzed, and then the improvement protocol is developed and implemented. The CPI strategy engages practitioners for evaluating baseline data, and guideline development is based on data gathered in their everyday practice. Next, published data must be integrated to measure current practice vs. the ideal, and guidelines can then be made. Each improvement project might not relate to all four indicator categories (economic, clinical, humanistic, and process), but it is best to have at least two types of quality indicator measures for the project.

Examples of clinical outcomes include measures such as reduced adverse reactions, reduced bleeding episodes, or goal laboratory value attainment. Process outcomes include indicators such as guideline compliance rate or capture rate of patient satisfaction surveys completed. Economic outcomes might include drug, equipment, or labor cost-savings, but can also measure more sophisticated data, such as length of stay and readmissions. Humanistic outcomes are often the most difficult to collect, but include patient satisfaction with care or quality-of-life measurement. Depending on the project, a mix of indicators is the best reflection of project impact. It is recommended to start with a clear, limited number of measurement indicators to evaluate program baseline practices and later monitor impact of changes made.[39] See Table 14.3 for sample CQI projects and indicators used to measure improvement.

Competency case application. For this competency CQI project, it was determined that two indicators would be used to evaluate practice: percentage of pharmacists meeting competency requirements and percentage average score on exams per pharmacist. Table 14.6 lists the defined parameters of both competency indicators.

Step 5: Analyze baseline data

Background. Once indicators are selected, baseline practice data must be measured in order to determine current practices. This step is important to objectively denote the current practice, make sure all major stakeholders are involved in the improvement process, and set the stage for problem solving. CQI should be data driven, so that measurement of current practice by collaboratively developing quality indicators clearly defines the extent of the problem. It is important to measure the baseline data at several time

Table 14.6 Competency Quality Indicators

	% Pharmacists Meeting Competency Requirements	% Average Score on Exams Per Pharmacist
Objective	Measure the percentage of pharmacists who have taken all required competency exams	Measure the average exam scores for pharmacists taking competency exams
Numerator	All pharmacists (staff, residents, clinical faculty) with the completed block of competency exams	Total correct point score for all exams for all pharmacists
Denominator	All pharmacists (staff, residents, clinical faculty)	Total possible point score for all exams for all pharmacists
Source of data	Competency database	Competency database
Threshold	100% pharmacists complete competency requirements	Average exam score ≥80%
Frequency of reporting	Quarterly	Quarterly
Reporting structure	Pharmacy administration Internal JCAHO compliance team Total quality council	Pharmacy administration Internal JCAHO Compliance team Total quality council

points before implementing change to establish that the problem is evident over time. Display of data graphically is an effective way to represent information. A variety of tools, e.g., bar charts, run charts, histograms, and statistical process control (SPC) charts, can be used to display data.[1,2] Bar charts are often used when there are less than three pre-implementation data points. A run chart is the simplest tool to use, and displays points on a line graph compared with the average or threshold to look at process change over time. A histogram can be used to display data and show its frequency distribution over time and degree of variation, e.g., showing exam scores and the commonly seen bell-shaped distribution of scores. The most comprehensive display is the SPC chart, which should be used only if there are at least 12 data points. It includes calculation of the mean and the upper and lower control limits of variation based on sample averages. The plot displays the practice compared with each of these parameters, and the data can be analyzed to find processes that are within the limits (in control) or consistently outside the limits (out of control).[1] Common causes of variation can be separated from special causes of variation. It is important with SPC charts to denote the threshold and monitor the stability of your process compared to your threshold. A stable, bad process might be occurring.

Competency case application.   For the two competency indicators chosen, the baseline data from the original assessment (at time of mock inspection) revealed that only 40 to 60% of pharmacists were caught up on requirements. This was well below the goal of 100% of pharmacists. Average exam scores were 88%, which was very encouraging and above the threshold at >80%. Baseline data graphics collected for this action step are combined with program results graphics and explained later.

Step 6: Review current practices

Background.   To review current practice, a flowchart is an effective visual way to define steps in the process. Flowcharts can help show all steps in what are sometimes complicated processes and educate the work team on the intricate steps that occur. Additional customers and team members can be identified through flowcharts, and inefficiencies and redundancies in current processes surface. The process must be clearly defined, and standard flowchart symbols should be used for process start and stop, process activity steps (rectangle or square), or decision (diamond).[1] Each activity box should have one output arrow, or a decision diamond should be considered.

Competency case application.   Figure 14.2 gives the current competency program flowchart. The work group brainstormed to discuss all process steps of the current complex competency program. Pharmacists are oriented to departmental operations and also to clinical programs. Competency exams are written and require manual grading and are distributed to

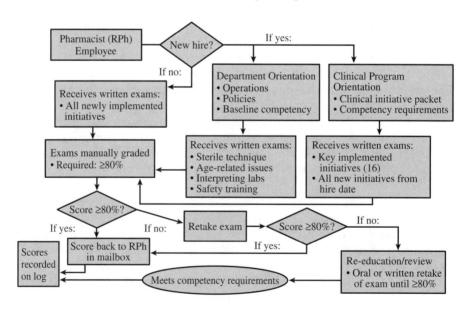

Figure 14.2 Baseline practice flowchart.

employee mailboxes. Notification of exam score also occurs through use of employee mailboxes. Scores are logged into a worksheet for later reference.

Step 7: Perform root cause analysis

Background. Baseline data and flowcharts denote the extent of the problem. The next challenge for the work team is to identify all possible causes for the problem and then prioritize them for action. The work team's experience and creativity are used to capture as many aspects of the problem as possible and create new potential solutions. Brainstorming is an effective tool to use in this action step to create numerous ideas in a short time frame. General rules for brainstorming include the following: (1) agree on the issue being brainstormed; (2) never criticize suggested ideas; (3) give each team member a turn to speak in sequence (no interjections); (4) write all suggested ideas on a flipchart or board in the words of the speaker; and (5) ensure that the total process takes no longer than 5 to 15 min.[1] Brainstorming can be structured or unstructured. If unstructured, the same rules apply, except that ideas can be contributed as they occur to the participants instead of members having to speak in sequence. At the end of the brainstorming session, all ideas should be grouped into common categories or major causes. A cause and effect diagram, also known as a fishbone or Ishikawa diagram, can be used to list all possible causes.[1,7,8] This diagram helps designate the relation between the effect (or problem) and brainstormed causes. For every problem, causes can be grouped into general major categories, such as materials, personnel, procedures, and technology.[1] Additional categories, depending on the problem, may include patients, place, and supplies. The diagram helps to organize the identified theories about problem causes, and the group should challenge itself to keep asking why the cause is occurring until the root cause is uncovered. To find the most basic causes of the problem, repeated causes should be determined. On the fishbone diagram, causes are listed as "bones" or minor causes related to the four or five major causes.

Once major causes are diagrammed, they can be priority ranked using a tool called the pareto chart.[1,8] Frequency of occurrence is listed on the left *y*-axis and cumulative percentage occurrence is on the right *y*-axis. Causes are graphed in order of frequency of occurrence, from high to low. The highest bar on the chart helps focus on what is most commonly causing the problem. The pareto principle, coined in the early 1900s, states that a vital few members of a group account for most of the total effect.[2,8] Most simply, this principle explains that the majority of problems are caused by a small number of causes; in other words, we should concentrate on defining the "vital few and the trivial many."[7,40] Use of the principle improves problem-solving efficiency. Ideally, all causes identified should be solved, but this is often not the most efficient use of time. Problem-solving attention is directed toward the few characteristics that account for the majority of the problem.

Competency case application.   Brainstorming identifies causes for competency program ineffectiveness. Causes include minimal computer support, clinical information not readily available, manual scoring of exams, and work prioritization issues. These causes were easily categorized into technology, material, personnel, and procedural categories. When ranked for priority, nearly 65% of the causes identified during brainstorming were traced to the inefficiencies of the current manual system. Also, access to educational materials was shown to be the next major cause. Using the cause and effect diagram and the pareto chart, the work team determined that the major cause of the competency requirements not being met was an inefficient manual system. Figure 14.3 and Figure 14.4 show application of these CQI tools.

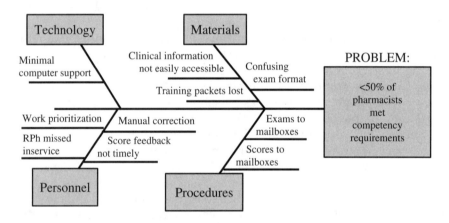

Figure 14.3 Cause and effect diagram.

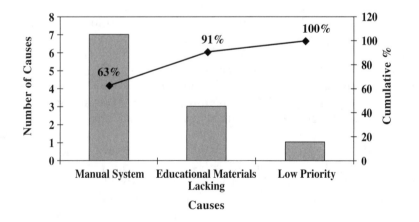

Figure 14.4 Pareto diagram. The major cause of competency requirements not being met was an inefficient manual system.

Step 8: Create the action plan for change

Background. The final step of the Plan phase is to create the action plan for change. Developing consensus on actions is essential. All work team members must contribute to the design of actions. The action plan should be results oriented and also realistic and measurable. Activities should be clearly defined, with timetables for improvement specified. Each work team member should have specific responsibilities for contributing to the completion of the project. From the brainstorming sessions and subsequent discussions, many ideas should be considered and solutions prioritized. Support for the best solution should be identified, with a project champion identified whenever possible. Potential resistance should also be identified, and those situations or persons should be engaged in the problem solving from the outset. For the action plan, the expected result should be defined clearly, and the activities listed to achieve the result outlined. For clinical improvements, actions that are grounded in the literature are important. Recommendations based in the literature or demonstrated successful projects from other benchmarks are strong statements. It is also important, based on the project, to gain necessary administrative or leadership approval for the project. This can help with resource deployment or dissemination of problem importance as implementation is planned. A consideration in planning is whether the project needs to be piloted, or trialed. Depending on the magnitude of the change, a pilot change might be helpful to work out initial problems before full implementation. Involvement of frontline staff is essential in not only developing the improvement project but also piloting the actions and implementing change.

Competency case application. In the root cause analysis, it was determined that the current manual competency assessment program was inefficient. Project interventions included (1) creating a Web-based competency program; (2) automating competency assessment exam scoring and grade notice; (3) giving electronic access to educational materials; and (4) creating a mechanism for staff feedback on the program. The Web-based competency program was housed on the hospital pharmacy's intranet Web site, and the structure of the program incorporated into a departmental policy. The current competency exams were reformatted into standard multiple-choice, true–false questions, and the computer support specialists were able to create a site on the pharmacy page for the competency program. Exams were posted on the developmental server and tested by the work team designee, and staff could access the password-protected site when exams were posted. The scores were automatically graded by the computer, and an electronic mail notice of the score automatically sent to the pharmacist and to the secretary maintaining the competency database. For each exam posted, the departmental teaching materials and the full clinical support documents were electronically linked for ease of access on the competency site. Finally, the competency site had a suggestion box wherein staff could offer suggestions for improvement or ask for guidance.

Do phase

Step 1: Implement recommendation

Background. A systematic approach must be taken to implement the recommendations or improvement actions. Implementing the guideline or policy is even more difficult than writing it.[41] A timetable should be created, denoting specific responsibilities, target dates, and groups that need to be educated. If the project is a large change in practice or process, it might be best to pilot, or trial, the improvement. A small area should be targeted, and detailed monitoring of process change should be performed to evaluate impact and modify approach before full expansion of the project. Many obstacles can be identified, and modifications can be easily tested.

The best strategies for implementation are multifaceted, i.e., a combination of written, verbal, and electronic approaches. Implementation should also be a multidisciplinary process, involving the team members and focusing on all stakeholders affected by the process changes.[2,12,13] Effectiveness of practice policies and care guidelines has been evaluated in the literature. It has been shown that three factors determine the success of guidelines and policies: (1) origin of development; (2) dissemination method chosen; and (3) implementation strategy.[42] Internally developed guidelines and policies were found to be more effective than external ones, because engaging local champions and experts was able to influence practice. Specific educational programs yielded better results than broad notices or mailings did. Concurrent, or active, intervention was more effective for implementation than retrospective reminders. Generally, effective strategies include practitioner reminders (e.g., computerized), focused educational outreach, interactive small group sessions (vs. classroom teaching), and their combinations.[41] Strategies found to be variably effective include audit with retrospective feedback, local consensus-forming meetings, and consumer education programs. Implementation strategies found not effective include passive educational programs (e.g., a single mass mailing or medical grand rounds), particularly if they are the only type of education used.[41]

Competency case application. Because the development of much of the Web site was new, the work team decided to pilot the competency site with a few core pharmacists. Also, because many pharmacists at the time were not familiar with the Internet, an educational program also was needed to explain access and help staff navigate through the site. An educational flyer was created that listed the steps to access the competency Web site and secure an area for exam taking. The flyer was distributed to mailboxes, posted in the pharmacy areas, and also sent via e-mail to staff with the link to the site in the mail message. Educational sessions were held for the pharmacists to introduce the Web site, and new pharmacists were tutored on this during their 4-week department orientation.

Four pharmacists were identified to pilot the program. Development of the site took roughly 2 months. Testing occurred for 1 month before full departmental implementation. Figure 14.5 shows the competency Web page.

Step 2: Ensure multidisciplinary, multifaceted education

Background. Focused efforts must be taken to educate all customers of the improvement project. Multidisciplinary, multifaceted education is essential. When surveyed, clinicians have reported that short executive summaries or synopses of recommendations and expected benefits are most preferred.[43] Involving the multidisciplinary teams to provide the education to their respective groups also can be very effective. Small group education sessions have been repeatedly shown to be very effective, and should be used to reinforce concepts presented at didactic sessions if large group programs are done. Ideally, one-on-one education should be performed also, because it has been shown to be very effective.[32,41,44]

Competency case application. The target audience for the competency program were pharmacists and pharmacy administration. Focused education was done in a group session to introduce the Web-based competency program and demonstrate how to access the site and link to topical educational material. Also, part of this education was a review of competency expectations for the pharmacists. The information shared was also e-mailed to the pharmacists and placed into a one-page fact sheet distributed to

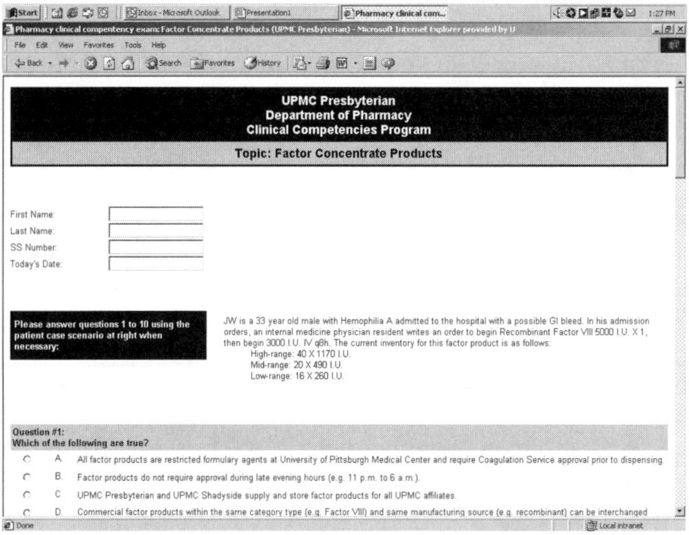

Figure 14.5 Competency Web site.

mailboxes. One-on-one education was also performed if pharmacists had problems with access and during new staff orientation. It was also important for the pharmacists to receive ongoing feedback on performance; therefore, as the exam score threshold was ≥80%, the program was designed such that if a pharmacist received a score lower than this after taking the exam twice, a one-on-one educational session on the topic would be held with a clinical pharmacist and the exam retaken. This reinforcement step was in place before the Web-based competency program, but it was essential that it continue, as not only the efficiency of the program was being changed, but also the quality of the program was to be maintained, and even improved by making educational materials much more accessible for pharmacists. Additionally, because the program was innovative, an additional outcome measure was added to gauge pharmacist satisfaction with the computerized competency program.

Check phase

Step 1: Reassess indicator progress

Background. During Step 4 of the Plan phase, measurement indicators were designed to monitor program impact. Baseline data was gathered to show current practice. In Step 1 of the Check phase, which is post-implementation of the improvement, data should be gathered again to monitor improvement. This data should be collected over time and compared with pre-implementation findings and improvement thresholds.[2] It is best to monitor progress frequently, e.g., weekly or monthly, at initiation of the project to get a sense of the impact of the change. A learning-curve phenomenon might occur, during which the first several months are difficult, particularly if the project is a big practice change — so monitor carefully during this time. Practice changes will settle out, and quarterly data should stabilize. It is important to measure continually practices against the indicators, track practice changes, and identify variances in practice that can be focused on. The reporting structure for the indicators must also be defined, and project improvements and lessons learned disseminated.

Displaying the indicator findings is important, particularly to audiences outside the development team. A simple way to show improvement steps is to modify the process flowchart from Step 6 of the Plan phase and insert new steps. New steps can be shown in a different color, displaying a visually evident change of process. Graphing the results post-implementation is also an effective way to view changes over time. In Step 5 of the Plan phase, bar charts, run charts, and SPC charts were suggested as formats to display baseline data. Post-implementation data should be added to these graphics not only to show improvement made but also to link pre-implementation data and the performance threshold goal. If benchmarking was used to gather baseline data, the national, regional, or local benchmark data can also be displayed on the outcome graphics to display progress related to these standards.

Competency case application. For the competency program, the CQI indicators were designed in Step 4 of the Plan phase and included measures of pharmacists completing all exams and exam scores. Additionally, satisfaction with the competency program was measured through a survey. The coordinator of the competency program gathered the indicator and survey data and prepared the graphic reports. The reports were prepared for the pharmacy director, and these indicators became part of the pharmacy performance improvement program. Especially with competency assessment, other departments in the hospital must have programs, so this Web-based approach might be sought after by other practice areas or groups.

Overall, compared to the manual competency program, the percent of pharmacists caught up on exams increased from <50 to 90% during the program. The learning curve was as expected, because it took pharmacists several months to become very familiar with the site. Exam scores were good at the baseline, and improvement was seen with the Web-based program. From the surveys, pharmacists reported satisfaction with the rapid score feedback, found it easier to meet deadlines, and found online training materials to be very helpful. Figure 14.6 shows the improved

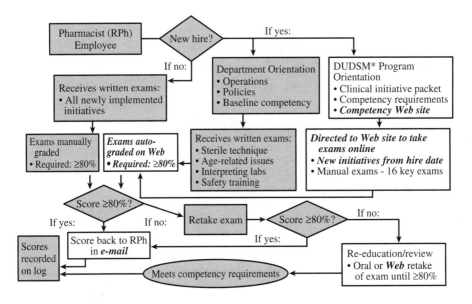

Figure 14.6 Revised competency process.
*DUDSM = Drug Use and Disease State Management Program.
Note: Revisions are shown in boldface within white boxes.

competency program flowchart of activities, and Figure 14.7, Figure 14.8, Figure 14.9, and Figure 14.10 show indicator results.

Step 2: Identify barriers to progress

Background. Barriers to progress are important to identify. Reasons why guidelines and protocols do not work have been studied in the literature.[21,45] One of the most important reasons why guidelines might not work is that the guidelines themselves are not accessible. If practitioners cannot easily access and become familiar with the guidelines, the guidelines will not be fully utilized. Especially for clinical practice guidelines, if practitioners doubt the validity or robustness of the guidelines, they will not be embraced. Grounding recommendations in the literature and ensuring multidisciplinary development can help avoid this barrier. Also, barriers within the

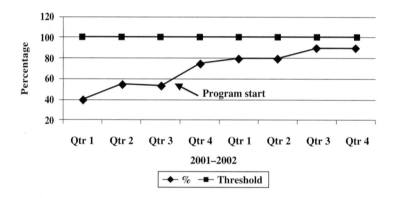

Figure 14.7 Indicator 1 results: percent of pharmacists completed with competency requirements.

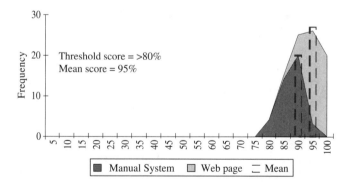

Figure 14.8 Indicator 2 results: average exam scores for Web site.

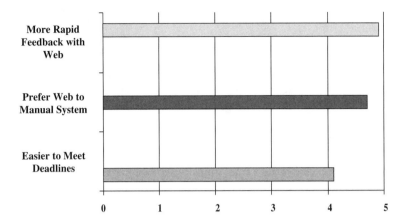

Figure 14.9 Overall staff satisfaction. Scale: 1 = strongly disagree; 5 = strongly agree.

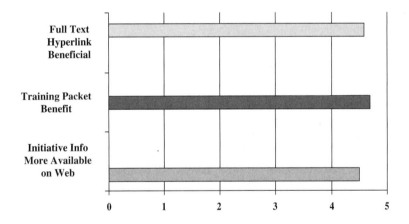

Figure 14.10 Ease of access to information. Scale: 1 = strongly disagree; 5 = strongly agree.

institution or practice, e.g., not allowing pharmacists to independently access the Web site with a passcode (in our case example), will inhibit their ability to complete the competency program. Other barriers to progress include end-user lack of confidence in carrying out the guidelines or protocol, unclear outcomes of improvement, and overcoming the "inertia of previous practice"[45] (practitioners being used to doing things a certain way and not comfortable with change). These barriers are well known and often seen when implementing CQI projects; therefore, the multidisciplinary development work team should focus on these barriers during guideline development and implementation to ensure end-user comfort level and confidence.

Recommendations for improvement that are very defined, clear, credible, and feasible work best.[46]

Competency case application.   Implementation of the Web based competency program was a success. Although not at 100% compliance for Indicator 1 (Figure 14.7), progress is moving toward that threshold. The learning curve has been a bit slower than expected, and with pharmacist turnover, the need to continually review the program with new and current pharmacists has become very important. Pharmacists have the ability to make suggestions for improving the program and have challenged the work team with ideas such as creating a Web-based "new pharmacist" case study series, expanding the Web program to pharmacy technician competency exams getting feedback on not only exam scores but also receiving clinical reasons why answers are right or wrong. None of these requests should be viewed as barriers, but as excellent continued improvements in the competency program. One additional challenge identified by the competency coordinator was the need to create a separate database for exam scores once the site automatically grades. How the Web site can automatically create a database to score and group exams is slated for future investigation.

Step 3: Identify lessons learned

Background.   During the pilot project, detailed records should be kept to identify barriers and how they were overcome. Before expansion, these lessons learned should be handled and integrated into implementation of the full program. Processes may need to be revised, education refocused, and measurement indicators added. The work team should continue to meet on a regular, although less frequent (than during development), basis to discuss successes and failures and determine course of action. Potential barriers to success, noted previously, should be focused on to make sure the improvement project is concise, readily accessible, and grounded in good science. Open communication mechanisms should be established in the form of regular work team meetings, e-mail input solicitation, a contact person for questions, and issue logs for work team meetings. As challenges arise, often immediate resolution can be achieved, and quick modifications should be made as long as the overall goals of the program are not compromised or changed excessively. The work team commitment and involvement with the project does not end once the project is implemented; it continues during outcome evaluation and while the program is in place.

Competency case application.   Lessons learned from the competency program were described in Step 2 of the Check phase. The work team should focus on lessons learned and continual improvements should be made, because the strategy for CQI used for this project will be adapted to other improvement projects in the future.

Act phase

Step 1: Design future plans

Background.   The foundation of CQI is the PDCA cycle. This cycling is essential to the project: the continued evaluation of practices, measurement of progress, trial of improvements, and expansion of efforts. The cycling repeats until improvement is sustained or threshold exceeded.[2] Part of the post-implementation actions of the work team include designing future improvements for the CQI project and setting a course for continual evaluation of the project in comparison with external innovations. Both organizational performance and outside practices should be evaluated by the work team, led by the project leader, to make sure the project is efficient in process and continues to be clinically pertinent.

Competency case application.   Feedback obtained during implementation sets the course for determining future plans for the competency program. Activities currently in process include designing the new pharmacist case-based assessment, expanding to the pharmacy technician competency program, providing feedback on missed answers, and creating active learning modules. Another future goal to pursue is having competency exams accredited for continuing education credits once screened by appropriate accreditation bodies. In addition, continuing to post new exams on the Web site is important to the growth of the competency program. New topics on the Web site include patient safety and medication errors.

Step 2: Establish a system for continued monitoring

Background.   The last step in the CQI process is to establish a regular reporting schedule for indicator results and continued work team meetings. Once CQI projects are underway, the indicators can expand from weekly to monthly and then to quarterly monitoring. Variance in compliance, if the indicator measures are consistently applied, can be identified through ongoing monitoring. By the daily feedback loops created through the contact person and the e-mail site, for example, additional variance and education gaps can be identified. In addition, the need for yearly review (maximum length of time) of the CQI project's clinical and process pertinence must be completed. Clinical pertinence involves reviewing the guidelines for new published evidence in the literature or new innovative national or regional practices. Primary literature, consensus papers, pharmacoeconomic studies, and meta-analyses should be reviewed at least annually for new practice. With clinical CQI projects, searchable indexes and journal tables of contents should be reviewed quarterly if possible, as health care is rapidly changing. National and regional benchmarks or best practice statements should also be reviewed to keep the guidelines or protocol current. Web sites, abstracts from national meetings, and queries of practice can be used to accomplish this.

Competency case application. For the competency program, the JCAHO is the primary source for direction on content and measurement indicators. Additionally, pharmacy literature contains examples of successful competency programs and newer certification programs, which might tie well to some of the internally developed programs. An information-sharing link has been established to the nursing and medical staff competency programs, both manual and Web-based, to gain insight into other discipline successes and lessons learned. Indicator measures continue to be monitored quarterly, with reports to the pharmacy director and the institution quality council, and practices at other institutions are queried to identify innovative successes.

Conclusion

CQI is an essential tool in health care and industry. The continual evaluation of practice, plan of project changes, monitoring of performance, multidisciplinary and multifaceted education, and modifications of activities will keep health care focused, competitive, and future-thinking. The methodology is straightforward, and the tools can be used to solve organizational performance issues and many other problems. Process improvements can be quickly identified and resolved, and more complicated practices (e.g., clinical practice guidelines) can be stringently evaluated and modified according to best practice in the literature and local expertise. CQI provides the methodology for a consistent approach and focused on outcome-driven success stories.

Acknowledgement

Ray Cefola, Pharm.D., and Colleen Culley, Pharm.D., are recognized for contributing to the online competency program at the University of Pittsburgh Medical Center.

References

1. Brassard M, Ritter D. *The Memory Jogger II: A Pocket Guide of Tools for Continuous Improvement and Effective Planning.* GOAL/QPC, Salem, NH, 1994.
2. Skledar SJ. *Continuous Quality Improvement in Managing the Patient-Centered Pharmacy,* Hagel H, Rovers JP, Eds. American Pharmaceutical Association, Washington, D.C., 2002.
3. Lynn ML, Osborn DP. Deming's quality principles: a health care application. *Hosp. Hlth. Serv. Admin.* 1991; 6(1): 111–120.

4. Shewart WA. *The Economic Control of Quality of Manufactured Product.* D. Van Nostrand Reinhold, New York, 1931. Reprinted by the American Society of Quality Control, 1980.
5. Deming WA. *The New Economics for Industry, Government, Education,* 1st ed. Massachusetts Institute of Technology Center for Advanced Engineering Study, Cambridge, MA, 1993.
6. Vermeulen LC, Beis SJ, Cano SB. Applying outcomes research in improving the medication-use process. *Am. J. Hlth.-Syst. Pharm.* 2000; 57(24): 2277–2282.
7. Walton M. *The Deming Management Method.* Putnam Publishing, New York, 1986.
8. Erickson SM. *Management Tools for Everyone: Twenty Techniques.* Petrocelli Books, New York, 1981.
9. Farris KB, Kirking DM. Assessing the quality of pharmaceutical care. II. Application of concepts of quality assessment from medical care. *Ann. Pharmacother.* 1993; 27: 215–223.
10. Donabedian A. Evaluating the quality of medical care. *Milbank Mem. Fund Q.* 1966; 44: 166–203.
11. Donabedian A. The quality of care: how can it be assessed? *JAMA* 1988; 260(12): 1743–1748.
12. Skledar SJ, Hess MM. Implementation of a drug use and disease state management program. *Am. J. Hlth.-Syst. Pharm.* 2000; 57 (suppl 4): S23–S29.
13. Skledar SJ. CQI process provides a template for designing clinical practice guidelines. *Formulary* 2001; 36: 230–233.
14. Langley GJ, Nolan KM, Nolan TW. The foundation of improvement. *Qual. Prog.* 1994; 27(6): 81–86.
15. Moen RD, Nolan TW. Process improvement. *Qual. Prog.* 1987; 20(9): 62–69.
16. Morris C, Cantrill J. Preventable drug-related morbidity indicators in the U.S. and U.K. *J. Manage. Care Pharm.* 2002; 8(5): 372–377.
17. Nau D. Evaluating medication use for continuous quality improvement in diabetes care. *J. Manage. Care Pharm.,* 2002; 8(5): 378–382.
18. Kerr EA, Krein SL, Vijan S et al. Avoiding pitfalls in chronic disease quality measurement: a case for the next generation of technical quality measures. *Am. J. Manage. Care* 2001; 7: 1033–1043.
19. National Committee for Quality Assurance. The state of managed care quality 2001, http://www.ncqa.org.
20. American Medical Association, Joint Commission on Accreditation of Healthcare Organizations, National Committee for Quality Assurance. Coordinated performance measurement for the management of adult diabetes, April 2001, http://www.ama-assn.org/ama/pub/category/3798.html.
21. Farmer KC. Methods for measuring and monitoring medication regimen adherence in clinical trials and clinical practice. *Clin. Ther.* 1999; 21: 1074–1090.
22. Gebhart F. When pharmacists have the final say on drug orders. *Drug Top.* 2002; 8: hse1.
23. Skledar SJ, Gross PR. Surgical antimicrobial prophylaxis: a comprehensive process for changing the standard of practice. *Formulary* 2000; 35(1): 53–64.

24. Matuschka PR, Burke JD, Cheadle WG et al. Improving the timing and documentation of antibiotic administration for surgical prophylaxis. *Hosp. Pharm.* 1998; 33: 293–296.
25. Carroll JCN, Schomberg R. Implementing an inpatient pharmacy-based pneumococcal vaccination program. *Am. J. Hlth.-Syst. Pharm.* 2001; 58: 1852–1855.
26. National Heart, Lung, and Blood Institute. Executive summary of the NAEPP expert panel report: guidelines for the diagnosis and management of asthma — update on selected topics 2002, http://www.nhlbi.nih.gov/guidelines/asthma/asthsumm.htm, accessed February 4, 2002.
27. Turk A. Understanding the impact of asthma in the 21st century. *J. Manage. Care Pharm.* 2002; 8(5): S3–S7.
28. Rischer JB, Childress SB. Cancer pain management: pilot implementation of the AHCPR guideline in Utah. *Joint Commis. J. Qual. Improv.* 1996; 22(10): 683–700.
29. King KM, Bungard TJ, McAlister FA et al. Quality improvement for CQI. *Prev. Med. Manage. Care* 2000; 1(30): 129–137.
30. Campion FX, Rosenblatt MS. Quality assurance and medical outcomes in the era of cost containment. *Surg. Clin. N. Am.* 1996; 76(1): 139–159.
31. *2003 Comprehensive Accreditation Manual for Hospitals (CAMH).* Joint Commission on Accreditation of Health Care Organizations, Joint Commission Resources, Oakbrook Terrace, IL, 2003.
32. Ellrodt G, Cook DJ, Lee J et al. Evidence-based disease management. *JAMA* 1997; 278: 1687–1692.
33. *Assessing Hospital Staff Competence.* Joint Commission of Accreditation of Health Care Organizations, Joint Commission Resources, Oakbrook Terrace, IL, 2002.
34. Marshall JM, Adams JP, Janich JA. Practical, ongoing competency-assessment program for hospital pharmacists and technicians. *Am. J. Hlth.-Syst. Pharm.* 1997; 54(12): 1412–1417.
35. Gallagher M. Home care pharmacist competency assessment program. *Am. J. Hlth.-Syst. Pharm.* 1999; 56(15): 1549–1553.
36. Merrigan D. Internal approach to competency-based credentialing for hospital clinical pharmacists. *Am. J. Hlth.-Syst. Pharm.* 2002; 59(6): 552–558.
37. Kozma CM, Reeder CE, Schulz RM. Economic, clinical, and humanistic outcomes: a planning model for pharmacoeconomic research. *Clin. Ther.* 1993; 15: 1121–1132.
38. Horn SD. Clinical practice improvement: a data-driven methodology for improving patient care. *JCOM* 1999; 6(3): 26–32.
39. Johnson, N. Assessing and reporting outcomes of a disease management program. *Formulary* 1999; 34: 455–460.
40. Juran JM, Godfrey AB. *Juran's Quality Handbook*, 5th ed. McGraw-Hill, New York, 1999.
41. Gross PA, Greenfield S, Cretin S et al. Optimal methods for guideline implementation: conclusions from the Leeds Castle meeting. *Med. Care* 2001; 39: II85–92.
42. Grimshaw JM, Russel IT. Effect of clinical guidelines on medical practice: a systematic review of rigorous evaluations. *Lancet* 1993; 342: 1317–1322.
43. Hayward RSA, Wilson MC, Tunis SR et al. Practice guidelines: what are internists looking for? *J. Gen. Intern. Med.* 1996; 11: 176–178.
44. Soumerai SB, Avorn J. Principles of educational outreach ("academic detailing") to improve clinical decision making. *JAMA* 1990; 263: 549–556.

45. Cabana MD, Rand CS, Powe NR et al. Why don't physicians follow clinical practice guidelines? A framework for improvement. *JAMA* 1999; 282(15): 1458–1465.
46. Grol R. Successes and failures in the implementation of evidence-based guidelines for clinical practice. *Med. Care* 2001; 39: II46–54.

chapter fifteen

Systems of pharmaceutical care

Brian J. Isetts

Contents

Introduction

The advent of pharmaceutical care has ushered in a new era of pharmacy practice based on a clear description of a pharmacist's patient care responsibilities and contributions to society. Before the era of pharmaceutical care, pharmacists engaged in professional activities often defined merely by a drug or disease state of interest. This potpourri of pharmacy activities previously referred to as a *practice* was inconsistent with the systems of care used by all other health care professions. This chapter presents and discusses

0-8493-1446-1/04/$0.00+$1.50
© 2004 by CRC Press LLC

the new professional practice of pharmacy as systems components of pharmaceutical care. The systems of pharmaceutical care presented in this chapter include:

1. The context of caring for another human within a patient's holistic, or biopsychosocial, system
2. The systematic process of caring for patients with drug-related needs
3. The management systems essential to a successful pharmaceutical care practice

Brief history of a new professional practice

There have been many changes in the ways pharmacists have functioned in the health care system. Throughout each transformation in our health care delivery system, pharmacists continue to be recognized as important health care professionals. Before the industrial era of premanufactured dosage forms, the family apothecary embraced an approach to care similar to the covenantal relationship established at present between a patient and pharmaceutical care practitioner. In addition, Gallup Poll surveys dating back to the mid-1980s have ranked pharmacists among the most respected professionals in terms of honesty, integrity, and ethical standards.[1]

The term *pharmaceutical care* was used in 1975 to generally refer to the care that a given patient requires and receives which assures safe and rational drug use.[2] At that point in time there was a renewed interest in returning to the days of caring for the patient rather than caring for the drug product. Unfortunately, the changes that occurred in the 1980s resulted in controls on the availability and distribution of the drug product rather than on meeting the needs of a specific patient within identifiable clinical parameters by using consistent processes of care.

The clinical pharmacy movement brought about recognition of pharmacists for their drug therapy knowledge expertise. Contributions of clinical pharmacists included drug use evaluations (DUE) and drug utilization reviews (DUR), and the emergence of specialty clinics and specialized clinical services such as warfarin clinics and diabetes education centers. Although the services provided to patients through disease-focused clinics have been beneficial to patients, only a small percentage of patients receive assistance from these services.

An important article published in 1990 provided a new direction for the profession of pharmacy.[3] This article provided pharmacists with a clear focus on patient care responsibilities, as opposed to merely serving as purveyors of a commodity. Although there has been general agreement that pharmacists should become involved in "the responsible provision of drug therapy for the purpose of achieving definite outcomes that improve a patient's quality of life," there has not been consensus on how this can or should be accomplished.

One of the first attempts to move the theory of pharmaceutical care into practice occurred in 1992. Pharmacists at 20 community pharmacies throughout Minnesota participated in a demonstration project to help determine what pharmaceutical care would look like in practice. The work of pharmacists providing care to patients in different clinical settings was used by the Minnesota project pharmacists to determine the nature of a pharmaceutical care practice. One of the most important contributions arising from the Minnesota project was implementation of a consistent and systematic process of care to guide pharmacists in delivering pharmaceutical care. Pharmacists have a long history of providing beneficial services to patients; however, no process of care could be universally applied, as seen in processes of care used by physicians in the differential diagnosis of disease or by dentists during an oral dental examination. This chapter presents this consistent and systematic process of delivering care that is pharmaceutical care.

Medication use systems failures

Patients have experienced unfortunate consequences attributable to the use of medicinal agents for thousands of years. When patients experience unfortunate medication consequences, three general reasons or systems-related causes are associated with these undesirable events:

1. Acts of commission (i.e., prescribing, dispensing, and medication administration errors)
2. Idiosyncratic causes (i.e., unpredictable adverse events)
3. Acts of omission (i.e., absence of systems and individuals to assume responsibility for patient medication outcomes)

Although it might be difficult to prevent adverse medication events attributable to idiosyncratic causes, there are systems to account for both the acts of commission and the acts of omission in the medication use process. For an excellent review of current and proposed actions to reduce medication errors from acts of commission, the reader is referred to the efforts and publications of the Institute for Safe Medication Practices.[4] This chapter focuses on acts of omission, or developing and implementing systems for the accountability of patient medication use outcomes.

Unfortunate medication use outcomes have been summarized as drug misadventuring or drug-related morbidity and mortality.[5,6] This is a serious concern in health care, a concern left unresolved for many years. In addition, data and information on the incidence and economic consequences of preventable drug-related morbidity continue to mount. About 3.2% of all hospital admissions in the U.S. and Europe might be caused by preventable drug-related morbidity in ambulatory care.[7] In 1995, the cost impact of these drug therapy problems in the U.S. health care system was estimated to be $76 billion, and a more recent update of this estimate for 2000 is $177 billion.[6,8]

As increasing numbers of people experience the ill effects of medication use and realize that this is not an inevitable consequence of our health care system, the public outcry for answers will intensify. Medication safety has been the driving force for many health care advances, such as the 1937 Elixir Sulfanilamide scandal (FD&C Act), the European thalidomide tragedy (1962 Kefauver Drug Amendments), and the incidence of adverse drug events in nursing homes (1974 Consultant Pharmacists' Law).[9]

In the airline industry, multiple systems are in place to promote safe travel.[10] If the air traffic control system resembled our approach to the use of medications, the results could be expected to be routinely catastrophic. When a true medication use system is in place, it will focus on the patient achieving therapeutic goals while avoiding or minimizing the consequences of drug therapy problems. All components of such a medication use system will be designed to support this purpose Although strict attention is paid to scientific design while conducting clinical trials, the question remains of how the scientific process is applied to the use of medications after a medication is approved for marketing. An exhaustive literature review combined with research conducted with physicians as part of a doctoral dissertation found that a rational, systematic approach to decisions made in the drug use process was not readily evident.[11]

Previous efforts to address the consequences of a nonexistent or haphazard medication use system include the work of early clinical pharmacy pioneers and consultant pharmacists. The clinical pharmacy movement focused on providing solutions to medication use problems occurring in the hospital setting. Consultant pharmacists have provided solutions to medication use problems occurring in the long-term care setting. Studies of adverse medication consequences experienced by patients in hospitals and nursing homes preceded the efforts of clinical pharmacy pioneers and consultant pharmacists. Demand for the services of these clinical and consultant pharmacists represented an early warning signal of a dysfunctional, or rather nonexistent, medication use system.

Experiences of clinical pharmacists have been important in developing pharmaceutical care practices. The implicit purpose of a clinical pharmacist's activities is the appropriate use of medications. Community pharmacists in the Minnesota project looked at the activities of clinical pharmacists to help establish a systematic patient care thought processes. Work of previous authors strongly supported moving back to basics in documenting the clinical pharmacists' activities and creating a problem-solving process applied to the use of drugs through a pharmacist's work-up of drug therapy.[12]

To help describe the development of pharmaceutical care practices, it is important to analyze the interrelated conditions, or environment, in which pharmaceutical care exists. The context of pharmaceutical care is systems failure related to the use of medications. In medicine there is a system in place to guide the physician's differential diagnosis, or in dentistry to guide the dentist's oral exam. When it comes to the use of medications, often it is only the most assertive and aggressive patients who can negotiate the health care maze to develop their own system for achieving positive drug therapy outcomes while avoiding the adverse consequences of medication use.

Overview of the practice

Before analyzing the interrelated systems of pharmaceutical care, a brief overview of this new professional practice will be helpful. The landmark pharmaceutical care article published in 1990 created the theoretical constructs for the responsible provision of drug therapy. This article set the foundation for the development of a new professional practice. Through efforts aimed at moving from theory into application, the definition of this new professional practice emerged. A pharmaceutical care practice then is defined as a practice in which the practitioner takes responsibility for all of a patient's drug-related needs and is held accountable for this commitment.[13]

Because there has not been a consistent, systematic, and rational medication use process, it is necessary to first describe the purpose of this systematic medication use process and then establish a new professional practice by clearly delineating the scope and domain of this practice. Defining the scope and domain of practice are essential to clarify how pharmaceutical care practitioners can address a problem better than other individuals or professions. The scope of pharmaceutical care is drug therapy problems and the domain is the practice environment in which a practitioner assumes responsibility for a patient's drug-related needs and is held accountable for this commitment.

The practice of pharmaceutical care was developed by using the rules governing all other health care practices. Although pharmacists have the ability to address drug therapy problems better than other health care professionals do, it might be necessary to create a new health care professional for the practice of pharmaceutical care to expand beyond the current cottage industry of selected pharmacy locations. The issue of creating a new health care professional would have profound implications on the mission and direction of pharmacy education.

Creating a new professional practice to address a problem for which no other professionals have assumed responsibility started by using the basic set of rules that apply to the care delivered by all other health care professionals. Consistent among all health care professions is their practices being viewed as the application of knowledge guided by a commonly held purpose or philosophy to resolve specific problems requiring special knowledge. In addition, health care professionals are expected to practice in a manner that is reviewed by professional peers and of a standard accepted by society.

All health care professions have a unique philosophy, process of care, and practice management system.[13] The commonly held purpose of a practice is its philosophy. The knowledge and expertise that a health care professional brings to care for a patient are done so within a common patient care process. The practice management system is vital to support the practice by facilitating application of the philosophy and process of care. By utilizing the common set of rules that apply to all other health care professions, the philosophy, process of care, and management system form the three essential components, or sets of rules, for constructing a practice.

The philosophy of care

All health care professions have a specific philosophy of care. The four components of the philosophy for pharmaceutical care are (1) the statement of social need, (2) a patient-centered need for meeting the social need, (3) the development of a therapeutic relationship to care for another human being, and (4) a description of the practitioner's specific responsibilities.[13] A philosophy of practice is a set of values that guide behaviors. This philosophy defines the rules, roles, relationships, and responsibilities of the practitioner.

This philosophy of practice is very important, particularly when hard decisions have to be made in practice, determining what is important, setting priorities in the care of patients, and managing ethical dilemmas. Although pharmacists might have their own philosophy of life, there can only be one philosophy of practice that practitioners uphold. This uniformity of practice philosophy results in standardization of practice behaviors applied to all patients. Each component of the pharmaceutical care philosophy of practice is briefly described next.

Stating the social need

A profession must meet a unique social need in order to be granted privileges by society. When a unique social need is met, professionals are rewarded with an implicit permit to provide services that apply specialized knowledge and skills to address patient problems. The problem of drug-related morbidity and mortality has reached such a magnitude that it is necessary for a specific individual to be held accountable for addressing and correcting this problem. The unique social need that this individual is to be held accountable is known as a drug-related need. Drug-related needs are defined as "those health care needs of a patient that have some relationship to drug therapy and for which the practitioner is able to offer professional assistance."[13]

Drug-related morbidity and mortality is the need that drives society to demand pharmaceutical care. Morbidity pertains to the incidence and prevalence of disease associated with, or attributable to, the use of drug therapies. Mortality is the incidence and prevalence of death associated with, or attributable to, the use of drug therapies. Although it has long been known that the use of medicinal agents can result in death and disease, the level of public acceptance of this risk is an issue of public concern and debate.

The need and demand for pharmaceutical care can be expected to intensify as society realizes that a significant proportion of drug-related morbidity and mortality is preventable. In 1995, it was widely disseminated that drug-related morbidity and mortality cost the U.S. $76 billion annually, and more recent estimates place this figure close to $200 billion annually.[6,8] Furthermore, 44,000 to 98,000 institutionalized patients fall victim to drug-related mortality.[14] It is now estimated that up to 60% of drug-related morbidity and mortality is preventable.[15,16] These statistics could be judged by society as an inherent consequence of using medications, or an unavoidable cost of doing business, if it were not for the concept of preventability. The preventability of many adverse drug-related consequences is an indication of a haphazard or nonexistent medication use system.

The patient-centered approach

All health care professions have a patient-centered focus as part of their philosophy of practice. This means that the patient is seen as a unique individual with rights, knowledge, values, and experience, and is not seen as a repository for drugs to be studied. Although this component of the philosophy of practice may appear obvious, it has not always been evident in the field of pharmacy. For instance, when a pharmacist engages in disease state management or provides services based on a specific drug of interest, patient centeredness may be violated if the patient's other drug-related needs are not systematically addressed.

This approach to patient care represents a paradigm shift for pharmacists moving away from providing simple information on how to take a dispensed medication to assuming responsibility for achieving intended therapeutic outcomes and resolving drug therapy problems impeding progress toward drug therapy treatment goals. The patient-centered approach focuses on the patient's needs, or in this case drug-related needs, being the responsibility of the practitioner. This component of the philosophy of practice has given rise to the development of pharmaceutical care as a generalist practice. As rational medication use systems are created, there will be a continuum of care between generalist pharmaceutical care practitioners and pharmacy specialists. The practical application of this rule to the profession of pharmacy is that there needs to be a generalist practitioner in place to address all of a patient's drug-related needs before there can be specialist practitioners.

Development of a therapeutic relationship

The third component of a philosophy of practice states that care is provided by establishing a therapeutic relationship between the patient and practitioner. The term *therapeutic relationship* has been adapted from the concept of a therapeutic alliance used in the mental health consulting professions. A therapeutic relationship is required to care for another human.

Within the context of pharmaceutical care, a therapeutic relationship is defined as "an alliance formed between the patient and the practitioner for the purpose of identifying the patient's drug-related needs."[13] When caring for another human within a therapeutic relationship, there are two complementary dimensions: (1) the technical dimension of taking care of a patient, and (2) demonstrating genuine concern for the well-being of another person. The technical dimension of caring for a patient relates to the pharmaceutical care knowledge base applied throughout the patient care process. Demonstrating genuine concern for the patient results in a covenant, or bond, between the pharmacist and the patient.

There certainly is an art to developing a therapeutic relationship. The experiences of numerous practitioners functioning within various pharmaceutical care demonstration projects, as well as those who have built practices through trial and error, provide us with insights regarding some of the basic dos and don'ts for establishing a therapeutic relationship. Some of the lessons learned from caring for thousands of patients are discussed in the section on the patient as a holistic system.

The practitioner's responsibilities

To address the social need of drug-related morbidity and mortality based on a patient-centered approach that is built on the establishment of a therapeutic relationship, there must be clearly defined practitioner responsibilities. In pharmaceutical care, the practitioner is responsible for all drug-related needs of a patient. As discussed in detail in the next section, this means that a practitioner seeks to ensure that all therapies are appropriately indicated and that all medical conditions of a patient are appropriately treated, and that all therapies in use are effective, safe, and convenient for the patient.

The scope of pharmaceutical care is drug therapy problems, defined as any aspect of a patient's drug therapy that is interfering with a desired, positive patient therapeutic outcome.[13] Before the advent of pharmaceutical care, there was no evidence of a consistent and systematic patient care process applied to the use of medications; therefore, pharmaceutical care practitioners' responsibilities are to ensure that therapeutic outcomes are achieved and to identify, resolve, and prevent drug therapy problems that hinder achievment of desirable therapeutic outcomes.

The patient as a holistic system

There are two equally important dimensions of providing pharmaceutical care: (1) the technical dimension of conducting an assessment and doing the work of a pharmaceutical care practitioner, and (2) the establishment of a therapeutic relationship. It does not matter how much drug knowledge practitioners might have or how many drug therapy problems they might have resolved in their lives if patients do not believe that practitioners genuinely care for their well-being. Demonstrating genuine concern for the patient is the foundation of a therapeutic relationship. Therefore, to discuss the essentials of establishing a therapeutic relationship, it is important to first view the patient as a unique individual influenced by a vast array of life experiences.

The purpose of this section is not to review existentialistic human theory, but to highlight some essentials and basics of the therapeutic relationship. A patient exists as a system within a microcosm. The individual patient system then interfaces with other human microcosms and global systems everyday. This interface and interaction between an individual and the environment is sometimes referred to as a patient's biopsychosocial system.

It is particularly useful to begin thinking about establishing a therapeutic relationship with the patient by avoiding one's own preconceived biases, not being prejudgmental, and not jumping to conclusions. A patient's perceptions of judgmental behavior exhibited by other health care professionals in previous encounters might influence how much information and how much trust a patient has in the current encounter with a pharmaceutical care practitioner. The merits, or success, of a pharmaceutical care practitioner depend on remaining nonjudgmental while demonstrating genuine interest in the beliefs and values of the patient.

The act of caring can be characterized by a state of responsiveness to others through a demonstrated willingness to become personally involved in meeting the individual's needs. When used as a verb, *to care* equates with showing genuine concern for the well-being of another human. In pharmaceutical care, this concern focuses on concern for meeting the medication-related needs of the patient. The product of this care is a covenantal bond or alliance between the patient and the practitioner for working together to achieve drug therapy treatment goals while minimizing the adverse consequences of medication use.

Although no two humans are alike, a few important aspects can improve a practitioner's ability to form an alliance with a patient. The most important aspect of building a therapeutic relationship is to find out what matters most to patients as it pertains to their health care in general and their use of medications specifically. Second is to show genuine concern for the patient. This means not interrupting patients when they are speaking, not forgetting to listen to them while thinking ahead to the next question, and not jumping to conclusions. Third is not to try to get every possible piece of information available from the patient during the initial assessment, or fearing that something might be missed.

Building a therapeutic alliance implies that the relationship will take shape over time, and such is the case with pharmaceutical care. Scheduled follow-up evaluations with the patient will permit the practitioner to obtain additional information and resolve drug therapy problems over time. Pharmaceutical care is a journey, not a destination or a one-stop shopping experience — enjoy the opportunity to meet a patient's drug-related needs at a pace comfortable to the patient. For students seeking to learn more about communications skills important to developing a therapeutic relationship within the practice of pharmaceutical care, there are reference texts available that discuss topics such as verbal and nonverbal communications, vocal intonation, facial expressions, and negotiating with patients to establish realistic therapeutic goals.[17,18]

The systematic patient care process

The patient care process clearly describes how a pharmaceutical care practitioner fulfills responsibilities outlined in the philosophy of care. The three steps in the patient care process are assessment, care plan, and evaluation. These three steps are continuous, or may be viewed as being cyclical in nature. The initial assessment helps the practitioner formulate a care plan in concert with the patient, and follow-up evaluation includes documentation of actual patient outcomes, leading back to assessment of new drug-related needs.

By using rules applied to health care professions, it is noted that all other health care professionals have a single patient care process guiding the care delivered. Although within any given health care profession the practitioner may execute the patient care process in a slightly different manner, there is still only one patient care process that helps the practitioner fulfill patient care responsibilities.

Pharmaceutical care practitioners have established patient care process criteria for providing pharmaceutical care, which were developed to help pharmacists learn this new approach to patient care as well as to help others determine how well a pharmacist does in delivering care to patients. The criteria used to evaluate performance within the patient care process include:[19]

1. Ascertaining and documenting the patient's understanding, concerns, and expectations about his or her drug-related needs
2. Linking each of the patient's active medication remedies to an appropriate medical indication
3. Determining the goals of therapy for each of the patient's medical conditions
4. Assessing the patient for the presence of drug therapy problems related to the indication, effectiveness, safety, and convenience of medications
5. Probing for additional drug-related needs and drug therapy problems through a review of systems
6. Establishing a mutually agreed-on care plan
7. Following up with an evaluation for every patient

The patient care process for providing pharmaceutical care is briefly described next.

Assessment

The pharmaceutical care practitioner always starts by assessing the patient's drug-related needs. Assessment is a systematic review of a patient's drug-related needs. Drug-related needs pertain to the intended use of all of a patient's medications, the effectiveness of each medication, the safety of use, and the convenience of use of all therapies. The assessment of drug-related needs provides the basis for identifying drug therapy problems.

When patients come to the Pharmaceutical Care Clinic at the University of Minnesota College of Pharmacy to receive care delivered by advanced standing pharmacy students in the presence of experienced faculty, students typically use a three-phase approach to conducting the initial assessment. The three phases of an initial assessment can be characterized as follows: building a therapeutic relationship, assessing all of a patient's existing medications and remedies, and conducting a verbal review of systems to make sure that no drug-related needs have been overlooked. This three-phase approach helps a student get organized and prepare for the first few complete and comprehensive assessments.[20]

Drug therapy problems

Identifying, resolving, and preventing drug therapy problems are the central focus of a practitioner's patient care responsibilities. The pharmaceutical care practitioner learns to fulfill this patient care responsibility better than any other health care professional. Table 15.1 presents a classification of drug therapy problems.

The order for identifying drug therapy problems is also critical. The practitioner always starts by determining whether there is an intended medical use for each of a patient's medications and remedies. If there is no

Table 15.1 Categories of Drug Therapy Problems

Indication
  1. The patient has a medical condition that requires the initiation of new or additional drug therapy.
  2. The patient is taking drug therapy that is unnecessary.

Effectiveness
  1. The patient has a medical condition for which an ineffective drug therapy is being used.
  2. The patient has a medical condition for which too little of the correct drug is being taken.

Safety
  1. The patient has a medical condition resulting from an adverse drug reaction.
  2. The patient has a medical condition for which too much of the correct drug is being taken.

Convenience (compliance)
  1. The patient has a medical condition resulting from not taking the correct drug appropriately.

Source: Adapted from Cipolle RJ, Strand LM, Morley PC. *Pharmaceutical Care Practice.* New York: McGraw-Hill, 1998. With permission.

medical reason for the use of a medication, then the drug therapy problem is resolved by discontinuing the therapy. If there is an intended medical reason but the medicine is not working, the practitioner must resolve this problem, usually by recommending a dosage increase or by using a more effective therapy. If the medication is indicated and working, the practitioner analyzes the safety of use in the patient. If the patient is experiencing undesirable effects or interactions, actions must be taken to resolve this problem.

Last — and always last — is to identify problems caused by noncompliance. This must be the last order of business when identifying drug therapy problems — imagine what will happen if the pharmacist starts by making sure that a patient is taking a medication that has no intended medical use, is not working, or is unsafe for the patient. Problems caused solely by noncompliance include such things as the patient forgetting to take the medication or not being able to afford the drug product.

Care plan development

A care plan is a detailed schedule outlining the patient's and the practitioner's activities and responsibilities to achieve therapeutic goals and resolve drug therapy problems. If the patient is achieving all goals of therapy and is not experiencing any drug therapy problems, the patient's pharmaceutical care plan might not be an elaborate document. The care plan is an agreement between the patient and the practitioner to describe who will do what to achieve therapeutic goals and to resolve and prevent drug therapy problems.

A care plan can be simplified by combining straightforward clinical condition endpoints with patient-specific goals of therapy. The care plan includes drug therapy treatment goals for each of the patient's clinical conditions. If the patient is achieving all therapeutic goals and has no unmet drug-related needs, such as an untreated medical condition, then the care plan might be very brief. A more detailed care plan is required when the patient is experiencing drug therapy problems and there needs to be an accounting of what the patient and practitioner will do to resolve and prevent the problems impeding progress and work toward desired, positive, therapeutic outcomes.

Evaluation

Evaluation is defined as the practitioner's determination of the patient's outcome and clinical status at planned intervals.[13] Evaluation represents accountability in the definition of a pharmaceutical care practice. This accountability is witnessed at the patient level by the practitioner assuming responsibility for finding out exactly what happens to the patient in the medication use process and documenting these results or outcomes.

The goals of conducting an evaluation are to evaluate achievement of therapeutic outcomes, resolve drug therapy problems, and establish time frames for conducting the follow-up evaluation. The follow-up evaluation may be conducted in person or over the telephone, depending on patient preferences and severity of the patient's drug therapy problems. Establishing a time frame for conducting the follow-up evaluation hinges on the expected amount of time to witness condition improvement and the potential for experiencing any unwanted medication effects. The practitioner works with the patient to set up a specific time and date for the follow-up encounter. The patient has responsibility for contacting the practitioner before the follow-up encounter if untoward medication effects occur.

The practice management system

A practice management system is the engine that drives a pharmaceutical care practice. The system for managing a pharmaceutical care practice is critical, and is probably the least understood of the three fundamental practice components (the other two components being the philosophy of practice and the patient care process). There is a temptation to launch out and start caring for patients and give little thought to developing systems that support long-term growth of the practice. This is a bad idea; having an explicit practice management system in place greatly enhances the prospects for success.

The remainder of this chapter is designed to first briefly discuss the evidence supporting the benefits of pharmaceutical care and then present the essentials of creating a practice management system. An important part of building a new practice is convincing others (as well as oneself) that pharmaceutical care improves clinical outcomes and reduces health care expenditures. Therefore, when the time comes to sell the service to others, there will be no hesitation or embarrassment about the value and worth of this health care innovation.

Evidence supporting the outcomes of pharmaceutical care

No other health care innovation or service has been held to a higher standard of evidence than the practice of pharmaceutical care. Few — if any other — health care professions have been required to demonstrate that their services not only improve care delivered to patients but also save money. Even when the debate over inclusion of chiropractic care services in health benefit plans transpired, it was more overwhelming public testimony rather than economic cost-savings data that persuaded third-party payers to begin covering these services. Although it is easy to say that this is unfair, the silver lining is that as pharmaceutical care becomes a more widely covered service, the profession of pharmacy will be well prepared to answer the call for accountability of outcomes.

The framework for presenting the evidence in support of a pharmaceutical care practice management system is clinical, humanistic, and economic outcomes data, which are described next.

Clinical outcomes evidence

Pharmacists working in collaboration with patients, physicians, and other health care providers through a redesigned medication use systems-approach can improve the achievement of therapeutic goals. A report released by the Medicare Payment Advisory Commission (MedPAC) states that "drug management is an evolving approach to care in which drug therapy decisions are coordinated collaboratively by physicians, pharmacists and other health professionals together with the patient." The MedPAC report also recommends that the secretary of the United States Department of Health and Human Services assess models for collaborative drug therapy management services in outpatient settings.[21]

In a two-year study of 397 ambulatory care patients with coronary heart disease, working collaboratively with pharmacists and physicians to promote persistence and compliance with prescribed dyslipidemic therapy, it was found that 62.5% of patients were at or below lipid management goals (National Cholesterol Education Panel specified LDL-C target levels) as of their last full lipid profile.[22] In the hospital setting, it was found that pharmacists working in collaboration with physicians through a redesigned medication use systems-approach can prevent errors and reduce drug costs.[23]

As regards achieving therapeutic goals, in a study of 2524 patients in pharmaceutical care plans from 1999 to 2002 it was found that the achievement of drug therapy treatment goals increased from 74% at patients' earliest encounters to 89% at their latest pharmaceutical care encounters.[24] Peer review by a panel of eight physicians and four pharmaceutical care practitioners, using 15 randomly-selected patient records, demonstrated that the panel agreed with 94.2% of all therapeutic determinations made by pharmaceutical care pharmacists.[24] In addition, a Cochrane database review examining the effects of expanding roles of ambulatory pharmacists on patient outcomes and health care use suggests that pharmacist intervention can improve patient behavior and adherence and also physician prescribing.[25]

Humanistic outcomes evidence

Patient satisfaction and quality of life are the two most common methods of measuring the humanistic outcomes of care. Improvements in patients' quality of life have not been consistently demonstrated; however, there is evidence that many of these studies purporting to provide pharmaceutical care were in fact disease state management or specific drug-focused programs in which pharmacists did not assume responsibility for all of the patients' drug therapy treatment goals.

One recent study provides a classic example of what will happen if a practice management plan is not in place clearly delineating pharmaceutical care from the business of dispensing medications. This study was unable to demonstrate that the provision of pharmaceutical care had a significant effect on Short Form-36 (SF-36) quality-of-life scores. In this program, pharmacists were extensively trained in the provision of pharmaceutical care; however, two of the five treatment pharmacies were unable to maintain implementation of pharmaceutical care.[26] Fortunately, patient satisfaction with the care delivered by pharmacists has been more consistently demonstrated.[26]

Economic outcomes evidence

Economic evidence supporting the practice of pharmaceutical care is substantial.[13,27–30] An evaluation of care delivered by pharmacists in a variety of health care settings reported an average benefit of $16.70 of value to the health care system realized for each $1 invested in clinical pharmacy services.[28] In the Minnesota Pharmaceutical Care Project, there was a benefit-to-cost estimate of $11 for every $1 invested.[13]

The latest and most convincing economic study is available from the Asheville Project. In patients with diabetes who received ongoing pharmaceutical care services, not only were improvements maintained in hemoglobin A1C levels over the 5-year study time frame, but also days of sick time decreased every year and estimated increases in productivity were $18,000 annually. In addition, total mean direct medical costs in the Asheville project decreased by $1200 to $1872 per patient per year compared with the baseline.[30]

Building the practice management system

A practice management system is the organizational framework that supports the practice. A practice management system represents an orderly approach to developing a system that enables practitioners to provide pharmaceutical care. A practice management system contains four elements: (1) a clear description of the service provided, (2) a list of resources required to deliver the service, (3) a practice evaluation process, and (4) a revenue stream.

After the organizational framework supporting a pharmaceutical care practice is in place, attention is focused on the job of building the practice. There are five steps to building a pharmaceutical care practice:

1. Preparing to build a practice
2. Focusing on patients' drug-related needs
3. Assembling necessary support staff
4. Creating an appropriate practice environment
5. Securing compensation

Building a practice requires careful thought and planning. Hence, there must be an individual responsible for managing the practice. The manager's job will be much easier if plans for building the practice are reduced to writing. The written plan for managing the practice is referred to as the practice management plan.

Creating a practice management plan

A practice management plan serves as the guide, or road map, when building a practice. The practice management plan begins with a mission statement, or a clear description of the service provided, patient care goals, and a growth schedule for the practice. All other health care practices have a statement of their mission, and this is true of pharmacists functioning as primary care generalists or in a specialized disease-focused service.

Mission statement. Without a statement of mission, there is no clear definition of the purpose to guide practitioners through their daily duties and responsibilities. The following is an example of describing the service as part of the mission for a pharmaceutical care practice:

1. Assess all the patient's drug-related needs in a systematic and com-
    prehensive manner for the purpose of achieving all therapeutic goals
    and to identify drug therapy problems.
2. Develop a care plan for the patient to achieve goals of therapy and
    resolve and prevent drug therapy problems.
3. Evaluate the actual patient outcomes and status.

Table 15.2 presents an example of a management plan for a pharmaceutical care practice located in an ambulatory care clinic.

Resource requirements. Resources required to deliver the service include physical, financial, and human resources. The business of managing a pharmaceutical care practice is much different than the business of dispensing medications. All resources required for operating a pharmaceutical care practice focus on delivering a service to the patient as opposed to a commercial product-focused business.

A successful pharmaceutical care practice must have a clear separation of resources between a product-focused business and the patient service business. A lack of clear resource separation between the two businesses manifests in patient confusion, as well as practitioner frustration when having to abandon patient care goals in the face of growing prescription-dispensing demands. Experiences from many attempted practices indicate that when the two businesses are indistinguishable to consumers, reimbursement for the provision of pharmaceutical care rarely occurs. A clear separation of services leads to an enhanced professional image and improves the opportunity to obtain reimbursement for services.

Evaluation of the practice. Evaluation of the practice means structured reflection of all phases of a practice. Evaluation includes periodic review of the clinical care delivered to patients (case presentations to peers), processes for delivering care (care team management meetings), and the flow of resources (balance sheet analysis). Scheduled meetings among fellow pharmacists is a good way to review cases, share experiences, and improve

Table 15.2 Sample Pharmaceutical Care Practice Management Plan[a]

Practice Plan	1 Month	3 Months	6 Months	12 Months
Mission				
Service provided	1. Assess all the patient's drug-related needs systematically and comprehensively to achieve all therapeutic goals and to identify drug therapy problems 2. Develop a care plan for the patient to achieve goals of therapy and resolve and prevent drug therapy problems 3. Evaluate the actual patient outcomes and status	Continue same service mission	Continue same service mission	Continue same service mission
Patients receiving care	Patients in the ACME insurance plan demonstration project	1. ACME plan patients 2. Patients from pediatric asthma clinic	1. ACME plan patients 2. Pediatric asthma clinic patients 3. Senior living facility patient appointments	1. ACME plan patients 2. Pediatric asthma clinic patients 3. Senior living facility patients 4. General clinic referrals
Number of patients	One new patient per day (M–F)	Two new patients per day plus follow-up evaluations	Three new patients per day plus follow-up evaluations	Four new patients per day plus follow-up evaluations
Growth schedule for practice	15–20 total patients in active care plans	75 patients in care plans	200 patients in care plans	500 patients in active care plans

Table 15.2 Sample Pharmaceutical Care Practice Management Plan[a] (continued)

Practice Plan	1 Month	3 Months	6 Months	12 Months
Resources				
Personnel/time	1. One pharmaceutical care practitioner at 0.5 FTE 2. One support technician at 0.2 FTE	1. One practitioner at 0.75 FTE 2. One support technician at 0.25 FTE	1. Two practitioners at 1 FTE 2. One support technician at 0.5 FTE	1. Two practitioners at 1.5 FTE 2. One support technician at 0.75 FTE
Physical plant	1. Modify patient consultation area in pharmacy 2. Assist clinic in preparing the old cast room for pharmaceutical care appointments	1. Add pictures and posters to consult area. 2. Install data port to clinic exam room 3. Install file cabinets	1. Install interactive Web-based kiosk 2. Schedule patient appointments in clinic room	Continue minor improvements on both patient interaction areas
Educational resources	Update reference textbooks	Add medical library Internet access	Obtain CD-ROM reference materials	Attend international pharmaceutical care retreat in Auckland, NZ
Documentation	Use paper charts for first 10 patients	Use Microsoft® Access to construct a patient database	Purchase pharmaceutical care software program	Link interactive kiosk to documentation system and patient home internet
Financial Goals				
Costs	$1500/mo	$2000/mo	$3000/mo	$4000/mo
Revenues	$250/mo	$500/mo	$2000/mo	Start 5-year business plan
Savings	Individual patient savings documented on paper	Prepare drug therapy problem database	Submit information to university for start of economic study	Start pharmacoeconomic study in ACME university analysis

Evaluation

Patient care	1. Review total number of drug therapy problems identified 2. Establish a patient advisory panel to discuss program impressions 3. Keep track of number of patients achieving desired therapeutic goals	1. Conduct monthly practitioner case presentations focusing on common drug therapy problems 2. Develop patient satisfaction survey items with advisory panel 3. Compare number of goals achieved at initial and follow-up appointments	1. Use monthly case presentations by practitioners to determine level of congruence with selected clinical practice guidelines 2. Administer patient satisfaction survey	1. Conduct independent, blinded practitioner reviews of cases to obtain feedback on patient feedback in relation to the care that has been documented 2. Use evening dinner meeting sponsored by local pharmaceutical company to launch postmarketing surveillance initiative
Practice	1. Review the number of patients receiving pharmaceutical care 2. Keep track of the most commonly encountered medical conditions in patients receiving pharmaceutical care. 3. Implement an accounts receivable system for introductory program payments	1. Compare patient enrollment goals to actual number of patients in care plans 2. Collect practitioner productivity statistics 3. Reconcile accounts receivable	1. Analyze process flow between clinic and pharmacy 2. Determine expansion opportunities for third-party reimbursement demonstration projects	1. Compare actual numbers of patients in care plans to program goals 2. Discuss patient satisfaction survey results 3. Compare actual revenues to initial program revenue goals 4. Commence 5-year business plan based on revised program revenue goals

[a] For an ambulatory pharmacy located in a primary care clinic.

Source: Isetts, BJ. *Pharmacotherapy Self-Assessment Program — The Science and Practice of Pharmacotherapy* I, 4th ed., Book 5. American College of Clinical Pharmacy, Kansas City, 2002, 147–182. With permission.

abilities to identify and resolve drug therapy problems. Care team management meetings are conducted to minimize personnel conflicts and discuss methods of improving service delivery. A review of the financial viability of the practice must be judged against goals set forth in the initial, and subsequently modified, management plan.

For the practice to thrive, an effective appointment scheduling system is required. An appointment scheduling system can be established by reviewing the successes, and avoiding the mistakes, of other health care practices. Although the technology used to support appointment scheduling is important, success is largely dependent on the personal touch applied to appointment scheduling by the people working together in a practice. Some patients like a reminder call the day before an appointment, some want their appointment at times that might be inconvenient to the practitioner, and some patients want to see the practitioner without having to make an appointment. Although there needs to be a certain amount of structure to the appointment scheduling system, there must also be room to adapt to the individual preferences of patients.

Another decision to be made in starting a new practice is which patient, or groups of patients, to take care of first. When learning the patient care process, there are no right or wrong answers for selecting the first few patients — it is important to provide care to obtain needed patient care experiences. After this initial learning phase, the practice management plan guides patient selection. When providing pharmaceutical care, there must be time for reflection, introspection, and evaluation. If there is not time for appropriate practice plan evaluation, there is a risk of developing bad habits, overwhelming limited resources, and alienating patients.

The practice management plan sets forth patient care goals. There is no magic formula for selecting patients to receive care, and this selection process can be related to compensation goals in the practice management plan. Initial groups of patients selected to receive care can be based on specific project goals, time of day, reimbursement, or some other form of selection. Selecting patients with specific medical conditions, or trigger diagnoses, is one way to start identifying initial groups of patients to begin receiving pharmaceutical care. This patient selection technique is contrasted to disease state management, in which the focus is on only one of a patient's many medical conditions. It is now recognized that when the patient is referred or entered into practice, the practitioner assumes responsibility for all drug-related needs.

It is important to continually monitor progress toward meeting practice plan goals. The value of continuously monitoring progress toward achieving practice plan goals occurs when scheduling, coordination, and resource allocations are modified in response to unmet practice development goals.

Promotion and marketing

Promotion and marketing of a pharmaceutical care practice requires persistence and patience. Whenever there is change, consumers express a certain amount of apprehension about the change. Practitioners must listen carefully to individual patients and to the collective needs of their community. An effective tool for gauging practice plan progress is through the use of a patient advisory panel.

A common marketing axiom states that consumers need to be exposed to something new, on average, seven different times before a decision is made to engage in that new experience or service or to buy the new product. This also applies to the practice of pharmaceutical care. Another marketing statement is that if people like a new service, they tell three other people about their experience.

To successfully generate consumer interest and demand in pharmaceutical care, it might be helpful to make the connection between the use of medications and preventable drug-related morbidity and mortality. Tag lines that can be used to generate consumer interest in a newspaper advertisement, promotional brochure, or radio public service announcement include: "Did you know that over 100,000 people die each year as a result of their medications?" or, "Are you wondering whether or not all your medications and supplements are working as well as possible?" or, "Are you, or a loved one, taking dangerous combinations of drugs or herbal preparations?" Another simple fact that can be used in a brochure to generate demand among consumers is that the number of drug therapy problems increase with the number of medications and remedies a patient takes.

Marketing tools are available for use in promoting a practice. If it is true that a consumer will be exposed to something new, on average, seven times before acting on this information, then a number of different methods can be employed to convey the pharmaceutical care message. It might require a combination of marketing tools to prompt a patient to utilize the services of a pharmaceutical care practitioner. Delivering the service and asking satisfied patients to tell their friends and colleagues about the new service is another marketing tool. In addition, the use of discount, complementary, or introductory coupons are a useful way to attract new patients.

Documenting a practice

The two aspects of documentation are documenting care delivered to patients and documenting progress toward meeting practice plan objectives. The problem-oriented medical record is used by health care professionals to convey information about patient care. The problem-oriented medical record is a means to organize observations into a systematic, problem-solving approach that can be conveyed to others. The problem-oriented approach to documentation is intended to streamline the amount of reading that practitioners must do to update themselves on a patient's status.

Similarly, pharmaceutical care documentation is intended to improve care delivered to patients and convey information to fellow practitioners. Three important purposes for documentation of the care delivered to patients in a pharmaceutical care practice are to (1) ensure continuity of patient care over the course of the therapeutic relationship, (2) evaluate actual patient outcomes, and (3) receive compensation for the delivery of care. When documenting care delivered to the patient, practitioners create a clear and concise account of the important aspects of the encounter, their assessment, the care plan, and evaluation of actual outcomes on follow-up.

Some computer software products in the market are designed to help pharmaceutical care practitioners document the drug therapy problems encountered by patients, interventions taken to resolve drug therapy problems, and actual patient outcomes. Documentation software products are available that have features such as creating a patient pharmaceutical care chart, tracking drug therapy problems, recording interventions taken to resolve drug therapy problems, scheduling patient follow-up appointments, maintaining a database of actual patient outcomes, and documenting progress toward meeting practice plan objectives.

It is also helpful to also include a brief progress note to describe additional aspects of delivering care to the patient or to convey information to a fellow practitioner. One notation format that can be utilized for structuring a progress note is the subjective, objective, assessment, and plan (SOAP) notation format. A SOAP note is typically oriented by each of the patient's medical conditions.

Practice-level documentation is the tool for evaluating practice plan progress. It is conducted for improving care delivered to all patients in a practice as opposed to the documentation, described previously, designed to improve care delivered to individual patients. This type of documentation includes a series of management reports.

Practice plan management reports include the number of patients seen each day, the amount of time spent with patients, common types of medical and drug therapy problems encountered, and resources used to care for patients. Management reports are used to understand the nature of the practice, generate data on efficiencies of the service, and submit compensation claims.

Management reports can also be used to continuously improve the quality of a pharmaceutical care practice. Quality improvement concepts are used in many service-oriented industries. Management reports are essential to improve pharmaceutical care services by integrating data from groups or populations of patients served to help make practice management decisions.

Collaborating with physicians and other providers

Collaborative practice relationships facilitate the integration of pharmaceutical care services into systems for delivering health care services.[31] Reasons for physician collaboration with pharmaceutical care practitioners include patient achievement of positive therapeutic outcomes and reductions in drug-related morbidity and mortality. Although some physicians might not be interested in collaboration, it has been observed that when physicians and pharmacists work together there are opportunities to decrease drug-related morbidity, improve patient outcomes, and improve efficiencies.[32] One of four recent suggestions for improving the quality of medication use in elderly patients includes a call for enhanced collaborations between those who prescribe drugs and those who know medications best (clinical pharmacists).[33]

Drug therapy management and *drug management* are terms used in proposed federal legislation and in federal government reports to describe contemporary models in which pharmacists and physicians work together to manage the complex medication needs of Medicare beneficiaries. The MedPAC report described earlier recommends that the secretary of the U.S. Department of Health and Human Services assess models for collaborative drug therapy management services in outpatient settings.[21]

The economic reward systems of pharmaceutical care

A practice cannot survive without a revenue stream. The most important revenue source is the cash-paying patient. If a service is of value to a patient, this value will be equated with the transfer of a monetary payment. This monetary payment can be in the form of either fee-for-service reimbursement paid directly to the provider by the patient, or as part of a health care benefit premium. There will therefore need to be standard procedures in place for collecting payment for providing pharmaceutical care.

When starting a new business, a 3- to 5-year business plan is a good tool for measuring the financial viability of a practice. A year zero is designated in the business plan as the initial start-up phase of the practice. It is anticipated that within a long-term business plan, the break-even point for revenues and expenses occurs sometime around Year 3. The categories of expenses within a business plan include practitioner and support personnel salary costs and benefits, utilities, rent, marketing, billing costs, software fees and reference expenses, capital equipment, and depreciation. Securing compensation for the practice of pharmaceutical care requires managers to convince patients, employers, and other payers of the value of this practice.

Other health care providers use a resource-based relative value scale to categorize compensation claims, and it is a method applicable to the practice of pharmaceutical care.

In 1992, the federal government adopted the resource-based relative value scale (RBRVS) method as the Medicare physician payment system. The RBRVS represents a ranking of services according to the relative costs of the resources required to provide the services. The system has three components: (1) the relative work involved in providing the service, (2) practice expenses, and (3) liability insurance costs. The system also permits the use of modifying factors, such as geographic differences and annual increases. A pharmaceutical care RBRVS system was developed as part of the Minnesota Pharmaceutical Care Project.

The pharmaceutical care RBRVS patient complexity schematic described in a 1998 reference text[13] was developed to account for varying resources required to care for patients with increasingly complex drug-related needs. In medicine, there are five levels of patient complexity based on the variables of patient history, physical exam, and complexity of decision making.[13] The five levels of patient complexity in pharmaceutical care were devised similar to the five levels of patient complexity in medicine. The variables to describe a patient's complexity in the practice of pharmaceutical care include the number of medical conditions a patient has that require drug therapy, the number of active medications the patient is consuming, and the number of drug therapy problems the patient is experiencing. A patient taking one or two active medications to treat a single medical condition with no drug therapy problems is characterized as Level 1, requiring the least amount of resources to meet pharmaceutical care needs. A Level 5 patient has nine or more active medications for four or more medical problems and four or more drug therapy problems, thereby requiring the greatest amount of resources.

The future of pharmaceutical care

There might be a relationship between the numbers (or critical mass) of pharmacists actually practicing pharmaceutical care and compensation. In tandem with training offered by the pharmaceutical society and the college, the Pharmacy Guild of New Zealand successfully negotiated government remuneration for prescription review services undertaken by pharmacists. Approximately 5% of New Zealand's community pharmacist workforce actively practices pharmaceutical care. The number of pharmacists actually providing pharmaceutical care has been cited as a reason for encouraging the government in the country to fund the process.[34]

There has been extensive professional discourse on the roles and responsibilities of pharmacists. Experiences of early clinical pharmacists paved the way for expanded professional responsibility. Pharmaceutical care emerged as a call for the responsible provision of drug therapy for achieving definite outcomes that improve a patient's quality of life. The experiences of pharmacists seeking to incorporate this philosophy into everyday practice have led to the definition of a pharmaceutical care practice as one in which the practitioner takes responsibility for all of a patient's drug-related needs and is held accountable for this commitment.

The unique social need that is compelling society to demand pharmaceutical care is drug-related morbidity and mortality. The magnitude of drug-related morbidity and mortality continues to escalate and a national policy debate on this subject has generated interest in the causes of medical errors. Information and data related to the preventability of drug-related morbidity and mortality indicate that drug misadventuring need not be an inevitable consequence of the medication use process.

Net results from over 50 years of reliance on the dispensing fee is that two generations of society have been left with an indelible image that pharmacists primarily count pills rather than fulfilling the caring apothecary functions of previous generations. The future of pharmaceutical care depends on pharmacists making an investment in providing pharmaceutical care. For society to recognize that there is a solution to the health care crisis of drug-related morbidity and mortality, an ample number of pharmaceutical care practices must exist.

Compensation for pharmaceutical care needs to be present for a practice to survive. Fortunately, new pharmacist compensation developments will enhance the effectiveness of pharmaceutical care management systems. The Medicare Prescription, Improvement, and Modernization Act of 2003 (Public Law No. 108-173) designates pharmacists as Medicare-eligible providers and includes coverage of medication therapy management. In addition, the profession of pharmacy has been granted representation on the American Medical Association's Health Care Professionals Advisory Committee of the CPT-Editorial Panel concerned with health care coding and reimbursement. The future of the profession can be as bright as those pharmacists who are willing to maintain their devotion to helping patients achieve desired drug therapy treatment goals while avoiding or minimizing the adverse consequences of medication use.

References

1. Anon. Public rates nurses as most honest and ethical profession. http://www.gallup.com/poll/releases/pr031201.asp, accessed December 29, 2003.
2. Mikeal RL, Brown TP, Lazarus HL, Vinson MC. Quality of pharmaceutical care in hospitals. *Am. J. Hosp. Pharm.* 1975; 32: 567–574.
3. Hepler CD, Strand LM. Opportunities and responsibilities in pharmaceutical care. *Am. J. Hosp. Pharm.* 1990; 47: 533–543.
4. Cohen MR, Ed. *Medication Errors.* Washington, D.C.: American Pharmaceutical Association, 1999.
5 Manasse HR Jr. Medication use in an imperfect world: drug misadventuring as an issue of public policy. *Am. J. Hosp. Pharm.* 1989; 46: 924-944, 1141–1152.
6. Johnson JA, Bootman JL. Drug-related morbidity and mortality. *Arch. Intern. Med.* 1995; 155: 1949–1956.
7. Hepler CD. Regulating for outcomes as a systems response to the problem of drug-related morbidity. *J. Am. Pharm. Assoc.* 2001; 41: 108–115.
8. Ernst FR, Grizzle AJ. Drug-related morbidity and mortality: updating the cost-of-illness model. *J. Am. Pharm. Assoc.* 2001; 41(2): 192–199.
9. Sonnedecker G, Ed. *Kremers and Undang's History of Pharmacy.* Philadelphia: Lippincott Williams & Wilkins, 1976.
10. Committee on Quality of Health Care in America, Richardson WC (Chair), *To Err is Human: Building a Safer Health System.* Washington, D.C.: Institute of Medicine-National Academy Press, 2000.
11. Strand LM. *Evaluation of the Drug Selection Process in the Treatment of Essential Hypertension.* Doctoral dissertation presented to the Graduate School of the University of Minnesota, 1984.
12. Strand LM, Cipolle RJ, Morley PC. Documenting the clinical pharmacist's activities: back to basics. *Drug. Intell. Clin. Pharm.* 1988; 22: 63–67.
13. Cipolle RJ, Strand LM, Morley PC. *Pharmaceutical Care Practice.* New York: McGraw-Hill, 1998.

14. Lazarou J, Pomeranz BH, Corey PN. Incidence of adverse drug reactions in hospitalized patients: a meta-analysis of prospective studies. *JAMA* 1998; 279: 1200–1205.

15. Winterstein AG, Sauer BC, Hepler CD, Poole C. Preventable drug-related hospital admissions. *Ann. Pharmacother.* 2002; 36: 1238–1248.

16. Bates DW. Frequency, consequences and prevention of adverse drug events. *J. Qual. Clin. Pract.* 1999; 19: 13–17.

17. Klein-Schwartz W, Isetts BJ. Patient assessment and consultation. In: Berardi, RR., Ed., *Handbook of Nonprescription Drugs*, 13th ed. Washington, D.C.: American Pharmaceutical Association, 2002, chap. 2, pp. 21–40.

18. Isetts BJ. Pharmaceutical care. In: Mueller B, Ed., *Pharmacotherapy Self-Assessment Program — The Science and Practice of Pharmacotherapy I*, 4th ed., Book 5. Kansas City: American College of Clinical Pharmacy, 2002, pp. 147–182.

19. Isetts BJ, Sorensen TD. Use of a student-driven, university-based pharmaceutical care clinic to define the highest standards of patient care. *AJPE* 1999; 63:443–449.

20. Isetts BJ. Evaluation of pharmacy students' abilities to provide pharmaceutical care. *AJPE* 1999; 63: 11–20.

21. Medicare Payment Advisory Commission, Hackbarth GM (Chair), *Report to the Congress: Medicare Coverage of Nonphysician Practitioners.* Washington, D.C., 2002, pp. 21–26.

22. Bluml BM, McKenney JM, Cziraky MJ. Pharmaceutical care services and results in project impact: hyperlipidemia. *J. Am. Pharm. Assoc.* 2000; 40: 157–173.

23. Leape LL, Cullen DJ, Clapp MD et al. Pharmacist participation on physician rounds and adverse drug events in the intensive care unit. *JAMA* 1999; 282: 267–270.

24. Isetts BJ, Brown LM, Schondelmeyer SW, Lenarz LA. Quality assessment of a collaborative approach for decreasing drug-related morbidity and achieving therapeutic goals. *Arch. Int. Med.* 2003; 163: 1813–1820.

25. Beney J, Bero LA, Bond C. Expanding the roles of outpatient pharmacists: effects on health services utilisation, costs, and patient outcomes (Cochrane Review). The Cochrane Library, Issue 1, 2002. Oxford, U.K.: Update Software.

26. Volume CI, Farris KB, Kassam R et al. Pharmaceutical care research and education project: patient outcomes. *J. Am. Pharm. Assoc.* 2001; 41: 411–420.

27. Hatoum HT, Akhras K. 1993 bibliography: a 32-year literature review on the value and acceptance of ambulatory care provided by pharmacists. *Ann. Pharmacother.* 1993; 27: 1106–1119.

28. Schumock GT, Meek PD, Ploetz, PA et al. Economic evaluation of clinical pharmacy service — 1988–1995. *Pharmacotherapy* 1996; 16: 1188–1208.

29. Schumock GT, Butler MG, Meek PD, Vermeulen LC, Bhakti-Arondekar MS, Bauman JL. Evidence of the economic benefit of clinical pharmacy services: 1996-2000. *Pharmacotherapy* 2003; 23: 113–132.

30. Cranor CW, Bunting BA, Christensen DB. The Asheville project: long-term clinical and economic outcomes of a community pharmacy diabetes care program. *J. Am. Pharm. Assoc.* 2003; 43: 173–184.

31. Ferro LA, Marcrom RE, Garrelts L et al. Collaborative practice agreements between pharmacists and physicians. *J. Am. Pharm. Assoc.* 1998; 38: 655–664.

32. Carmichael JM, O'Connell MB, Devine B et al. Collaborative drug therapy management by pharmacists. *Pharmacotherapy* 1997; 17: 1050–1061.

33. Gurwitz JH, Rochon P. Improving the quality of medication use in elderly patients: a not-so-simple prescription. *Arch. Intern. Med.* 2002; 162: 1670–1672.
34. Isetts BJ, McKone BJ. Practice changes facilitated by pharmaceutical care. In: Knowlton CH and Penna RP, Eds., *Pharmaceutical Care*, 2nd ed. Bethesda, MD: American Society of Health-System Pharmacy, 2003, chap. 12, pp. 213–231.

chapter sixteen

Medication errors

Patricia C. Kienle

Contents

Medication errors

In 1999, the Institute of Medicine published *To Err Is Human*, which brought medical and consumer attention to medication errors. The report stated that in the U.S., at least 44,000 and as many as 98,000 people are killed each year as a result of medical errors. An estimated 7,000 of these deaths can be attributed to medication errors.[1]

The discussion of medication errors is not new. An 1857 British regulation mandated that bottles of poisons have specific colors and tactile letters.[2] For years, pharmacists have been warned to read the label three times when dispensing a prescription: when removing it from the shelf, when dispensing it, and when returning it to the shelf or discarding the container. Nurses have been cautioned to be aware of the five rights of medication administration: the *right* drug to the *right* patient at the *right* dose by the *right* route at the *right* time. However, in the last decade, research has concentrated on seeking the cause and prevention of medication errors. There is a realization that the root of errors is the fault of systems — not people — and that recognition of potential errors increases the likelihood of developing tools to prevent errors.

Definition

A medication error is any preventable event that might cause or lead to inappropriate use or patient harm while the medication is in the control of the health care professional, patient, or consumer. Such events can be related to professional practice, health care products, procedures, and systems, such as prescribing; order communication; product labeling, packaging and nomenclature; compounding; dispensing; distribution; administration; education; monitoring; and use.[3] A near miss is an error caught before administering medication to the patient. Each of the phases of the medication use system presents its own challenges for prevention of errors. Table 16.1 presents examples of medication errors.

Why medication errors occur

Medication errors occur primarily because of two reasons: lack of knowledge or lapse in performance. In either case, if safety systems are not in place to prevent the error from going forward, an error can result. The more safety systems are in place, the greater the chance of the error being trapped before it gets to the patient. Leape and colleagues identified a number of proximal causes of medication errors in their study of causes of adverse drug events (Table 16.2).[4]

Table 16.1 Examples of Medication Errors

- Wrong drug
- Wrong patient
- Wrong dose
- Wrong route
- Wrong rate of infusion
- Wrong dosage form
- Wrong date
- Wrong time
- Dose administered outside parameters
- Patient has stated allergy to the drug
- Drug not ordered
- Extra dose
- Omission of a dose
- Expired drug
- Contraindicated drug

Table 16.2 Causes of Medication Errors

- Lack of knowledge of the drug
- Lack of information about the patient
- Violation of rules
- Slips and memory lapses
- Transcription errors
- Faulty identity checking
- Faulty interaction with other services
- Faulty dose checking
- Infusion pump and parenteral delivery problems
- Inadequate monitoring
- Drug stocking and delivery problems
- Preparation errors
- Lack of standardization

Source: From Leape LL. In Cohen MR, Ed., *Medication Errors,* Jones and Bartlett, Sudbury, MA, 1999.

Human factors of errors

Human factors involve the study of interrelationships among humans, the tools they use, and the environment in which they live and work.[5] Aviation and nuclear power industries have realized for years that humans make errors and systems must be designed to minimize human consequences. The health care industry has been slow to recognize these human factors. Environmental and other human factors influence how and when errors are likely to occur.

Reason divides errors into two general types: (1) slips, which involve errors in mechanical issues; and (2) mistakes, which involve errors in problem solving.[6] A slip is an unintentional departure from an otherwise adequate plan of action. It is an unconscious glitch. Stress, interruption, and fatigue can lead to a slip. Generally, a slip occurs when an individual knows what to do but performs the task incorrectly. A mistake is an error made in solving a problem and involves an inadequate plan of action. Generally, a mistake occurs when decisions are based on inadequate information or a lack of knowledge. As with slips, mistakes can result from external factors.

Complex systems such as the medication use system create an environment that allows these errors to occur. Slips or mistakes can apply to any of the steps in the medication use system. The volume of existing and new medications, therapies, and nuances used in medical practices is overwhelming. Systems that prevent the need to depend on memory improve medication safety.

Types of medication errors

Omission errors, incorrect doses, and prescribing errors were the top three causes of medication errors reported by health systems in 2002.[7] The Joint Commission on Accreditation of Healthcare Organizations (JCAHO) tracks sentinel events submitted to it by accredited heathcare facilities. A sentinel event is an unexpected occurrence involving death or serious physical or psychological injury, or the risk thereof.[8] Table 16.3 lists the root causes of medication errors reported by JCAHO-accredited organizations.[9]

How errors are detected

Some errors are detected by the persons who make the errors and others by chance observation. However, many errors are not identified because there is no reliable method for detecting them. Errors are generally detected by

Table 16.3 Causes of Medication Errors

Issue	% of Errors
Orientation and training	60
Communication	56
Availability of information	26
Standardization	23
Storage and access	21
Competence and credentialing	21
Supervision	18
Staffing levels	18
Labeling	17
Distraction	13

Source: From *JCAHO Comprehensive Accreditation Manual for Hospitals: The Official Handbook,* Update 4, November 2000, GL-22.

voluntary reporting, direct observation, or through pharmacy procedures, such as those that identify missing or unadministered doses.

Voluntary reports are usually made by the person who detects the error. In many organizations, individuals are afraid to report errors, because there is fear that they might be associated with disciplinary actions. An anonymous reporting program may promote better error reporting.

Direct observation of medication administration is sometimes called a med pass observation. This method allows review of the entire administration process and is likely to result in a greater number of error reports, because a separate individual can directly observe errors.

Pharmacy procedures can identify some errors. Requests for missing doses or evaluation of returned (unadministered) doses could identify breaks in the system that might have caused errors.

Issues of culture

Some organizations respond to errors by punishing the individuals involved in the errors. However, punitive methods present a number of negative issues:

- Do little to prevent reoccurrence of error
- Might ignore significant root causes of the error
- Might hold the wrong person responsible
- Are difficult to apply fairly
- Expose the organization to risk if needed system improvements are not made

A proactive approach for medication safety promotes a nonpunitive culture, wherein errors and near misses can be reported and safety improved. Practitioners need to be assured by their organization that reporting errors is encouraged, individuals will not be punished for system failures, and improvements will be made to prevent future errors.

The medication use system

The medication use system can be divided into five areas: selecting, ordering, dispensing, administering and monitoring. Error potential is prevalent in each area. Some causes of errors transcend segments of the medication use system and occur in two or more phases. In particular, violations of rules and slips, or memory lapses, are seen in each of the five areas of the medication use system.

Systems that are well thought out include clear policies and procedures to guide practitioners. Deliberate violations of these guidelines can lead to errors. Pharmacists can prevent errors and increase patient safety by using safe practices.

Errors involving selecting medications

The formulary process encompasses the objective evaluation, selection, and use of medicinal agents in the facility.[10] Most systems have a formal approval process, by which pharmacists, physicians, and other health care and administrative practitioners evaluate medications for admission to a system's formulary. Recently, it has been identified that safety issues need to be included in this review. Important characteristics include:[11]

- Recognition of look-alike and sound-alike medications, such as dopamine and dobutamine, morphine and hydromorphone, or Lantus and lente insulins
- Limiting use of abbreviations and symbols, such as using u for unit, or chemical abbreviations such as MSO_4 and $MgSO_4$
- Poor packaging, such as single- and multiple-dose vials that look alike
- Poor or absent labeling and confusing dosing, such as fosphenytoin
- Multiple salts, such as calcium and phosphate

In some cases, the offending drug or package type must be added to the formulary if no alternative exists. In that case, education, use of auxiliary labels, and other safety steps must be added to enhance patient safety.

Lack of patient information

Sometimes, medications are selected for patient use without the complete knowledge of important patient parameters. Important characteristics include:

- Age of the patient
- Comorbid conditions
- Knowledge of allergy status
- Ability to administer medications properly

Standardization of medications can be an effective method to reduce errors. High-risk medications can often be standardized to minimize confusion, streamline ordering, and allow preprinted rate charts to be available to staff. Insulin, heparin, cardiovascular agent infusions, and other high-risk medications lend themselves to this safety step.

Errors involving ordering medications

Most orders and prescriptions are transmitted via verbal and written requests. Though automation of prescribing is increasing dramatically, manual methods are still prevalent.

Automation introduces its own set of challenges. Dispensing accuracy can be increased by using a series of automated steps, such as machine-readable coding (bar codes). Automation can introduce redundancies in a system, which exceed human ability to be accurate. However, blind acceptance of medications provided through automated systems violates a basic safety step. Medications ordered, dispensed, and administered through automated systems still require safety steps to assure that the process is intact and that the medication is correct.

Verbal orders

Verbal orders are oral communications between senders and receivers in person or by telephone or other similar devices. The National Coordinating Council for Medication Error Reporting and Prevention (NCC MERP) developed recommendations to reduce errors related to verbal orders. Table 16.4 notes the elements that should be included in a verbal order. Table 16.5 outlines NCC MERP's additional recommendations.[12]

Abbreviations and dose expressions cause medication errors. The handwritten or printed *u* intended to abbreviate *unit* can easily be misinterpreted as a zero, causing a 10-fold overdose. Decimal points can be difficult to read on prescriptions or orders, causing a 10-fold dose error. Decimals less than 1 should always be preceded by a zero (use 0.2, not .2) and a whole number should not be followed by a zero (use 2, not 2.0). The Institute for Safe Medication Practices (ISMP) has additional recommendations on abbreviations and dose expressions (Table 16.6).[13]

Errors involving dispensing medications

Pharmacists are most cognizant of avoiding dispensing errors. Dispensing errors can be traced to a number of system failure points, including com-

Table 16.4 Verbal Order Elements

- Age and weight, when appropriate
- Drug name
- Dosage form
- Exact strength or concentration
- Dose, frequency, and route
- Quantity or duration, or both
- Purpose or indication, unless disclosure is considered inappropriate by the prescriber
- Specific instructions for use
- Name and telephone number of prescriber
- Name of individual transmitting the order, if different from the prescriber

Source: From NCC MERP council recommendations to reduce medication errors associated with verbal medication orders and prescriptions, adopted February 20, 2001.

Table 16.5 Reducing Errors Associated with Verbal Orders and Prescriptions

- Verbal orders should be limited to urgent situations.
- Organizations should establish policies and practices that promote safe order writing.
- Leaders should promote a culture to encourage staff to question unclear or potentially unsafe verbal orders.
- Verbal orders for antineoplastic agents should not be permitted.
- The content of verbal orders should be clearly communicated.
  - The name of the drug should be confirmed by spelling, providing both the brand and generic name as well as the indication for use
  - Numbers should be dictated with clarity, e.g., "fifty milligrams ... five zero milligrams" to avoid confusion between 50 and 15.
  - Instructions should be provided without abbreviations, e.g., "take one tablet three times daily" rather than "1 tid."
- The verbal order should be repeated.
- All verbal orders should be immediately reduced to writing and signed by the individual receiving the order.
- Verbal orders should be documented in the patient's medical record, reviewed, and countersigned by the prescriber as soon as possible.

Source: From NCC MERP council recommendations to reduce medication errors associated with verbal medication orders and prescriptions, adopted February 20, 2001.

Table 16.6 Dangerous Abbreviations

Abbreviation/ Dose Expression	Intended Meaning	Misinterpretation	Correction
Apothecary symbols	Dram Minim	Can be read as 3 or ml	Use only the metric system
U	Unit	Read as a zero, causing a 10-fold overdose	
CPZ	Compazine (prochlorperazine)	Chlorpromazine	Use the complete spelling for drug names
MgSO₄	Magnesium sulfate	Morphine sulfate	
MSO₄	Morphine sulfate	Magnesium sulfate	
Nitro drip	Nitroglycerin infusions	Sodium nitroprusside infusion	
TIW	Three times a week	Three times a day	
q.d.	Every day	Four times a day	
SC	Subcutaneous	Sublingual	

Source: Adapted from ISMP, Special issue: Do not use these dangerous abbreviations or dose designations. Available at www.ismp.org/msarticles/dangerousabbrev.htm.

pounding, miscalculations, poor label printing, workload, distractions, inadequate references, labeling, and faulty dose-checking. The USP outlines recommendations for pharmacists to improve dispensing medication safety (Table 16.7).[14]

Errors involving administering medications

In hospitalized patients, generally the nursing staff is responsible for administering medications. However, many other health professionals, including physicians, dentists, podiatrists, pharmacists, respiratory therapists, radiology technologists, paramedics, perfusionists, physical therapists, and patients, administer medications in institutions. In the ambulatory setting, the patient or a caregiver generally administers medications. A comprehensive program promoting medication safety should include all disciplines that administer medications. In all cases, the individuals who administer medications need to be knowledgeable about:[15]

- Indication for use of the medication
- Precautions and contraindications
- Expected outcome from the medication
- Potential adverse drug reactions (ADRs) and interactions with food or other medications
- What action to take if an ADR or interaction occurs
- Storage requirements

Administration errors can also occur with devices used to administer and monitor medications. Metered-dose inhalers, nebulizers, infusion pumps,

Table 16.7 Improving Dispensing Safety

- Prescriptions and orders should always be reviewed by a pharmacist before dispensing. Any orders that are incomplete, illegible, or of any other concern should be clarified using established processes for resolving questions.
- Patient profiles should be current and contain adequate information.
- The dispensing area should be designed to prevent errors. Environmental conditions (lighting, temperature, noise level, ergonomic fixtures), minimization of distractions, clutter and sufficient resources must be considered.
- Inventory should be arranged to help differentiate medications from one another.
- A series of checks should be established to assess the accuracy of the dispensing process before the providing medication to the patient. Whenever possible, an independent check by a second individual should be done.
- Labels should be read three times — when selecting the product, when packaging the product, and when returning the product to the shelf.
- Patients should be counseled.
- Pharmacist should collect data regarding potential and actual errors for continuous quality improvement.

Source: From *USP Qual. Rev.*, June 1999, No. 67. With permission.

PCA devices, blood glucose monitors, and other devices must be working properly and used correctly for safe medication use.

Errors involving monitoring medications

A patient should be monitored for each medication used. Nurses or other practitioners administering medications to hospitalized patients, and patients or caregivers for ambulatory patients, need to be aware of basic medication safety related to their therapy. Patient counseling should include:

- Name of the medication
- What effects to expect
- Directions for use
- Precautions (side effects, contraindications)
- How to store the medication

Table 16.8 presents some additional monitoring tips.[16]

Branches dealing with special populations, such as pediatrics and oncology, require additional vigilance to promote monitoring for patient safety. Many of the products for such populations have narrow therapeutic indices. Small changes in dosage can result in disastrous effects. Additional checks of these agents should be built into the medication use system.

Error points can occur throughout the medication use system. As systems and technology evolve, pharmacists must adapt new methods to promote medication safety. For example, potential medication errors might evolve, depending on the sophistication of the medication system used and the patient's level of care (Table 16.9).

Emphasis on patient safety

Accrediting organizations emphasize patient safety as a fundamental issue. The federal Centers for Medicare and Medicaid Services includes monitoring of medication errors as part of their conditions of participation, noting that "the medical staff is responsible for developing policies and procedures that minimize drug errors. This function may be delegated to the hospital's

Table 16.8 Checklist for Monitoring Medications

• Monitor patients on medications with narrow therapeutic range.
• Review all serum drug levels reported and intervene as appropriate.
• Monitor and report all drug misadventures (ADRs and medication errors).
• Establish protocols and guidelines for use with critical or problem-prone medications.

Source: From Breland BD. *Hosp. Pharm. Rep.*, August 2000: 56–65.

Table 16.9 Potential Medication Errors

Phase of the Medication Use System	Bed Patient in an Institution	Ambulatory Patient
Selecting	Poor formulary system	Lack of knowledge when self-selecting medication
Ordering	Wrong drug selected from computerized prescriber order entry system	Physician prescribed new medication with contraindication
Dispensing	Look-alike medication dispensed in error	Illegible prescription
Administering	Medication administered to the wrong patient	Dose omitted
Monitoring	Laboratory results not communicated in a timely manner	Poorly calibrated blood sugar monitoring device

organized pharmaceutical service."[17] Facilities must demonstrate during surveys that their medication safety program is functioning and appropriate.

The JCAHO has a major focus on patient safety, including medication safety. As facilities report internal sentinel events to JCAHO, they are reviewed and analyzed. JCAHO has issued a number of sentinel event alerts, notifying health care organizations and consumers to specific safety issues and practice recommendations to improve them. Several have addressed medication issues such as potassium chloride and other concentrated electrolytes, insulin, heparin, injectable opiates and narcotics, infusion pumps, and look- and sound-alike medications and abbreviations. Table 16.10 summarizes the recommendations for these sentinel event alerts.[18–22]

The JCAHO annually publishes six national patient safety goals and surveys the accredited organizations related to them. The initial six goals include several medication-related safety improvements:[23]

- Improve the accuracy of patient identification, such as using at least two patient identifiers (neither to be the patient's room number) whenever administering medications.
- Improve the effectiveness of communication among caregivers, such as implementing a process for taking verbal or telephone orders that require a verification read-back of the complete order by the person receiving the order.
- Standardize the abbreviations, acronyms, and symbols used throughout the organization, including a list of abbreviations, acronyms, and symbols not to use.
- Improve the safety of using high-alert medications, such as removing concentrated electrolytes (including, but not limited to, potassium chloride, potassium phosphate, sodium chloride >0.9%) from patient care units.

Table 6.10 Medication-Related JCAHO Sentinel Event Alerts

Topic	Recommendations	Reference
Potassium chloride	• Keep concentrated potassium chloride in the pharmacy only	18
High-risk drug: insulin	• Double check • Store separately from heparin • Spell out *unit* • Establish independent check system for pump rates and concentration settings	19
High-risk drugs: opiates and narcotics	• Limit floor-stock availability, double check patient-controlled analgesia (PCA) pumps • Remove from floor stock	
High-risk drug: concentrated potassium	• Use premixed solutions or prepare drug in pharmacy • Standardize and limit drug concentrations	
High-risk drug: heparin	• Use only single-dose containers • Standardize concentration and use premixed solutions • Store separately from insulin	
High-risk drug: Sodium chloride >0.9%	• Remove from floor stock • Standardize and limit concentration • Double check	
Infusion pumps	• Eliminate pumps that allow free flow[a]	20
Look- and sound-alike medications	• Do not store problem medications alphabetically by name • Place the purpose of the medication on the prescription • Establish a safe policy and practice for verbal orders • Use both the generic and brand name of the drug • Provide patients with written information about their medications	21
Abbreviations	• Develop a list of unacceptable abbreviations and ensure that they are not used • Develop a procedure to verify orders containing an unacceptable abbreviation	22

[a] Free flow occurs when the solutions are under the force of gravity, and not controlled by the pump. This can occur in some pumps when the set is removed from the pump without performing some other function, such as engaging a clamp.

- Standardize and limit the number of drug concentrations available in the organization.
- Improve the safety of using infusion pumps, such as ensuring free-flow protection on all general-use and patient-controlled analgesia (PCA) intravenous infusion pumps used in the organization.

Analyzing errors

Several methods of analyzing medication errors exist. Two common methods are root cause analysis and failure mode and effects analysis.

Root cause analysis

A root cause analysis is an examination of an error after it occurred, to detect what went wrong to cause the mistake. The error is dissected and an attempt made to improve situations wherein problems occurred. A multidisciplinary review of an error often identifies issues missed by one person or a group from the same department.

Failure mode and effects analysis

A failure mode and effects analysis (also known as failure mode and criticality analysis) examines a high-risk process in advance of an error to detect potential problems. The problems can then be fixed before an error occurs. It is used to discover the potential risk in a product or system. It involves examining a product or system to identify all the ways in which it might fail and allows for a proactive approach to fixing problems before they occur.

Although the root causes of medication errors are thought to be system errors, there are some unfortunate situations wherein intentionally unsafe acts cause an error. Not all misadventures are errors. Intentionally unsafe acts are any events that result from a criminal act, a purposefully unsafe act, an act related to alcohol or substance abuse by an impaired provider, or events involving alleged or suspected patient abuse of any kind.[24] Although errors that result from such acts should be reported through existing medication error reporting systems, these egregious acts are also appropriately dealt with through an organization's disciplinary policies.

Measuring errors

The NCC MERP medication error index classifies errors according to the severity of patient outcome. Near misses are also classified as potential errors that deserve a system-wide approach to improvement. Figure 16.1 shows the NCC MERP risk levels.[25] Some organizations categorize errors from NCC MERP risk levels A and B as near misses. Practitioners are often more likely to report these because these are errors caught before reaching the patient.

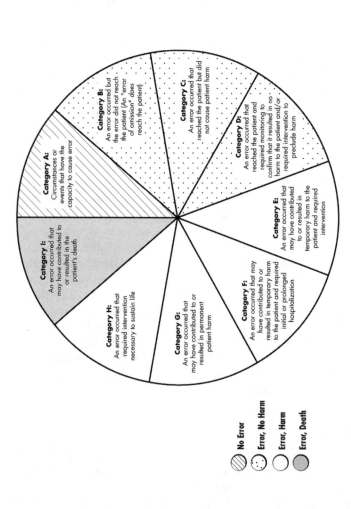

Definitions

Harm
Impairment of the physical, emotional, or psychological function or structure of the body and/or pain resulting therefrom

Monitoring
To observe or record relevant physiological or psychological signs

Intervention
May include change in therapy or active medical/surgical treatment

Intervention Necessary to Sustain Life
Includes cardiovascular and respiratory support (e.g., CPR, defibrillation, intubation, etc.)

Category A: Circumstances or events that have the capacity to cause error

Category B: An error occurred but the error did not reach the patient (An "error of omission" does reach the patient)

Category C: An error occurred that reached the patient but did not cause patient harm

Category D: An error occurred that reached the patient and required monitoring to confirm that it resulted in no harm to the patient and/or required intervention to preclude harm

Category E: An error occurred that may have contributed to or resulted in temporary harm to the patient and required intervention

Category F: An error occurred that may have contributed to or resulted in temporary harm to the patient and required initial or prolonged hospitalization

Category G: An error occurred that may have contributed to or resulted in permanent patient harm

Category H: An error occurred that required intervention necessary to sustain life

Category I: An error occurred that may have contributed to or resulted in the patient's death

No Error
Error, No Harm
Error, Harm
Error, Death

PS0306

Figure 16.1 NCC MERP index for categorizing medication errors. (From www.nccmerp.org.)

Practitioners and consumers often want to know the acceptable medication error rate. There is no benchmark. A zero error rate is desired, but unattainable because of human factors. If organizations can determine measuring points and consistently follow them, it might be possible to determine an internal benchmark to be used for quality improvement purposes. However, because the parameters of the measurement are unlikely to be duplicated elsewhere, use of the number for external comparisons is not valid.

Reporting systems

The Medication Error Reporting Program (MERP) is a voluntary program administered by the U.S. Pharmacopeia (USP) in conjunction with the ISMP. This confidential reporting system improves patient safety by alerting practitioners and the industry to potential or actual problems. Practitioners are asked to report errors and near misses to this program so that others learn from errors and prevent similar errors in the future.

How to respond to an error

Organizations need to establish a policy to follow when a medication error occurs. Although pharmacists strive for 100% accuracy, human failures do not allow that level of accuracy. Mistakes will happen, and need to be dealt with appropriately and professionally. Table 16.11 outlines suggestions for dealing with a medication error.[26]

Pharmacist's role to improve medication safety

A continuous process of accessing medication safety should be a part of every pharmacist's position. Improvements will be possible, based on assessment of past errors and near misses, improvements in technology, and

Table 16.11 Dealing with a Medication Error

- Be aware of, and follow, your organization's policy concerning errors.
- Take seriously all comments and questions that hint of an error.
- Be honest with patients and treat them with respect and concern.
- Minimize any potential ill effects for the patient. Give the patient your immediate attention.
- Move to a private area, and get details of the situation.
- Check the original prescription or order as well as computerized records.
- Contact the prescriber, explain the situation, and discuss the best course of action.
- Explain the error to the patient, without excuses. Correct the mistake, and, if possible, retrieve the incorrect prescription.
- Document the occurrence and your actions. Know the terms of your malpractice insurance.

Source: From Palacioz K. *Pharm. Lett.* 2001; 17(170601).

sophistication of error-prevention techniques. There should be an attempt to minimize calculations, reliance on memory, unnecessary steps, and transcriptions.

Continuous improvement techniques should include:

- Double-checking all processes
- Assuring competence
- Assuring complete patient data
- Standardizing orders and products when appropriate
- Automating processes

Lee developed a set of principles of a fail-safe medication use system striving for a system that is patient centered, based on respect for others, and requires an acceptance of responsibility and a collaboration of interests.[27]

These principles set the tone for characteristics of a fail-safe medication use system that:

- Is seamless
- Operates with the principle of logical process flow
- Makes proper use of all resources at each function and logical talent
- Includes all drugs
- Is the same at all sites
- Reflects consistent pharmacy practice
- Ensures that all necessary information is provided to all professionals responsible for patient care
- Is secure
- Is time sensitive
- Ensures strict accountability
- Is fail-safe

Pharmacists in health care systems are key to coordinating an effective medication safety program. An awareness of patient safety and collaboration among health professionals will improve medication safety for patients.

References

1. Kohn L.T., Corrigan J.M., Donaldson M.S., Eds. To err is human: building a safer health system. National Academy Press, Washington, D.C., 1999. Available at www.nap.edu/catalog/9728.html, accessed July 3, 2002.
2. Leape L.L. A systems analysis approach to medical error. In Cohen M.R., Ed., *Medication Errors.* Jones and Bartlett, Sudbury, MA, 1999, p. 37.
3. The National Coordinating Council for Medication Error Reporting and Prevention (NCC MERP), 1995. Available at www.nccmerp.org, accessed August 5, 2002.
4. Leape L.L. et al. Systems analysis of adverse drug events. *JAMA* 1995; 274: 35–43

5. Weinger M.B. et al. Incorporating human factors into the design of medical devices [letter]. *JAMA* 1998; 280: 1484.

6. Reason J. *Human Error.* Cambridge University Press, Cambridge, 1990.

7. MedMARx 2002 Data Report Highlights, Press Release, December 8, 2002. Available at http://www.onlinepressroom.net/uspharm/, accessed December 24, 2003.

8. *JCAHO Comprehensive Accreditation Manual for Hospitals: The Official Handbook,* Update 4, November 2000, GL-22.

9. *Joint Commission Perspectives* 22(8), 2002, p. 5.

10. ASHP statement on the formulary system. Available at www.ashp.org/best-practices/Formulary/Statement, accessed July 28, 2002.

11. Gordon, B.M. *Making the Formulary Safe: General Strategies for Reducing Risks.* ASHP Medication Use Safety Learning Community, Baltimore, June 2002.

12. NCC MERP council recommendations to reduce medication errors associated with verbal medication orders and prescriptions, adopted February 20, 2001. Available at www.nccmerp.org/council2001-02-20.html, accessed January 9, 2004.

13. ISMP, Special issue: Do not use these dangerous abbreviations or dose designations. Available at www.ismp.org/msarticles/dangerousabbrev.htm, accessed August 5, 2002

14. Recommendations for avoiding error-prone aspects of dispensing medications, *USP Qual. Rev.,* June 1999, No. 67.

15. NCC MERP recommendations to reduce errors related to administration of drugs, adopted June 29, 1999. Available at www.nccmerp.org, accessed July 28, 2002.

16. Breland B.D. Strategies for prevention of medication errors, *Hosp. Pharm. Rep.* 2000; 56–65.

17. Centers for Medicare and Medicaid Services, Conditions of participation, Pharmaceutical Services (482.25). Available at cms.hhs.gov/cop/default.asp, accessed August 4, 2002.

18. JCAHO Sentinel Event Alert No. 1: Medication error prevention — potassium chloride, February 27, 1998. Available at www.jcaho.org, accessed August 5, 2002.

19. JCAHO Sentinel Event Alert No. 11: High-alert medications and patient safety, November 19, 1999. Available at www.jcaho.org, accessed August 5, 2002.

20. JCAHO Sentinel Event Alert No. 15: Infusion pumps — preventing future adverse events, November 3, 2000. Available at www.jcaho.org, accessed August 5, 2002.

21. JCAHO Sentinel Event Alert No. 19: Look-alike, sound-alike drug names, May 2001. Available at www.jcaho.org, accessed August 5, 2002.

22. JCAHO Sentinel Event Alert No. 23: Medication errors related to potentially dangerous abbreviations, September 2001. Available at www.jcaho.org, accessed August 5, 2002.

23. Joint commission announces national patient safety goals, July 24, 2002. Available at www.jcaho.org, accessed August 5, 2002.

24. *VHA National Patient Safety Improvement Handbook,* section 4d, January 30, 2002. Available at www.patientsafety.gov, accessed July 3, 2002.

25. NCC MERP risk levels. Available at www.nccmerp.org, accessed August 5, 2002.

26. Palacioz K. How to respond to medication errors, *Pharm. Lett.* 2001; 17(170601).
27. Lee P., Ideal principles and characteristics of a fail-safe medication use system, *Am. J. Hlth.-Syst. Pharm.,* 2002; 59: 369–371.

Bibliography

ASHP guidelines on preventing medication errors in hospitals. Available at www.ashp.org/bestpractices, accessed July 28, 2002.
Cohen M.R., Ed. *Medication Errors,* Jones and Bartlett, Sudbury, MA, 1999.
Schneider P.J. Applying human factors in improving medication-use safety. *Am. J. Hlth.-Syst. Pharm.* 2002; 59: 1155–1159.

chapter seventeen

The role of the pharmacist in disease management

*Laura T. Pizzi, Jaime B. Howell, and Jennifer H. Lofland**

Contents

Introduction

The practice of pharmacy is continuing to undergo a paradigm shift from a dispensing-focused to a patient-care-focused profession. With the advances in technology and the increased supply of pharmacy technicians, pharmacists have more time to provide clinical services. One area in which pharmacists have seized the opportunity to become involved in patient care is disease management.

* Dr. Lofland's work was supported by the Agency for Health Care Research and Quality K-08 00005 Mentored Clinical Scientist Award and a PhRMA Foundation grant.

Definition of disease management

In its current understanding, the term *disease management* (DM) was first given broad exposure in a 1993 report by the Boston Consulting Group.[1] Since then, the term has taken on various definitions in different practice settings, such as managed care organizations (MCOs), the pharmaceutical industry, and academia. Within MCOs, DM has been described as involving "aspects of case and outcomes management, but the approach focuses on specific diseases, looking at what creates the costs, what treatment plan works, educating patients and providers, and coordinating care at all levels: hospital, pharmacy, physician, etc."[2] The term *care management* is sometimes used interchangeably with DM, especially when referring to the management of conditions rather than diseases (e.g., pain).

The Disease Management Association of America (DMAA) defines DM as "a system of coordinated health care interventions and communications for populations with conditions in which patient self-care efforts are significant."[3] DM has also been defined as a "systematic management tool applied to specific diseases with an emphasis on prevention and 'best practices' to provide high quality care at a reasonable cost with an ongoing process of monitoring and continuous improvement."[4] In general, organizations either choose to develop and build their own DM programs or hire a vendor to perform services.[5]

DM programs involve an intervention or series of interventions aimed at improving the patient outcomes associated with specific diseases or conditions that have a high prevalence or high treatment costs (e.g., diabetes).[6] Although DM is applicable to all conditions, programs have typically been focused on chronic illnesses,[7] because they account for a disproportionately high percentage of all medical expenditures.[8] In the U.S., chronic illnesses affect over 100 million people and account for 75% of the nation's annual health care costs and are the major cause of death, disease, and disability.[7,9]

The intervention component of a DM program can consist of clinical practice guidelines; case management by nurses, pharmacists, or other health professionals; patient education programs; and administrative interventions aimed at avoiding duplicative services and ensuring appropriate timing of visits.[10] The targeted outcomes of DM programs generally include clinical goals that, if achieved by a sufficient number of patients, will result in a savings that equal or exceed the financial costs of the program itself.[11] However, from a pharmacist's perspective, it is important to note that medication use (and costs) can increase as a part of a DM program if the drug treatments are necessary to avert outpatient visits or hospitalizations.[12] A key element of DM programs is the ability to collect and analyze data by using computerized information systems[10] and interpret whether increased drug costs are offset by the benefits of improved patient outcomes.

Both interventions and outcomes are usually developed using the best practices that are identified through the literature, discussions with clinical experts in the disease or condition, government agencies (e.g., the National

Institutes of Health), and professional organizations (e.g., American Diabetes Association). Table 17.1 summarizes key characteristics of disease management programs.

Organizations that offer disease management programs

The growth of DM has paralleled the evolution of managed health care. The types of organizations that currently offer DM services now encompass virtually every stakeholder in the provision of health care, including health benefits administrators, health care providers, information managers, finance experts, and patients.[12] Although managing disease has always been a part of medical care, the growth of structured DM programs did not accelerate until the early 1990s.[13]

MCOs and pharmacy benefit management (PBM) firms are considered the originators of the DM movement.[5] DM later gained the attention of pharmaceutical companies, large employers, and DM companies.[14] More recently, other organizations, such as device and laboratory companies, medical product wholesalers and distributors, physician groups, and community pharmacies have developed DM capabilities.[14] In addition, health care purchasers, such as Medicaid (see Chapter 18), have begun to use DM tools as a means to effectively manage patients.[8] There are now companies that specialize in selling DM services to health care providers who choose not to develop programs with their own staff. In fact, the DM industry has been among the fastest-growing investment segments in health care.[15]

The role of pharmacists in disease management

History of pharmacists' involvement in patient care

The origin of pharmacists' involvement in DM can be traced back to the hospital environment. In this setting, clinical pharmacy practice is believed

Table 17.1 Characteristics of a Disease Management Program

- Targets specific patient populations suffering from a disease.
- Integrates health care services directed toward the chosen disease by various components of the health care system, providing a seamless system of prevention and care.
- Bases health care services on consistent application of the best scientific information available on treatment and evaluation of care, with constant updating and improvement through use of quality improvement techniques.
- Links care to the outcomes of interest to consumers of health care, taking into account the multidimensional nature of quality by including clinical, economic, and humanistic outcomes.

Source: Adapted and reprinted from Holdford, D et al. *Clin. Ther.* 1998; 20(2): 328–339. With permission.

to have begun during the 1960s.[16] In an effort to demonstrate their value, clinical pharmacists began recording and tracking pharmacy interventions. In the late 1960s and early 1970s, literature regarding clinical pharmacy practice began to discuss direct patient contact and clinical involvement of the pharmacist.[17] During this early period, pharmacists' interventions were reactive, as opposed to proactive; that is, the bulk of the interventions focused on correcting existing problems with drug therapy, rather than preventing them.[14]

The 1990s marked the beginning of a new paradigm within the profession, the concept of pharmaceutical care. First defined by Hepler and Strand in 1989, pharmaceutical care refers to "the responsible provision of drug therapy for the purpose of achieving definite outcomes that improve a patient's quality of life."[16,18] Holdford and colleagues described pharmaceutical care as a component of DM by stating that "pharmaceutical care targets those with risk factors for drug-related problems, a history of non-adherence, and frequent changes in medication regimens."[6]

In practicing pharmaceutical care, a pharmacist is expected to assume greater responsibility for patients' medication-related outcomes.[19] For example, pharmacists have taken on roles to help assess patients' therapeutic needs, prevent adverse drug reactions, individualize drug therapy, manage chronic disease, and monitor follow-up care.[20] However, note that the extent to which pharmacists may actually practice pharmaceutical care is highly variable. For example, a 1996 study of Virginia pharmacists found that community pharmacists who practiced in rurally located, independently owned pharmacies filled less than 150 prescriptions per day and had a good rapport with patients, and local physicians were more likely to deliver pharmaceutical care.[21] Although these findings might be attributable to geographic and patient mix differences, results suggest that higher-volume retail chains were less likely to provide pharmaceutical care. However, these findings might not be relevant currently, because recent technological advancements (e.g., electronic prescriptions) help expedite prescription processing, making it more difficult to determine whether there is an association between high prescription volume and the inability to provide pharmaceutical care.

With expertise in pharmacotherapeutics and pharmaceutical care, pharmacists are uniquely qualified to participate in DM programs.[12] Pharmacists have been involved in developing and implementing many DM programs currently existing. Some have contributed through their positions in non-clinical settings, such as PBMs, health plans, and pharmaceutical companies, whereas others have participated in clinical settings such as long-term care facilities, hospitals, home health care providers, integrated delivery systems, and community pharmacies.

Research suggests that the potential impact of a pharmacist's intervention in patient care is significant. In a well-publicized study, Johnson and Bootman calculated the annual cost of drug-related morbidity and mortality at $76.6 billion.[22] In a follow-up project, they estimated that pharmacist intervention and pharmaceutical care could reduce the annual expense of drug-related problems by $45.6 billion, a savings that would occur even if pharmacists were paid an additional $10 for every patient encounter.[23]

Factors influencing pharmacist involvement in disease management

Patient access

Pharmacists are uniquely positioned to become involved in DM activities for several reasons.[14] First, within the community, pharmacists practice at the interface of care and therefore have the ability to interact directly with patients. In addition, public opinion polls reveal that pharmacists are consistently ranked among the most trusted professionals.[24] Figure 17.1 illustrates how the drug prescribing process places pharmacists at the interface of patient care. Because pharmacists, like physicians, have the ability to directly deliver DM services, they can serve as conduits for implementing DM programs developed by health insurance providers, PBMs, pharmaceutical companies, wholesalers and distributors, and employers.

Community pharmacies are particularly accessible for patients: some are open 24 hours a day, 7 days a week. As of this writing, there are more than 55,000 pharmacies in the U.S. and more than 130,000 pharmacists practicing at these sites.[25] Furthermore, no appointments or insurance preapprovals are required to receive one-on-one professional consultations with pharmacists.

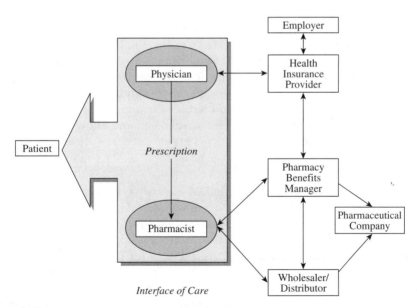

Figure 17.1 The prescribing process empowers pharmacists to deliver pharmaceutical DM services. *Note*: Circles represent the infrastructure in which pharmacists and physicians practice (e.g., group or clinic for physicians and corporate chain for pharmacists). (From Pizzi LT, Menz JM, Graber GR, Suh DC. *Dis. Manage.* 2001; 4: 143–154. With permission.)

Finally, patients with chronic conditions are likely to visit their pharmacy regularly in order to obtain refills.

Consistency between sites

Another factor promoting pharmacists' involvement in DM is the organization and structure of pharmacies (e.g., chain drug stores), which allow the administration of a program through pharmacists practicing at different locations. This feature, most obvious to chain pharmacies and hospital networks, provides the infrastructure required to implement programs across large or geographically dispersed patient populations. There are also some practical benefits to implementing DM within these settings. For example, outcomes data may be available through a single repository, and there is likely to be a process in place for communicating within and between the sites. For chain pharmacies, the structural layout of the stores might be similar, which could be important if a patient counseling area is required to administer DM services.

Expanding the role of pharmacy technicians

Another factor that has fostered pharmacists' involvement in DM is the expansion of the roles of pharmacy technicians. Greater use of technicians might allow pharmacists to devote more time to patient care.[26] In 1995, the American Society of Health-System Pharmacists (ASHP), American Pharmaceutical Association (APhA), and two state organizations, the Michigan Pharmacists Association and the Illinois Council of Health-System Pharmacists, jointly created the Pharmacy Technician Certification Board (PTCB),[26] which "develops, maintains, promotes and administers a ... certification and re-certification program for pharmacy technicians."[27] By 2002, over 100,000 pharmacy technicians were certified through this program.[27] It is expected that advanced training of technicians will reduce the amount of time that pharmacists typically devote to medication dispensing and allow more time for pharmacists to provide pharmaceutical care.

Legislative efforts

Pharmacists' involvement in specific DM efforts has been fostered through legislative efforts. In July 1998, the approval of a Medicaid waiver granted reimbursement for pharmacists providing DM services in the state of Mississippi. Under this legislation, pharmacists with appropriate training can be reimbursed for providing cognitive services for patients with diabetes, asthma, lipid disorders, and anticoagulation under patient-specific treatment protocols approved by a physician.[28] To qualify as a provider under the waiver, pharmacists must be credentialed in each of the therapeutic areas included. Table 17.2 provides the requirements for pharmacist reimbursement under this law.

As of this writing, legislation is before the U.S. Congress of proposing reimbursement of pharmacists' services delivered to Medicare beneficiaries.

Table 17.2 Requirements for Pharmacist Reimbursement under the Mississippi Medicaid Waiver

- The pharmacist must complete a credentialing program that is approved by the state Board of Pharmacy.
- The pharmacist must obtain a written referral from the patient's physician.
- The pharmacy at which the credentialed pharmacist practices must have a private counseling area.
- A record of services provided to the patient must be maintained in the pharmacy.
- The pharmacist must obtain a provider number from the state Medicaid department.

Source: Adapted from National Associations of Boards of Pharmacy. Answers to questions on DSM exams/credentialing. *NABP Newslett.* September 1998.

Currently, pharmacists receive Medicare reimbursement for providing education to patients with diabetes. To illustrate how this legislation could build on the experience with pharmacists in disease and drug therapy management (collective drug therapy management, CDTM) to improve the quality of care delivered in the U.S., issues surrounding atrial fibrillation and stroke will be discussed.

In the future, the Centers for Medicare and Medicaid Services could mandate that in order to receive reimbursement, a pharmacist would need to be certified in anticoagulation management. Currently, the American College of Clinical Pharmacy through selected training sites offers anticoagulation certification across the country.[29] Medicare could then reimburse pharmacists for the management of warfarin therapy for patients with atrial fibrillation. As a Medicare provider, pharmacists would be held to the same standards and provisions for reimbursement as other providers. By utilizing ubiquitous community-based health care professionals such as pharmacists as a means for primary stroke prevention, disease management can be delivered and the quality of care for Medicare beneficiaries will improve (see Chapter 18).

In response to this legislation and the need for pharmacists across the country to receive advanced training to qualify as DM providers, the National Association of Boards of Pharmacy (NABP), APhA, National Association of Chain Drug Stores (NACDS), and the National Community Pharmacists Association (NCPA) collaborated to form the National Institute for Standards in Pharmacist Credentialing (NISPC). The NISPC currently offers pharmacists certifications in the areas of asthma, diabetes, dyslipidemia, and anticoagulation.[20]

Impact of the pharmacist in managing specific diseases

Most DM efforts have focused on chronic conditions that are common or have high associated treatment costs, or both. Some specific disease states for which the impact of the pharmacists has been demonstrated are asthma, cardiovascular conditions (hypertension, hyperlipidemia, and anticoagulation), and diabetes. Research supporting these contributions is described here. Although the interventions and outcomes measured might differ considerably according to the specific disease or condition, pharmacists' have demonstrated their ability to improve patient outcomes.

Asthma

Asthma is a prevalent disorder affecting an estimated 15 million people in the U.S., and the total annual costs (direct and indirect) of the disease are approximately U.S.$12.7 billion.[30] Pharmacists dispense more than 30.5 million prescriptions annually to treat asthma.[31] Given these frequent patient encounters, pharmacists have a unique opportunity to provide patient care, which may lead to improved patient outcomes. The National Asthma and Education Program recognized the potential of pharmacist interventions and created a guide that describes the role of the pharmacist in asthma care.[32] Table 17.3 presents pharmacist responsibilities delineated in this guide. These guidelines provide a framework for defining the pharmacist's role in asthma DM.

An asthma DM program can assist pharmacists in providing education to patients with asthma. Hunter and Bryant developed an educational intervention administered by pharmacists and targeted at pediatric asthma patients and their parents.[34] The educational intervention consisted of a 45-min presentation, a demonstration of drug delivery devices, and a discussion session for participants to ask questions and share experiences. All the participants indicated on a questionnaire that they had received enough information to safely and effectively administer asthma medications.

However, does enhanced patient understanding about medication use translate into improved patient outcomes? A study of a physician-directed, pharmacist-managed asthma program evaluated the impact of attending a

Table 17.3 National Asthma Education Program Guidelines for Pharmacist Responsibilities in Asthma Disease Management

- Educate patients about the role of each medication.
- Instruct patients about the proper techniques for inhaling medications.
- Monitor medication use and refill intervals to help identify patients with poorly controlled asthma.
- Encourage patients purchasing nonprescription asthma inhalers or tablets to seek medical care.
- Help patients use peak-flow meters appropriately.
- Help patients discharged from the hospital after an asthma exacerbation to understand their asthma management plan.

Source: Adapted from National Institutes of Health (NIH). The role of the pharmacist in improving asthma care. NHLBI, NIH 1995; 95-3280, 1–16.

special asthma clinic designed for patients with frequent asthma exacerbations.[35] The program consisted of regular telephone contact between the patient and the pharmacist, as well as follow-up through the clinic. During the study period, the patients experienced fewer emergency room visits for asthma exacerbations as compared with what they did the same 6 months of the year before enrolling in the study. As a result, the program saved between $30,683 and $68,393.[35]

Cardiovascular disease

Hypertension

Unlike asthma, hypertension is a largely asymptomatic disease. As with other asymptomatic diseases, patients with hypertension are often noncompliant with their therapy.[9,36] This presents a challenge for health care practitioners, because chronic uncontrolled hypertension can lead to serious sequelae such as stroke, coronary disease, and cardiac failure.[37] Pharmacists have been shown to have an impact in improving the clinical and humanistic outcomes among patients with hypertension.

A randomized controlled study was conducted to determine the clinical value of comprehensive pharmacy services for hypertensive patients in a chain pharmacy setting.[38] Patients were enrolled into either a control or an intervention group. Intervention patients participated in four scheduled monthly visits, during which they received drug therapy monitoring (e.g., heart rate, blood pressure, medication history) and patient education. Control patients received traditional pharmacy services, which were defined as screening for prescribing errors, prescription filling, limited patient education (i.e., drug regimen), and monitoring patient-volunteered adverse drug reactions. Both groups of patients completed quality-of-life questionnaires on entering and completing the study. Results from the study showed that blood pressure and quality of life were significantly improved in the intervention group.

A second study evaluated the effectiveness of pharmacists in a rural hypertension clinic.[39] Before the study, the pharmacists participated in an intensive skill-development program. Fifty-one patients with controlled or uncontrolled hypertension were randomized to either the pharmacist intervention group or the control group. All patients completed the Short Form 36 to assess quality of life. Control-group patients received traditional pharmacy services, such as brief counseling and prescription review for errors. Intervention patients were scheduled to see the pharmacist every 3 to 5 weeks to have their blood pressures and heart rates measured and to be questioned regarding their compliance, adverse drug reactions, and understanding of present drug regimens and lifestyle modifications. The impact of the pharmacist intervention was positive, with blood pressure reduction and increased quality-of-life scores in the areas of physical functioning, physical role limitations, and bodily pain.[39]

Another hypertension DM program at Cedars-Sinai Health System evaluated a pharmacist–physician comanagement approach at reducing both blood pressure and treatment costs.[40] Patients with uncontrolled hypertension were randomized to an alert group (primary care physicians received a letter informing them of the patient's uncontrolled status) or an intervention group (patients were enrolled in a pharmacy clinic, where a pharmacist comanaged the patients with the physicians until the patients' blood pressure goals were achieved). Interim results demonstrated that blood pressure reductions were more substantial in the intervention group, decreasing from a baseline systolic pressure of 157.7 mmHg to 148.9 mmHg and 139.6 mmHg at 6 months and 1 year, respectively. At 6 months, the total cost of treatment per member per month (PMPM) for the intervention group increased because of an increased number of patient visits. However, at 1 year, cost savings were observed in the area of laboratory tests, office visits, and medications, resulting in an average savings of $6.40 PMPM. Results of this program demonstrated that pharmacists can contribute to containing costs within the health care system.

Hyperlipidemia

According to the American Heart Association, approximately 41.3 million U.S. adults have high cholesterol.[41] Effective management of cholesterol is known to reduce cardiovascular events. With this evidence, cholesterol treatment guidelines were developed and updated by the National Cholesterol Education Program Expert Panel (NCEP).[42] As a result of the new guidelines, it is estimated that the number people in the U.S. who are candidates for cholesterol-lowering medications will triple.[43] This projection points to an increased need for pharmacist involvement in lipid management.

Several studies have evaluated the effectiveness of pharmacist-administered lipid management programs.[44-46] Ellis and colleagues examined the effectiveness of pharmacist intervention in the management of dyslipidemia among veterans administration (VA) patients.[44] Patients in the intervention group were scheduled for drug assessments by ambulatory care pharmacists, whereas patients in the control group received usual medical care. Results demonstrated that the intervention group achieved a statistically significant reduction in both total cholesterol and low-density lipoprotein compared with the control group.

A smaller study by Faulkner and colleagues assessed the impact of pharmacist telephonic follow-up in patients who had recently undergone cardiac surgery and were receiving lipid-lowering therapy.[45] Patients in the intervention group were telephoned by a pharmacist once a week for 12 weeks to emphasize the importance of lipid-lowering therapy, assess refills, and identify potential issues related to compliance (drug cost, side effects, overall well-being). Results showed that the intervention provided no short-term benefit during the first 12 weeks of therapy, but compliance and lipid-lowering results were better in the intervention group in the long term (measured 2 years after the start of therapy). These results provided mixed evidence of the effectiveness of the intervention, but the authors suggest that the pharmacist telephonic follow-up might be a useful alternative when face-to-face counseling in a lipid clinic is either impractical or impossible.

Carson investigated the effectiveness of pharmacist consultation notes added to the charts of hyperlipidemic patients. The older guidelines, NCEP II, served as the basis for identifying risk factors and recommending treatment regimens. Results demonstrated that patients who received the pharmacist intervention were more likely to be prescribed lipid-lowering therapy, suggesting that pharmacist chart notes might help increase physician compliance with guidelines for prescribing lipid-lowering therapies.[46]

An earlier study by Bogden and colleagues measured the impact of a pharmacist–physician team on the ability to reach lipid-lowering goals.[47] Patients in the control group received usual care, whereas the intervention group received routine pharmacist–patient consultations and pharmacist–physician interaction, including recommendations on dosage, appropriate drug treatments, and monitoring. The NCEP II guidelines were used to guide the appropriate initiation of therapy as well as to set lipid-lowering goals. Results revealed that twice as many intervention patients reached their lipid-lowering goals compared with patients in the usual care group.[48]

Anticoagulation

In various settings such as the VA outpatient clinics, Kaiser Permanente outpatient services, hospital-based outpatient clinics, physician offices, and community pharmacies, pharmacists have been successfully managing patients' warfarin therapy.[48–53] Research demonstrates the positive outcomes associated with and the cost-effectiveness of pharmacist-run warfarin clinics.[50,51]

Wilt and colleagues studied the benefits of a pharmacist-managed anticoagulation monitoring service (AMS).[51] Outcomes (based on number of thromboembolic and hemorrhagic events, unplanned clinic visits, emergency room visits, and hospital admissions) of patients followed by AMS were compared with those of control-group patients (patients receiving warfarin but followed only by their physicians). Results of the study showed that the control group was 20 times more likely than the study group to experience any event. In addition, analysis of costs of hospital admissions, emergency room visits, and participation in the AMS indicated that a potential cost avoidance of $4072.68 per person-year of follow-up might have been possible if the control group had been followed by AMS.[51]

A second study by Mamdani and colleagues was conducted to evaluate clinical and economic effectiveness of a pharmacist-managed anticoagulation service.[50] The study examined clinical and economic endpoints for 50 patients in a usual care group vs. 50 patients in a pharmacist-managed group. Although no significant differences were noted between groups for the primary therapeutic end point, the pharmacist-managed group exhibited earlier initiation of warfarin therapy and shorter hospital stay with significantly lower total hospital costs ($1594 vs. $2014). Given the complexity of titrating warfarin therapy, the severity of potential adverse events, and demonstrated benefits in terms of cost savings, pharmacist involvement in this DM area is particularly warranted.

Diabetes mellitus

In addition to asthma and cardiovascular conditions, pharmacists have also demonstrated a positive impact in the management of diabetes. Two studies[56,57] evaluated the impact of pharmacist management on the outcomes of patients with diabetes. Jaber and colleagues[56] examined the impact of interventions that consisted of pharmacist-provided diabetes education, medication counseling, and evaluation and adjustment of the medication regimen in noninsulin-dependent diabetes mellitus (NIDDM) patients. After 4 months, patients who received the interventions were found to have significant improvements in their hemoglobin A1c and fasting plasma glucose. The study did not assess the overall impact of the intervention on the total health care costs of diabetes.

The second study compared a control group of patients with diabetes mellitus receiving standard pharmacist education to an intervention group receiving education via small group or individual instruction.[57] Patients in the intervention group had significantly lower average weekly blood glucose levels, a decreased incidence of hyperglycemic events, and demonstrated a significant increase in their understanding of diabetes medications as well as a positive difference in their perception and attitude toward communication with the pharmacist. Both studies demonstrated that intensive diabetes education involving pharmacists was associated with improved patient outcomes.

In summary, the results of studies assessing DM with pharmacist involvement demonstrate that pharmacists are capable of improving patient outcomes and reducing health care costs. Pharmacists' expertise has been shown to be particularly beneficial for diseases in which outcomes heavily rely on medications.

Future directions

In 2000, prescription drugs accounted for approximately 10% of the total spending on health care in the U.S.[58] This data represents a 17% growth from the previous year and indicates that prescription-drug spending is growing faster than any other health care service.[59] In the face of these increasing costs, pharmacists' expertise will be sought to ensure appropriate drug utilization and costs. Although the management of utilization and costs alone does not qualify as DM, it is likely that insurers and employers will attempt to manage drug costs as a part of broader initiatives.

Furthermore, it has been estimated that traditional prescription processing utilizes only about 10% of the technological potential that computers offer to pharmacists.[60] Software applications to assist pharmacists in DM have been developed and will continue to be improved. Ultimately, pharmacy information systems will support the processes of drug dispensing; prescription processing; and the task of outcomes data collection, documentation, and monitoring.[61] As these technology advances are realized, pharmacists will increasingly become more involved in managing chronic diseases and providing DM services, which will hopefully lead to improved quality of patient care.

It is extremely important that pharmacists be provided with the knowledge and skills necessary to contribute to DM. Two organizations that have emerged as leaders in providing disease management education to pharmacists are the NISPC and the National Institute for Pharmacist Care Outcomes (NIPCO). The NIPCO, initiated by the NCPA, has designed an educational curriculum aimed at educating community pharmacists on how to "provide an expanded level of patient care" related to disease management and wellness activities.[62] In addition to the efforts of these two organizations, the advanced clinical training provided by pharmacy schools, major health care providers, and accrediting bodies will better prepare pharmacists with the knowledge and skills required to contribute to DM. Lastly, it is essential that outcomes data surrounding these DM activities be collected to continue to substantiate the value of pharmacists' contributions to patient care.

Conclusion

The profession of pharmacy has undergone dramatic changes over the past decade. The DM movement, along with technological improvements in prescription processing, has fostered pharmacist involvement in patient care. Pharmacists in a variety of practice settings are participating in DM and are beginning to demonstrate their value in the management of several high-cost diseases, including asthma, cardiovascular disease, and diabetes. For the movement to be sustainable, pharmacists will have to demonstrate that the costs of developing and administering DM services do not exceed the benefits of improved patient outcomes. As employers and government purchasers continue to face pressures to reduce the cost of prescription benefits, pharmacists will be presented with opportunities to demonstrate their impact in providing DM.

Acknowledgments

Portions of this chapter were adapted with permission from the following article: Pizzi LT, Menz JM, Graber GR, Suh D-C. From product dispensing to patient care: The role of the pharmacist in providing pharmaceutical care as part of an integrated disease management approach. *Dis. Manage.* 2001; 4: 143–154. The authors of this chapter wish to thank Jean M. Menz, Geneen R. Graber, and Dong-Churl Suh for their contributions to the original article.

References

1. Disease management background. *Med. Market. Media (MM&M)* 2002: 1.
2. *MCOL Managed Care E-Dictionary: MCO Operations Terms.* 2002, pp. 1–20. Available at www. mcareol.com.
3. Disease Management Association of America (DMAA). Definition of disease management. 2002, p.1.
4. John Deere Health Care, National Managed Healthcare Congress Meeting, Washington, D.C., May 1997.
5. National Pharmaceutical Council (NPC). *Disease Management: Balancing Cost and Quality.* An annotated bibliography of studies on the benefits of disease management services for the treatment of asthma. National Pharmaceutical Council, Reston, VA, 2002, pp. 1–51.
6. Holdford D, Kennedy D, Bernadella P, Small R. Implementing disease management in community pharmacy practice. *Clin Ther.* 1998; 20: 328–339.
7. Nash, D, Clark, JL. Disease management. *Issue Brief* 2002; 1(2): 1–23.
8. Wheatly, B. Medicaid disease management seeking to reduce spending by promoting health. *State Coverage Initiatives Issue Brief*; August 2001: 1–6.
9. Dezii CM. A retrospective study of persistence with single-pill combination therapy vs. concurrent two-pill therapy in patients with hypertension. *Manage. Care* 2000; 9 (suppl.): S2–S6.
10. Kesteloot K. Disease management: a new technology in need of critical assessment. *Int. J. Technol. Assess. Hlth. Care* 1999; 15: 506–519.
11. Doyle J. Health outcomes: measuring and maximizing value in disease management. In: Todd W, Nash D, Eds., *Disease Management: A Systems Approach to Improving Patient Outcomes.* American Hospital Publishing, New York, 2002, pp. 61–86.
12. Gurnee, MC and Da Silva, RV. Constructing disease management programs. *Manage. Care Mag.* 1997: 1–9. Available at www.managedcaremag.com/archives/9706/9706.disease_man.shtml, accessed August 5, 2002.
13. Zitter M. A new paradigm in health care delivery: disease management. In: Todd W, Nash D, Eds., *Disease Management: A Systems Approach to Improving Patient Outcomes.* American Hospital Publishing, New York, 1997, pp. 1–26.
14. Pizzi LT, Menz JM, Graber GR, Suh DC. From product dispensing to patient care: the role of the pharmacist in providing pharmaceutical care as part of an integrated disease management approach. *Dis. Manage.* 2001; 4: 143–154.
15. Wollschlaeger, B. Disease management: utilize the Web for healthcare delivery. *Dis. Manage.* 2002: 1–4. Available at www.miamimed.com/MiamiMed%20article%20archive/disease_management.htm.accessed August 23, 2002.
16. Hepler CD, Strand LM. Opportunities and responsibilities in pharmaceutical care. *Am. J. Hosp. Pharm.* 1990; 47: 533–543.
17. Angaran D, Hepler CD, Bjornson D, Hadsall R. Career patterns of pioneer clinical pharmacists. *Am. J. Hosp. Pharm.* 1988; 45: 101–108.
18. Glossary. *Manag. Med.* 2002. Available at www.managingmedicines.com/print.php?page=glossary, accessed August 21, 2002.
19. American Society of Health-System Pharmacists. ASHP guidelines on a standardized method for pharmaceutical care. *Am. J. Hlth.-Syst. Pharm.* 1996; 53: 1713–1716.
20. Keely JL. Pharmacist scope of practice. *Ann. Intern. Med.* 2002; 136: 79–85.

21. Sisson EM. Extent of community-based delivery of pharmaceutical care in Virginia. *Pharmacotherapy* 1996; 16: 94–102.

22. Johnson JA, Bootman LJ. Drug-related morbidity and mortality: a cost-of-illness model. *Arch. Intern. Med.* 1995; 155: 1949–1956.

23. Johnson JA, Bootman LJ. Drug-related morbidity and mortality and the economic impact of pharmaceutical care. *Am. J. Hlth.-Syst. Pharm.* 1997; 54: 554–558.

24. Stergachis A, Maine L, Brown L. The 2001 national pharmacy consumer survey. *J. Am. Pharm. Assoc.* 2002; 42: 568–576.

25. National Association of Chain Drug Stores (NACDS). Industry statistics 2001. Available at www.nacds.org., accessed January 27, 2003.

26. Zellmer WA. The role of pharmacy organizations in transforming the profession: the case of pharmaceutical care. *Pharm. Hist.* 2001; 43: 75–85.

27. Pharmacy Technician Certification Board. PTCB and NABP working together fact sheet, 2002, pp. 1–3. Available at www.ptcb.org/releases/PTCB%20NABP%20Q&A.html, accessed August 20, 2002.

28. National Associations of Boards of Pharmacy. Answers to questions on DSM exams/credentialing. *NABP Newslett.* September 1998. Available at www.nabp.net.

29. American College of Clinical Pharmacy. Anticoagulation Training Program 2002. Available at www.accp.com/ClinNet/ri02anti.pdf, accessed May 11, 2002.

30. Weiss KB, Sullivan SD. The health economics of asthma and rhinitis. I. Assessing the economic impact. *J. Allerg. Clin. Immunol.* 2001; 107: 3–8.

31. The Asthma Picture. NIH and Allergy and Asthma Network/Mothers of Asthmatics. Pediatric Health Web site, pp. 1–4. Available at www.pediatrichealth.org/asthma.html, accessed December 29, 2003.

32. National Heart, Lung and Blood Institute (NHLBI). National Asthma Education and Prevention Program: Program Description. NHLBI, NIH, 2002: 1–5. Available at www.nhlbi.nih.gov/about/naepp/naep_pd.htm.

33. National Institutes of Health (NIH). The role of the pharmacist in improving asthma care. NHLBI, NIH 1995; 95-3280, 1–16. Available at www.nhlbi.nih.gov/health/prof/lung/asthma/asmapmcy.pdf, accessed December 29, 2003.

34. Hunter KA, Bryant BG. Pharmacist provided education and counseling for managing pediatric asthma. *Pat. Educ. Couns.* 1994; 24: 127–134.

35. Pauley TR, Magee MJ, Cury JD. Pharmacist-managed, physician-directed asthma management program reduces emergency department visits. *Ann. Pharmacother.* 1995; 29: 5–9.

36. Dezii CM. Medication noncompliance: what *is* the problem? *Manage. Care* 2000; 9 (suppl.): S7–S12.

37. NIH. The Sixth Report of the Joint National Committee on Prevention, Detection, Evaluation, and Treatment of High Blood Pressure. National High Blood Pressure Education Program, NHLBI, NIH 1997; 98-4080: 1–70.

38. Park JJ, Kelly P, Carter BL, Burgess PP. Comprehensive pharmaceutical care in the chain setting. *J. Am. Pharm. Assoc.* 1996; NS36: 443–451.

39. Carter BL, Barnette DJ, Chrischilles E, Mazzotti GJ, Asali ZJ. Evaluation of hypertensive patients after care provided by community pharmacists in a rural setting. *Pharmacotherapy* 1997; 17: 1274–1285.

40. Cedars-Sinai hypertension programs sees savings, lower BP. *Rep. Med. Guide.Outc. Res.* 1997; 8: 1–5.

41. Centers for Disease Control and National Center for Health Statistics. National Health and Nutrition Examination Survey Phase III (NHANES III): Cholesterol statistics, 2002, pp. 1, 2. Available at www.americanheart.org/presenter.jhtml?identifier=536, accessed December 29, 2003.

42. Expert Panel on Detection EaToHBCiA. Executive summary of the third report of the National Cholesterol Education Program (NCEP) expert panel on detection, evaluation, and treatment of high blood cholesterol in adults (Adult Treatment Panel III). *JAMA* 2001; 285(1a): 2486–2497.

43. Kolata G. U.S. panel backs broader steps to reduce risks of heart attacks. *NY Times Late Ed.* p. 1, May 16, 2001.

44. Ellis S, Carter B, Malone D, Billups S, Okano G, Valuck R et al. Practice insights: clinical and economic impact of ambulatory care clinical pharmacist in management of dyslipidemia in older adults: The IMPROVE Study. *Pharmacotherapy* 2000: 1508–1516.

45. Faulkner MA, Wadibia EC, Lucas BD, Hilleman DE. Impact of pharmacy counseling on compliance and effectiveness of combination lipid-lowering therapy in patients undergoing coronary artery revascularization: a randomized controlled trial. *Pharmacotherapy* 2000; 20: 410–416.

46. Carson JJ. Pharmacist-coordinated program to improve the use of pharmacotherapies for reducing risk of coronary artery disease in low-income adults. *Am. J. Hlth.-Syst. Pharm.* 1999; 56: 2319–2324.

47. Bogden PE, Koontz LM, Williamson P, Abbott RD. The physician and pharmacist team. *J. Gen. Intern. Med.* 1997; 12: 158–164.

48. Kroner BA. Anticoagulation clinic in the VA Pittsburgh healthcare system. *Pharm. Pract. Manag. Q.* 1998; 18: 17–33.

49. Conte RR, Kehoe WA, Nielson N, Lodhia H. Nine-year experience with a pharmacist-managed anticoagulation clinic. *Am. J. Hosp. Pharm.* 1986; 43: 2460–2464.

50. Norton JL, Gibson DL. Establishing an outpatient anticoagulation clinic in a community hospital. *Am. J. Hlth.-Syst. Pharm.* 1996; 53: 1151–1157.

51. Knowlton CH, Thomas OV, Williamson A, Gammaitoni AR, Kirchain WR, Buttaro ML et al. Establishing community pharmacy-based anticoagulation education and monitoring programs. *J. Am. Pharm. Assoc. (Wash.)* 1999; 39: 368–374.

52. Dager WE, Branch JM, King JH, White RH, Quan RS, Musallam NA et al. Optimization of inpatient warfarin therapy: impact of daily consultation by a pharmacist-managed anticoagulation service. *Ann. Pharmacother.* 2000; 34: 567–572.

53. Dedden P, Chang B, Nagel D. Pharmacy-managed program for home treatment of deep vein thrombosis with enoxaparin. *Am. J. Hlth. Syst. Pharm.* 1997; 54: 1968–1972.

54. Mamdani MM, Racine E, McCreadie S, Zimmerman C, O'Sullivan TL, Jensen G et al. Clinical and economic effectiveness of an inpatient anticoagulation service. *Pharmacotherapy* 1999; 19: 1064–1074.

55. Wilt VM, Gums JG, Ahmed OI, Moore LM. Outcome analysis of a pharmacist-managed anticoagulation service. *Pharmacotherapy* 1995; 15: 732–739.

56. Jaber L, Halapy H, Fernet M, Tummalapalli S, Diwakaran H. Evaluation of a pharmaceutical care model on diabetes management. *Ann. Pharmacother.* 1996; 30: 239–243.

57. Veldhuizen-Scott MK, Widmer LB, Stacey SA, Popovich NG. Developing and implementing a pharmaceutical care model in an ambulatory care setting for patients with diabetes. *Diab. Educ.* 1995; 21:117–123.
58. Heffler S, Smith S, Won G, Clemens MK, Keehan S, Zezza M. Health spending projections for 2001–2011: the latest outlook. Faster health spending growth and a slowing economy drive the health spending projection for 2001 up sharply. *Hlth. Aff. (Millwood)* 2002; 21: 207–218.
59. Levit K, Smith C, Cowan C, Lazenby H, Martin A. Inflation spurs health spending in 2000. *Hlth. Aff.* 2002; 21(1): 172–181.
60. Felkey BG, Barker KN. Technology and automation in pharmaceutical care. *J. Am. Pharm. Assoc.* 1996; NS36: 309–314.
61. West DS, Szeinbach S. Information technology and pharmaceutical care. *J. Am. Pharm. Assoc.* 1997; NS37: 497–501.
62. National Community Pharmacists Association. National Institute of Pharmacist Care Outcomes. www.ncpanet.org/nipco/nipco.shtml, accessed November 13, 2002.

chapter eighteen

The U.S. health care system: health insurance

Barbara J. Plager

Contents

0-8493-1446-1/04/$0.00+$1.50
© 2004 by CRC Press LLC

Introduction

This chapter gives an overview of health insurance in the U.S. It begins with an overview of how the U.S. approach to health insurance differs from that of other advanced nations. This is followed by a discussion of *public* and *private* health care and how these terms are not as clear and distinct as commonly assumed. A brief history of health insurance in the U.S. follows, tracing the early forms of health insurance, efforts to achieve universal health insurance, and major reforms that cover significant numbers of people. This is followed by a description of the structure of health insurance at the beginning of the 21st century, with an explanation of the major types of coverage and key health insurance concepts. Next is an overview of the types of managed care organizations and the tools of managed care that are commonly applied to achieve cost savings and improve quality. This overview includes the role of pharmacy benefit management (PBM) firms. The chapter ends with a summary of proposals to cover persons who are currently uninsured.

Health insurance in the U.S. vis-à-vis other countries

All advanced industrialized nations except the U.S. have a system of universal health care coverage. The coverage is a form of social insurance that assures that all citizens have access to health care services and are protected from financial devastation as a result of illness or injury. Under these systems, the national government assures that its citizens have health care coverage. Beyond assuring that all citizens are covered, universal health care takes a different form in each country. There is wide variation in the forms of financing, administering, and delivery of health care.

The U.S. is unique among advanced nations in that it has resisted the implementation of a system of universal health care and instead has gradually built a system in which employers are the primary sponsors of health care coverage for the majority of the population. Medicare and Medicaid cover the elderly, disabled, and very poor. According to data from the U.S. Census Bureau, a small proportion of people, less than 7% of the population under 65 years of age, purchase health insurance on their own. In 2002, the remaining 41 million persons were uninsured. The uninsured represent 14.6% of the total population, 16.5% of the population under 65 years. Those with adequate resources pay out of their pockets for health care. The others go without care, delay care, or seek health services from a fragile and incomplete system of charity care and safety-net providers.

Public vs. private health care in the U.S.

Many people in the U.S. make a strong distinction between private and public health care. They perceive employer-sponsored plans as private health care and Medicaid and Medicare as public. This rigid distinction is not accurate. While Medicaid and Medicare are funded by general taxes, employer-sponsored health plans are heavily financed through tax subsidies. The employee does not pay taxes on the value of the health care benefits, and employers deduct as expenses their contributions to health care premiums and flexible spending accounts. Government employees (local, state, and federal) might be enrolled in private health plans, but taxpayers pay for their health insurance. Although health care services might be ultimately paid by a public source, such as Medicaid or Medicare, the delivery system in the U.S. is almost entirely private. The exceptions to this are the veterans administration health system, military hospitals, and local public hospitals and public health clinics.

History of health insurance in the U.S.

In 1789, Congress established the first type of health insurance in the U.S. by creating the U.S. Marine Hospital Service and funding it through compulsory contributions from seamen's wages. In the 1870s, the first forms of employer-sponsored health benefit programs developed in specific industries, such as railroads and mining, under which company doctors, funded by deductions from workers' wages, were made available to workers.

During the reform period of the early 20th century, there were efforts to protect workers generally against the financial devastation caused by unemployment, illness, or injury. Theodore Roosevelt endorsed a program of health insurance to cover medical expenses, combined with compensation for lost wages, in his 1912 Progressive Party bid for the presidency. Although he lost the election, the movement for national health insurance gathered some steam through alliances with physician organizations, union leaders, and moderate businessmen. However, as differences and divisions arose, this tentative support collapsed and solidified into strong opposition. Efforts to establish compulsory health insurance programs in several states also failed. Entry into World War I diverted attention away national health insurance and other social reforms.

There were, however, a few developments in the business and industrial sector. In 1910, Montgomery Ward & Company entered into one of the earliest group insurance contracts. More physician service and industrial health plans were established in the Northwest and remote areas. In 1913, the International Ladies Garment Workers Union (ILGWU) formed the first union medical service.

The Depression Era engendered deep fears in people about becoming unemployed or being unable to work and at the same time having medical bills to pay. In 1929, a group of schoolteachers in Dallas, TX, arranged for a local hospital to provide room, board, and other services at a predetermined monthly cost. This plan is considered the forerunner of Blue Cross plans.

The Blue Cross Commission was established in 1937. Throughout the New Deal, however, national health insurance was always on the periphery. It was omitted from Social Security and was never strongly endorsed by President Franklin D. Roosevelt.

One of the most significant and far-reaching developments in health insurance in the U.S. occurred during World War II. The National War Labor Board froze wages, and employers began using health insurance as a way to attract and retain scarce workers. Health benefits were a means to get around wage controls. Because workers' health benefits were not subject to income tax or Social Security payroll taxes, as were cash wages, unions joined in the support of this form of compensation.

In 1945, Harry Truman was the first president to advocate for universal health insurance. He pushed for a single health insurance system that would cover all classes of people, and he supported investment in hospitals, medical research and education, and public health programs. In an effort to gain the support of organized medicine, Truman promised physicians higher incomes and no changes in the organization of medical practice. The American Medical Association (AMA) proposed instead an expanded system of voluntary insurance and mounted a campaign exhorting physicians to resist the Truman plan as an attempt to make doctors subservient to government-controlled medicine. The AMA was able to turn public opinion, which initially supported the concept of universal compulsory insurance, against Truman's proposal.

Once employer-sponsored health insurance began to cover more people in the U.S., it became increasingly popular. As medical expenses increased, insurance became a greater necessity. Expanded insurance coverage increased compensation without additional taxes, and it provided vital financial protection if hospitalization was necessary. The benefits to employers became codified as well. The Revenue Act of 1954 defined employers' contributions to health plans as tax-exempt and clarified that these were deductible business expenses. Recognizing that the burgeoning system was leaving out many workers, President Eisenhower proposed, but failed to achieve, market reforms in 1956.

These developments formed the foundation of the U.S. system of health insurance — a voluntary system under which employers offer health insurance as a strategy to attract and retain employees, and employees are given the choice of participating or not in their employer's plan. In the unionized workplace, unions negotiate employer support for health benefits. In some cases, union members must join the health plan operated by their union.

Although the burgeoning system of employer-sponsored coverage addressed the needs of employed persons and often their dependents as well, it left uncovered the elderly and the nonworking population. Services to uninsured persons were sometimes available through a patchwork of public health facilities and charity health organizations. Hospitals received some payment from federal welfare grants channeled through the states for this purpose.

President John F. Kennedy made Medicare a major election issue in 1960, but it was not until Lyndon Johnson achieved a landslide victory, accompanied by Democratic control of Congress, that another defining step was taken in the history of health insurance coverage. In 1965, Congress amended the Social Security Act to implement Medicare for the elderly and Medicaid to help states pay for health services for their very low-income parents and children.

After the implementation of Medicare and Medicaid, President Richard Nixon proposed a Comprehensive Health Insurance Plan that would cover all citizens under one of three programs: a mandated employer-sponsored insurance, an improved Medicaid program, or a new Medicare program. His plan failed to pass, although he did succeed in signing into law the Health Maintenance Organization (HMO) Act of 1973, which accelerated the development of HMOs. President Jimmy Carter proposed phasing in health insurance coverage with new requirements for employers and a new federal program to replace Medicaid to cover all low-income individuals in addition to the elderly and disabled. Debated during an economic downturn, this plan also failed. In 1992, Bill Clinton was elected with an apparent mandate to reform the system of health care coverage in the midst of a recession and an expanding uninsurance epidemic. His complicated plan to reform the health care system and to implement universal coverage was attacked by a broad range of health care special interest groups and sank under its own weight.

In 1997, Congress, skittish about the politics of proposals for large-scale change, enacted the State Children's Health Program (SCHIP) to address what it considered a very vulnerable group among the uninsured — 10 million children who did not have coverage through their parents.

With the course set by the rapid growth of employer-sponsored health insurance after World War II and the implementation of public programs for the elderly, poor, and disabled in the 1960s, the U.S. took a distinctly different direction from Canada, Australia, New Zealand, Japan, and the European welfare states. In the postwar period, other advanced countries implemented a variety of models of health care delivery and financing, all with universal coverage and all planned and guided by their version of a Ministry of Health. In contrast, the U.S. fostered growth of an employer-sponsored system with tax incentives that are out of view of public debate and limited the authority of the Secretary of Health and Human Services to the public programs (Medicare, Medicaid, and SCHIP). Compared with the systems of other advanced countries, the U.S. performs better in terms of personal choice (for those with coverage) and the development and dissemination of technological and scientific advances. However, the U.S. performs more poorly in terms of cost and the number of people covered.

Throughout the 20th century, universal health insurance emerged as a possibility only to be defeated. Although the circumstances vary with each try, a combination of resistance by powerful health care interest groups and disagreement among the advocates contributed to failure to forge the legislation necessary to make it a reality.

Health insurance at the beginning of the 21st century

Health insurance is financed by purchasers. In the U.S., purchasers are employers, government (federal, state, and local), and individuals. Figure 18.1 is a chart displaying the sources of health insurance for people in the U.S. in 2001.

Many persons report more than one type of coverage. For example, Medicare beneficiaries often have supplemental retiree health benefits as well as Medicare, and a disabled child might be covered under both a parent's employer-sponsored coverage and Medicaid. The following sections discuss each of the major types of health insurance coverage.

Employer-sponsored health insurance

In the U.S., employer-sponsored health insurance covers 175 million people, and is therefore the most common form of health insurance. This is the source of health insurance for two thirds of the population under 65 years of age. Employer-sponsored insurance includes coverage of workers and their dependents, early retirees, and retired Medicare beneficiaries.

No federal or state laws require that private employers provide health insurance to their employees. Employers offer health insurance in order to attract and retain employees, and union contracts typically require that

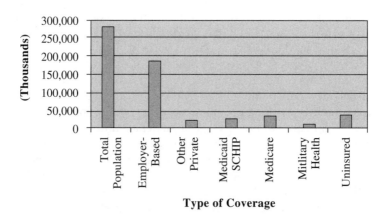

Figure 18.1 Health insurance coverage in the U.S., 2001. (From the U.S. Census Bureau, *Health Insurance Coverage: 2001*, September 2002.)

employers heavily subsidize union member health benefits. Consequently, because of the infinite variety of types of employers and employees, employer-sponsored health insurance varies according to each company or business. Each employer determines which employees to cover, whether to cover the employee's dependents, whether to cover retirees, the type and scope of benefits to pay for, and how much of the cost of the insurance the employee (active or retired) should bear. Because health insurance is regulated by the states, different states have specific requirements regarding benefit packages, marketing of health plans, handling of consumer complaints, and a variety of other factors related to financial stability and quality assurance.

The largest companies (5000 or more employees) typically have a department of specialists to analyze employees' utilization of health services; create different benefit packages; and negotiate with hospitals, physicians, and other professionals to provide care. Large employers (1000 or more employees) are large enough to have health benefits managers who make the decisions about health benefits for employees. Most large companies, however, split the administrative responsibilities between their in-house benefits department and insurance companies. Often with the assistance of employee benefits consulting firms, the in-house staff determines the benefit packages to offer, establishes the cost-sharing options for employees, and explains the choices to employees. It hires insurance companies to administer the health benefits: send out identification cards, answer questions, and pay claims. Employees receive an identification card with the logo of a large insurance company, but, in fact, their own employer may assume the risk for whatever claims their employees incur, plus an administrative fee. Companies that assume this risk self-insure. By assuming the financial risk for their employee's health benefits, they are exempt from state insurance regulations and are subject to less onerous federal regulations applicable to employee benefits generally.

Midsize companies (200 to 999 employees) usually cannot afford this overhead and level of financial risk, and they rely on insurance companies to assume the risk for their employee health benefits. Health insurance companies charge for assuming this risk and adjust premiums accordingly. Consequently, premiums are higher for midsized companies than for larger ones. Midsized employers usually have a health benefits manager who negotiates with insurance companies licensed to market in their geographic area to offer one or more products to their employees. The health plans typically have a menu of basic plans, consisting of a standard benefit package with options related to a having a restricted choice of providers (less costly) or greater choice of providers (more costly). The negotiations focus on the options the health insurance company offers for the employer to split the cost of coverage with employees. Midsize employers also negotiate whether to offer a rider, an additional benefit, such as prescription drugs, dental care, or eyeglasses, not included in the basic benefit package.

Employees typically contribute toward the cost of their health benefits through cost sharing. Because of the rising cost of health insurance, and to increase awareness of the cost of health insurance among employees, employers of all sizes are having their employees contribute more toward the expense of health care coverage. These contributions are in the form of premium payments, deductibles, and copayments. Under premium payments, an employee contributes toward the monthly premium usually through a payroll deduction. Under deductibles, the employee (or an insured dependent) must incur a fixed dollar amount for specific services (such as hospitalization or physician visits) before the insurance pays the remaining cost of services. A copayment is an amount that the provider collects from the insured every time services are rendered. Common examples are copayments for every physician visit, home health visit, or emergency room visit.

Small employers (2 to 99 workers) rely on brokers to fulfill the administrative functions filled by human resource departments at midsize and larger employers. Brokers are independent agents who receive commissions from insurers whose products they sell. Brokers obtain quotes from insurers for different benefit packages, assist in explaining the benefit packages and cost-sharing options to employees, and help enroll employers in plans. They often assist with solving problems such as denied claims.

When a company offers health insurance, not all workers get covered. Employers often set waiting periods for new employees and minimum work hours for established workers before they can be covered. Some workers choose not to enroll because they consider their share of the premium to be prohibitive, or they might be covered through a spouse who works for a different employer.

The cost of employer-sponsored health insurance continues to escalate. According to the Kaiser Family Foundation's employer health benefits annual survey in 2002, the average monthly premium for insuring workers was $255 for single coverage ($3060 annually) and $663 for family coverage ($7954 annually). This was a 12.7% increase over the previous year. Coverage is more expensive for small employers than larger ones. The smaller the employer, the less likely it is for employees to have a choice of plans. Employees pay more toward their health insurance and health care in the form of contributions toward premiums, deductibles, and copayments. When the economy weakens and health insurance premiums rise, more employers drop health insurance coverage for their workers.

The system of employer-sponsored coverage profoundly influences job decisions by U.S. workers. Employer-sponsored health insurance is not portable; that is, employees cannot keep the same health coverage at the same price when they leave an employer. Many employees find themselves in a job lock because they or a family member has a serious medical problem. Leaving the workforce or changing jobs can mean facing a waiting period for coverage, denial of coverage for preexisting conditions, or the inability to obtain any coverage. Many workers postpone retirement until they can be covered by Medicare at 65 years of age.

The federal Health Insurance Portability and Accountability Act (HIPAA) attempts to address some of the lapses in coverage faced when employees change or lose their jobs. HIPAA requires health insurers to limit preexisting condition exclusion periods that exclude coverage of preexisting health conditions for new enrollees. HIPAA requires health insurance companies to make all the small group products available to small employers, regardless of their claims experience or health status of employees. HIPAA also requires health insurance companies to accept certain individuals for individual policies, regardless of their health status and without any exclusion period for preexisting medical conditions. Finally, HIPAA expanded protections against loss of coverage due to high utilization of medical services by prohibiting the termination of group or individual coverage except in cases of fraud or failure to pay premiums.

The impact of HIPAA on access to insurance coverage has been severely limited because it does not regulate the premiums that can be charged by health insurance companies. Although coverage may theoretically be accessible to persons regardless of their claims history, health status, or preexisting conditions, the premiums set by health insurers for new and renewing enrollees are often unaffordable.

There has been a dramatic shift in the type of plans in which workers with employer-sponsored health insurance are enrolled. Figure 18.2 displays the change that has occurred since the late 1980s, when the majority of covered workers were enrolled in conventional indemnity insurance plans.

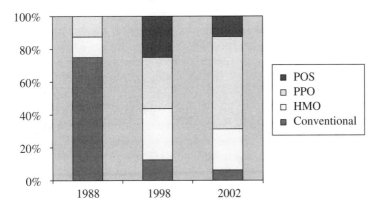

Figure 18.2 Type of health plan for workers with employer-sponsored coverage (From the Kaiser Family Foundation and HRET, *Employer Health Benefits, 2002: Annual Survey,* Menlo Park, CA: The Henry J. Kaiser Family Foundation, 2002.)

Under indemnity insurance, insurers pay a predetermined portion of the providers' fees. There are few restrictions on what a provider can charge and what the insurer will pay for. More than half the workers are now enrolled in preferred provider organizations (PPOs), a less restrictive form of managed care. About one quarter of workers select HMOs. Only 5% are enrolled in conventional indemnity insurance plans.

Individual coverage

In the U.S., over 16 million people purchase their basic health coverage on their own. These purchasers include individuals who are self-employed, unemployed, and not eligible for a public health insurance program. They also include persons who are not eligible for their employer's coverage or their employer does not offer health insurance.

Nearly half of the individual purchasers have access to group coverage through professional organizations, nonprofit associations, or former employers. An estimated 8.6 million persons purchase this coverage in what is called the individual health insurance market.

Because the states regulate the health insurance industry, there are 50 different markets for individual health insurance. The extent of regulation in each state determines the number and types of policies that can be sold to individuals. The more types of policies allowed, the more insurers tend to segment the market and target groups with different expectations of their use of services. The result is high premiums for people who expect to have high medical costs and low premiums for persons who consider themselves healthy. For example, a policy might exclude maternity care or prescription drugs, or both, to keep the premium low. Alternatively, a policy that offers unlimited hospitalization, physician visits, home health care, and prescription coverage will be considerably more expensive.

Insurance carriers that serve this market are afraid of adverse selection, the situation that occurs when people who expect to have high medical costs are more likely to purchase health insurance than people who expect to have low costs. If an insurer enrolls a disproportionate number of high-cost people relative to the premium charged, it can spell financial ruin for the company. Insurance companies compete by minimizing their risk of enrolling high-cost members or charging higher premiums to compensate for the expected risk. To the extent possible within the state's regulatory environment, insurance companies implement a variety of measures to avoid high-cost enrollees. These strategies include refusing to issue policies to persons with a history of medical problems, excluding coverage for preexisting conditions, and emphasizing relatively inexpensive preventive services while limiting other services (e.g., mental health and substance abuse treatment). Insurers tailor deductibles to different groups, and they actively market to persons likely to be at lower risk (e.g., the self-employed) vs. those with anticipated higher costs (e.g., the unemployed or early retirees).

In states where there are regulations to limit risk selection of individuals, there might be requirements for some form of community rating. Pure community rating sets premium rates based on the actual cost of health care for all subscribers in a specific geographic area (e.g., a state or region of a state). The purest form of community rating prohibits any variation in insurance premium rates based on an individual's or one employer group's claims experience. Modified forms of community rating allow premium rate setting based on age, sex, family composition, and industry classification, still prohibiting setting rates for a particular individual or employer group based on their anticipated claims experience. Forms of community rating attempt to pool more people with varying kinds of risks and reduce premiums for persons with greater expected medical expenses. However, the result is typically that persons who perceive themselves as being low risk believe the insurance is priced too high for their needs and drop out of the market, leaving the market composed of higher-cost individuals. Similarly, experiments by states to create pools for high-risk individuals have not been successful in making insurance more available to low-income individuals with chronic illness. The funds are usually underfunded and unable to reduce premiums to an affordable level.

Despite some reforms, many states allow insurers to medically underwrite enrollees and experience rate premiums. Underwriting involves the process of selecting, classifying, and pricing premiums for groups of people with the same expected medical costs. Experience rating involves setting premiums based on historical utilization of medical services. The combination of selection practices and experience rating allows insurers in most states to charge low premiums to younger, healthier people while older or chronically ill people usually face rates they cannot afford.

With the dramatic changes in the labor market, particularly the shift from manufacturing to retail and service jobs and from lifelong positions with a single company to freelance and independent contract work, there is increasing interest in making individual health insurance more comprehensive and affordable for persons who are self-employed or whose employer does not offer health insurance. However, policy analysts who study the individual market propose several mechanisms to balance the interests of low-risk and high-risk people as well as persons of varying income levels. These include regulating the number and type of policies that can be offered, subsidies for individuals to purchase insurance, and payments to insurance companies to compensate for individuals with high medical costs. The goal of these proposals is to have general taxpayers assume the risk of persons with higher medical costs and not low-risk persons with low costs who purchase their health insurance in the individual market.

Medicaid

Medicaid has evolved far beyond its original concept in 1965, which was to provide federal support for state medical welfare programs. At present,

Medicaid covers over 40 million people in the U.S. and accounts for more than 15% of national health care spending. Medicaid is the largest health insurance program in the U.S. in terms of the number of enrollees. In 1998, Medicaid paid for one third of all births, half of nursing home care, and the health care for 25% of children under the age of five.

In addition, Medicaid has become the financing mechanism for many persons and conditions considered uninsurable by the commercial market (employer-sponsored or individual). Medicaid covers persons living with HIV/AIDS, persons infected with tuberculosis, and the chronically disabled. Medicaid provides support for managed care systems and community-sponsored, long-term care arrangements for persons with physical and mental disabilities. It provides supplemental insurance coverage for low-income Medicare beneficiaries and coverage for persons with disabilities who are able to work if they have adequate medical support.

Medicaid is a joint federal–state program. Each state administers its own program within broad guidelines established by Congress and monitored by the Center for Medicare and Medicaid (CMS). Within federal parameters, the states set their own financial eligibility criteria for enrollment, and the scope, type, amount, and duration of services covered in their Medicaid program. There is tremendous variation among the states along all these dimensions. A few states have fairly generous eligibility criteria and have expanded significantly on the minimum set of benefits that must be offered. Most states have very stringent criteria for eligibility, and each state's Medicaid benefits package reflects the state's approach to limit benefits within statutory and regulatory protections for beneficiaries.

Medicaid is funded by both the federal government and the states. The federal government pays each state according to a formula, covering 50 to 80% of a state's approved Medicaid program expenditures. The funding is open ended: the more the state spends, the more federal matching dollars it draws down. Medicaid is the second largest budget item in state budgets.

Medicaid is an entitlement program, meaning that any individual who meets the eligibility criteria must be allowed to enroll immediately and receive prompt medical assistance. Eligibility is both categorical and means tested. Individuals must fit into a category of persons eligible for Medicaid, as well as demonstrate their lack of means by disclosing personal financial information. Categories of eligibility include persons whom Congress has historically viewed as deserving of public medical welfare. These include the lowest-income families with dependent children on cash welfare programs, families in which a parent is making the transition from welfare to work, low-income pregnant women, low-income children, and low-income elderly and disabled. Single adults, childless couples, illegal immigrants, and many legal immigrants are excluded from state Medicaid programs unless the state chooses to fund their coverage without federal support.

The income standard often used by the federal and state governments to determine eligibility for Medicaid is the federal poverty level (FPL).

Income eligibility standards for various categories of Medicaid are set as percentages of the FPL, e.g., 100% FPL, 125% FPL, or 250% FPL. In 2002, the FPL for a family of three was $15,020. Some categories of Medicaid also require that individuals meet an asset test, which measures the value of savings accounts and personal property. Together, the income test and the asset test constitute means testing for many categories of Medicaid.

Since 1997, when Congress separated Medicaid from the cash benefit welfare program, no one is automatically enrolled in Medicaid. Individuals must apply to be covered by Medicaid. Besides falling into one of the eligible categories, individuals who apply for Medicaid must meet financial eligibility criteria established by their state within federal guidelines. In many states, these criteria are extremely restrictive. Parents who work full time at the minimum wage and have dependent children are eligible for Medicaid in only one third of the states. Although Medicaid is the main insurance program for low-income persons, it in fact covers only 44% of persons below the FPL ($15,020 for a family of three in 2002).

By law and regulation, each state Medicaid program must provide more extensive coverage than that provided by commercial insurance plans. Medicaid prohibits, or severely restricts, almost all the mechanisms used by commercial insurers to control costs, such as cost sharing, exclusions for preexisting conditions, limitations on mental health and substance abuse services, and denial of services if significant improvement cannot be demonstrated. For children, state Medicaid programs must cover services that foster growth, development, and the prevention of disability, and not only the treatment of illness or injury.

Since the 1980s, to control Medicaid expenditures and to obtain more value for public funds, states have required that Medicaid beneficiaries enroll in managed care plans. In 2001, 57% of Medicaid beneficiaries were enrolled in some form of managed care. Because Medicaid payments to managed care organizations are based on historically low provider payments under the fee-for-service Medicaid program, states find it increasingly difficult to attract and retain commercial managed care organizations as contractors. Commercial managed care organizations, whose primary focus is to market to employer groups and organize services for an employed population, often have difficulty managing services for the Medicaid beneficiaries, who frequently have more complex health and social needs as well as literacy and linguistic barriers. Almost half the Medicaid beneficiaries enrolled in managed care are served by plans that specialize in organizing services for the Medicaid population.

State Children's Health Insurance Program (SCHIP)

Although a separate program, the SCHIP is closely linked to Medicaid. In 1997, Congress passed SCHIP to address the glaring problem of 10 million children in the U.S. being uninsured. Created shortly after the failure of the Clinton health plan, SCHIP was designed to cover uninsured poor and near-poor children whose parents earn too much to qualify for Medicaid.

Like Medicaid, SCHIP is administered by the CMS. It is also a joint federal–state program, with the federal government matching state expenditures at a rate more favorable than under the Medicaid program. Similar to Medicaid, SCHIP is administered by the states under broad federal parameters.

With SCHIP, Congress was intent on not creating another entitlement program and on giving states greater flexibility with benefits and cost sharing than they have under Medicaid. Consequently, states were given the option of participating in SCHIP by expanding their Medicaid programs, creating a separate child health program, or a combination of the approaches. During the implementation of SCHIP, states decided to develop SCHIP as an expansion of their Medicaid program or to create SCHIP more along the lines of a commercial insurance product. States choosing to expand their Medicaid program must follow all the Medicaid rules regarding eligibility determination, benefits, and prohibition of cost sharing. States choosing to implement a separate program can offer a more limited benefit package, require cost sharing from parents, and impose a cap on enrollment.

Therefore, like Medicaid, there is tremendous variability among the states in the reach, scope, and success of SCHIP in covering previously uninsured children. Nearly all states now cover children at least to 150% of the FPL, with a few states expanding coverage to 350% of FPL. SCHIP has also equalized coverage among children of different ages, so that all children under the age of 19 years have the same benefit package. Previously, under Medicaid, only the youngest children were eligible for coverage but slightly older school-age children in the same family were not. Some states have also taken advantage of a special provision under SCHIP and cover the parents of children enrolled in SCHIP. As of 2002, nearly 4 million children were enrolled in SCHIP. This enrollment has reduced the number of uninsured children by about 1 million. SCHIP enrollment has facilitated the enrollment in Medicaid of more Medicaid-eligible children and has buffered the erosion of family coverage under many employer-sponsored health plans.

Taken together, SCHIP and Medicaid are the health insurance safety net for children in the U.S. According to the Kaiser Family Foundation, the majority of children in low-income families (below 200% of the FPL) are eligible for either Medicaid or SCHIP. As of 2001, 8.5 million children remain uninsured, nearly all being eligible for SCHIP or Medicaid. Special challenges exist with the enrollment of immigrant children and simplifying the enrollment and reenrollment processes for all eligible children.

Medicare

Medicare is the federal health insurance program that covers U.S. people over age 65 and persons with permanent disabilities. In 2001, it covered 39 million persons. The vast majority (87%) of the 39 million Medicare beneficiaries are 65 years and older. Five million Medicare beneficiaries are younger adults with disabilities or end-stage renal disease.

Medicare is an entitlement program and serves all eligible beneficiaries regardless of income or medical history. Like Social Security, Medicare is based on a system of social insurance. Medicare is composed of two programs. Medicare Part A covers inpatient care in hospitals and skilled nursing facilities. It also covers hospice care and some home health care. Part A is financed by a 1.45% payroll tax paid by both employees and employers (2.9% for self-employed persons). Current employers and employees pay for the health care of current Medicare beneficiaries, with the expectation that when they reach age 65 they will receive the same benefits. In the U.S., when people turn 65 years of age, they are automatically eligible for Medicare's Part A, and they do not have to pay for the hospital insurance if they, or a spouse, paid Medicare taxes when they were working.

Medicare Part B is a voluntary form of insurance, and beneficiaries choose whether to enroll in this part of Medicare. Part B is financed partly by a premium charged to the beneficiary ($54/mo in 2002) and typically is deducted from the beneficiary's Social Security check. The rest of Part B funding comes from general federal tax revenues. Medicare Part B helps cover physicians' services, outpatient hospital care, and some other medical services not covered under Part A. Nearly 95% of Medicare beneficiaries choose to enroll in Part B because the federal government pays for 75% of the premium cost. Medicaid pays the Part B premium for low-income elderly.

Medicare covers a broad range of basic health care services. However, its benefit package has changed little since it was first implemented, except for the addition of some preventive services. Medicare does not cover outpatient prescription drugs or long-term care. Both Part A and Part B have high cost-sharing requirements (deductibles and copayments). Most beneficiaries have some form of supplemental coverage to help pay for the gaps in coverage. Sources of supplemental coverage include employer retiree benefits, Medicaid for low-income beneficiaries, or purchase of an individual, private Medigap policy. All these forms of supplemental coverage cover expenses not paid by Medicare. Despite the commonness of supplemental coverage, 27% of Medicare beneficiaries lacked prescription drug coverage in 1998. Medicare beneficiaries over 65 years of age spent an average of 22% of their income on health insurance premiums and health care services in 2000. The elderly with no supplemental coverage spent about 44% of their income on health care in 2000.

Medicare has played a key role in reducing poverty among the elderly since it was established in 1965. However, the growing role of medications in preventing and treating illness results in high out-of-pocket spending or unfilled prescriptions for beneficiaries without adequate prescription coverage. Further, drug coverage is predicted to decline further with the erosion of retiree health benefits and the rise of Medigap premiums. A major challenge facing Medicare is the expansion of benefits while controlling the costs of the program.

Medicare has had mixed success with encouraging HMOs to participate in Medicare and encouraging beneficiaries to select an HMO over the original Medicare program. The Medicare + Choice (also called Part C) program allows Medicare beneficiaries to enroll in a managed care plan. By joining a Medicare + Choice plan, beneficiaries usually have reduced cost sharing and often receive extra benefits, such as more preventive services, case management or care coordination, or prescription drugs. Under the Medicare + Choice, beneficiaries allow Medicare to collect the monthly Part B premium, and they may pay a premium charged by the plan in exchange for additional benefits. Medicare pays the plan a monthly premium for each beneficiary enrolled.

During most of the 1990s, Medicare enrollment in HMOs expanded rapidly. However, in 1999, plans began to withdraw from Medicare + Choice, forcing 500,000 beneficiaries to return to the original Medicare by 2002. Plans stated that they withdrew because of inadequate payment and heavy administrative requirements. In 2001, 14% of Medicare beneficiaries were enrolled in Medicare HMOs.

There is widespread agreement that Medicare needs to be modernized in terms of its benefits, administration, and financing. Designed to meet acute medical needs, the program requires restructuring to promote prevention, address the prevalence of chronic illness, and coordinate services for beneficiaries with multiple chronic conditions. Many administrative reforms have been recommended to allow Medicare to expand its customer service capacity (to beneficiaries, providers, and health plans), update purchasing strategies, promote evidence-based clinical practices, offer multiple products, improve quality, and take greater advantage of the Internet and other technological innovations.

From its inception in 1966, Medicare's eligible population doubled in size by 2000, and is projected to double again by 2030. This growth places enormous pressure on the two trust funds that finance Medicare. Congress has the challenge of improving benefits and protecting Medicare's most vulnerable beneficiaries while restricting overall program expenditures and securing financing of the program. The options facing Congress include some combination of cutting payments to providers, raising taxes, reducing benefits, and asking beneficiaries to pay more. Because of the popularity of the Medicare program with beneficiaries and the power of elder voters, Congress has tended to insulate beneficiaries from greater out-of-pocket costs and chosen to reduce provider payments and freeze payments to health plans.

Managed Care

Managed care is the complex mix of organizational, clinical, and financial activities that ensure the provision of appropriate health care services in a cost-effective manner. The term has taken on many meaning to patients, providers, and politicians. However, in its ideal form, managed care works to ensure that the appropriate service is provided at the appropriate time in the appropriate place. There are types of managed care organizations and delivery systems, and there are also specific managed care tools that can be applied in traditional settings to move a service, program, or delivery system further along the continuum from fee-for-service to managed care.

Managed care was initially embraced to counter the escalating costs and distorted incentives in the fee-for-service system. Under the fee-for-service health care, a physician, hospital, or other health practitioner charges separately for each patient encounter or service rendered. Expenditures increase if the fee itself increases, if more units of service are provided, or if more expensive services are substituted for less expensive ones. In the U.S., the fee-for-service system has historically favored institutional care over community-based care, acute care over preventive care, and medical intervention over patient education and self-care.

The best-known form of managed care, HMOs, evolved to give greater emphasis to early and preventive care and to control costs. With varying degrees of success, HMOs have implemented the original ideal of early identification of health concerns, reducing financial barriers to preventive care, and coordination of care when illness or injury occurs. In their ideal form, HMOs take a population-based approach to health services delivery, proactively assessing the health needs of enrollees and promoting services at the individual, provider, and community level.

HMOs implement this model by requiring that members select a primary care physician to coordinate their care, including referrals to specialists and other health practitioners. They typically put in place financial incentives to physicians for providing health screenings and other preventive services. HMOs also limit their provider networks in order to channel referrals to practitioners and facilities that agree to certain criteria related to access, cost, and quality. The HMO itself takes active responsibility in identifying enrollees' health needs, reminding enrollees when they are due for preventive health services, coordinating care, and providing health education directly to members.

The backlash that has occurred in the U.S. against managed care resulted when some managed care organizations emphasized cost containment almost exclusively. Highly publicized stories about denied care and patients being forced to leave the hospital before it was safe for them to do so have engendered support for a Patient's Bill of Rights and have slowed the growth of enrollment in HMOs in employer-sponsored plans. In 1996, 31% of covered workers selected HMOs, and by 2002 this percentage dropped to 26%, a level that appears to have stabilized.

Preferred provider organizations

Preferred provider organizations (PPOs) are now the most popular form of health insurance among persons with employer-sponsored health insurance.

More than half (52%) of covered workers are enrolled in PPOs. PPOs are entities composed of hospitals, physicians, and other providers that market themselves to purchasers (typically employers). PPOs offer some of the advantages of HMOs, particularly coverage for preventive services, but enrollees do not have to select a primary care physician and can refer themselves to specialists. PPOs are less expensive than indemnity insurance plans, because there is a defined network of providers that offer discounted rates. Enrollees have a choice of using the PPO network or going outside the network, but there are financial incentives to use PPO providers.

Point of service plans

Point of service (POS) plans are available with some large employers who offer employees a choice of plans (e.g., HMO, PPO, and fee-for-service). Subscribers can select among different plans when they need health services rather than locking themselves into one model. The cost-sharing arrangements differ with each plan, with the costs associated with care through the HMO being lowest and costs under fee-for-service being highest.

Primary care case management

Primary care case management (PCCM) is a form of managed care used in Medicaid. It is most common in sparsely populated areas where there are no HMOs available to contract with the state. PCCMs are physicians or groups with arrangements with physicians that contract with the state Medicaid agency to coordinate and monitor the use of primary care services by enrolled beneficiaries. PCCM contracts cover less than the full set of Medicaid benefits and typically involve minimal financial risk.

Managed care tools

Despite widespread dissatisfaction with tight restrictions on care and provider choice under managed care, private managed care organizations have developed many innovative tools that are considered promising both to control costs and improve quality for selected patients, procedures, or diagnoses. Many of these tools can be adapted by any purchaser, insurer, or provider of health care services.

Managed care financial incentives

Managed care organizations intentionally implement payment mechanisms to achieve predictable and stable expenditures. Capitation is the method of paying providers a fixed monthly amount for each enrollee. The payment amount does not change according to the amount or type of services provided. Capitation payments can be made to primary care physicians for primary care services, to specialty groups for specialty services, or to entities providing laboratory, radiology, or behavioral health services. While capitation protects against over-utilization, it raises concerns about under-utilization. Increasingly, capitation arrangements are accompanied by additional payment for achieving other indicators success, e.g., high immunization rates, mammography rates, extended office hours, participation in continuing education programs.

Other financial incentives include bonuses for conservative practice style, usually in conjunction with incentives for quality, access, and patient satisfaction. Still another mechanism is for physicians to share some of the financial risk for hospital care.

The appropriateness of financial incentives to control health care costs and improve quality is a subject of great interest to health policymakers and health services researchers. A consensus on appropriateness of types and degrees of financial incentives is still evolving.

Managed care administrative cost controls

If there are no incentives in the method of payment for providers to practice conservatively, managed care organizations typically implement forms of administrative oversight to control costs. This usually involves prior authorization of elective admissions to hospitals; ongoing review of the hospital stays; and prior authorization of expensive services, e.g., radiology scans, or services particularly sensitive to provider-generated demand, such as pain management clinics. Much of the criticism about managed care has centered on the manner in which prior authorization has been practiced, i.e., applying it to all referrals to specialists. Most managed care entities have cut back on the use of prior authorization and now target this tool to certain conditions, procedures, or providers in which data indicate the potential for unnecessary utilization.

Culture of physician practice

Some medical groups have developed a culture of efficiency as an alternative to financial incentives and administrative controls. Building or transforming the practice culture requires a tight knit medical group wherein there is a willingness to incorporate cost efficiency throughout the entire practice.

Demand management

Demand management is an evolving managed care tool. Usually implemented at the health plan level, the techniques include strategies to identify enrollees with specific problems or conditions and intervene early with education, referrals, and coordination of care to assure appropriate use of health services. Some plans operate telephone or computer helplines staffed by health professionals and use incoming calls as an opportunity to screen for health needs or remind patients about preventive health practices. Another technique is to conduct outgoing calls to new members to identify those with pregnancy, disabilities, or chronic illness to facilitate early intervention and case management. These contacts may be followed by mailing health educational materials, video or audio tapes, or enrolling in a specific disease management program in which arrangements are made for home visits or nurses call enrollees at home to assure that they are completing specific self-care activities.

Data analysis and provider profiling

Managed care plans have learned to "mine" claims data, looking for members who have elevated lead blood levels, pregnancy tests, diagnoses of chronic disease, or are filling medications no longer considered efficacious. These are opportunities to intervene with both members and providers to improve access to preventive services, educational programs, and state-of-the-art clinical care.

Many managed care entities have developed a system of profiling physicians in which their patterns of providing and ordering services is compared to a benchmark, usually other physicians of the same type participating in the plan. Typically, these are used to encourage physicians to alter their practice patterns through the influence of peer review and evidence. In some cases, the profiles may be used to require participation in continuing medical education as a condition for continuing participation in the plan.

Clinical practice guidelines

As managed care tools evolved, many health care entities began to develop clinical practice guidelines, usually specific to a specific disease or condition. This responsibility has been increasingly assumed by task forces on various health issues organized by the federal government and national specialty organizations. These are now widely available through professional organizations and the Internet. Most health plans now rely on this national work and focus their resources on disseminating these guidelines and adapting as standards for their own plans.

Pharmacy benefit managers

Pharmacy benefit management companies (PBMs) are private firms hired by health plans, unions, and employers to administer outpatient drug benefits. In the present environment of rising drug costs and utilization and the introduction of new and costlier medications, most purchasers and health plans have turned to PBMs to perform this responsibility. Developing rapidly in the mid-1990s, PBMs now set the standard for management of drug benefits. In the U.S., nearly 200 million Americans, 70% of the population, have their drug benefits managed through a PBM.

PBMs reduce administrative costs of managing drug benefits by using a highly automated environment. According to a study sponsored by the Health Care Financing Administration (HCFA), over 99% of all claims are processed electronically at the pharmacy where the prescription is dispensed, at an average cost of $0.30 to $0.40 per claim.

PBMs use a variety of mechanisms to reduce drug costs, and the following strategies are elaborated in Chapter 19:

- Retail pharmacy discounts
- Formulary development
- Manufacturer rebates
- Therapeutic substitution
- Generic substitution and tiered copayments
- Mail order and internet pharmacy services
- Drug utilization review
- Prior authorization of high-cost drugs or drugs subject to misuse

PBMs produce substantial savings, value, and efficiency in drug benefit programs. Most criticisms of PBMs focus on the use of formularies. There is concern that PBMs select drugs based more on their rebates from pharmaceutical manufacturers than on the efficacy of specific drugs. There is also criticism about the use of therapeutic substitution to enforce formulary compliance. The practices of PBMs are under particular scrutiny because of the prominence they have in managing drug benefits and the potentially even greater role under Medicare and Medicaid programs.

Covering the uninsured

The number of uninsured in the U.S. has persisted and grown during periods of both economic growth and downturn. With workers and their dependents accounting for 80% of the uninsured, there is now broader recognition that the system of employer-sponsored health insurance will not on its own provide coverage to all working people. There are several proposals for expanding health insurance coverage in the U.S. All the proposals attempt to address the challenge of increasing coverage for persons who earn too much to qualify for public programs, who cannot afford individual coverage or cost-sharing requirements of their employer, or whose employer does not offer coverage. The proposals cover the range of strategies and mechanisms, including enrollment in public programs, expanded access to coverage through employers, and tax credits or subsidies to purchase health insurance individually.

Expansion of public programs

Typically, these options propose building on the extensive infrastructure that already exists for Medicare, Medicaid, and the SCHIP and expanding the number of persons covered by these public programs. The options include expanding income thresholds for eligibility, lowering age limits for eligibility (Medicare), raising the age limits (SCHIP), and allowing persons to purchase coverage through these programs at subsidized premiums. They also call for streamlining enrollment in Medicaid and SCHIP so that currently eligible yet uninsured persons obtain coverage. Because Medicaid and SCHIP are operated by the states under federal guidelines and are jointly funded by the state and federal government, these proposals emphasize the involvement and capacity of state governments to design, administer, and support financially.

Proposals to expand employer-sponsored coverage

Because the majority of people in the U.S. obtain their health coverage through their employers, there are many proposals to build on this infrastructure and increase access to employer-sponsored coverage. These proposals include a wide range of suggestions, including both requiring and implementing incentives for employers to offer health insurance, extending access to employer-sponsored coverage for the unemployed and early retirees, forming purchasing pools for small employers, and providing subsidies to small employers and employers with large number of low-wage workers. Also included are proposals that allow the uninsured to buy in to large employer group systems, such as the Federal Employees Health Benefits Program.

Incentives to individuals to purchase health insurance

Because of the problems with job lock, continuity of coverage through employer-sponsored coverage, low eligibility levels for Medicaid and SCHIP, and the inequities perpetuated by the favorable tax treatment of employer-sponsored insurance, several health policy analysts have proposed expanding individuals' ability to select and purchase their own health insurance. These proposals cover a broad range of strategies, including completely delinking employment and the purchase of health insurance, supplementing the expansion of public programs with a system of tax credits for middle-income people, trying to reach all the uninsured through tax credits, and making group insurance rates available to individuals by establishing local or state purchasing pools, health insurance exchanges, or Internet-based brokers. The proposals vary considerably in the extent to which they call for reform of the current individual health insurance market, which is plagued with difficulties.

The problem of underinsurance

An estimated 30 million people in the U.S. are underinsured, i.e., having health insurance coverage less than adequate. As a consequence, these individuals and families experience high out-of-pocket costs (e.g., premium payments, deductibles, and copayments) and maximum benefit limits. Many policies exclude specific services, such as maternity services, mental health services, long-term care, or prescription drugs. Although their problems are not as severe as those without any insurance, the underinsured experience many of the same problems of barriers to care and financial hardship.

Influence of cultural values

Each nation that has implemented universal health insurance has created its system in the context of cultural, political, and economic values. The values held by other advanced countries that support universal health care include a sense of national and community responsibility, social solidarity, universality, equity, acceptance of the role of government, and skepticism about markets in addressing social and human needs. Political and economic values shape the administrative and financial dimensions of their health systems. As a result, each system is unique in its balance of central and local decision-making, the power and role of hospitals and physicians, and the extent to which market forces allocate resources.

In contrast to people in other advanced nations, people in the U.S. value choice, competition, individual and family accountability, and volunteerism, and are skeptical of the government. As in other nations, political and economic forces have further shaped the U.S. health system, specifically the system of health insurance. As a result, people in the U.S. tolerate a three-tiered system of coverage: those with private health insurance, those with public insurance, and those without any coverage. Any reforms are likely to reflect the core values of individual accountability, voluntary participation, and a level of confidence in market forces.

Bibliography

AcademyHealth (2003). *Glossary of Terms Commonly Used in Health Care*. Washington, D.C.: AcademyHealth.

Center for Studying Health System Change (2002). The individual health insurance market. In *Issue Brief: Findings from HSC*. Washington, D.C.: Center for Studying Health System Change.

Claxton, G. (2002). *How Private Insurance Works: A Primer*. Menlo Park, CA: The Henry J. Kaiser Family Foundation.

Conwell, L.J. (2002). *The Role of Health Insurance Brokers*. Washington, D.C.: Center for Studying Health System Change.

Davis, K. (2001). *Universal Coverage in the United States: Lessons from Experience of the 20th Century*. New York: The Commonwealth Fund, p. 4.

Dubay, L., Hill, I. et al. (2002). *Five Things Everyone Should Know about SCHIP*. Washington, D.C.: The Urban Institute.

EBRI (2002). *History of Health Insurance Benefits*. Washington, D.C.: EBRI.

Economic and Social Research Institute (2001). *Covering American: Real Remedies for the Uninsured*. Washington, D.C.: Economic and Social Research Institute, p. 215.

Fronstin, P. (2002). *Sources of Health Insurance and Characteristics of the Uninsured: Analysis of the March 2002 Current Population Survey.* Washington, D.C.: EBRI, p. 30.

Helms, R.B. (1999). The tax treatment of health insurance: early history and evidence, 1940–1970. In *Empowering Health Care Consumers through Tax Reform,* G.-M. Arnett, Ed. Washington, D.C.: American Enterprise Institute, pp. 73–100.

Iglehart, J.K. (1999). The American health care system: Medicaid. *New Engl. J. Med.* 340(5): 403–408.

Iglehart, J.K. (1999). The American health care system: Medicare. *New Engl. J. Med.* 340(4): 317–332.

Institute of Medicine (2001). *Coverage Matters: Insurance and Health Care.* Washington, D.C.: National Academy Press.

Kaiser Commission on Medicaid and the Uninsured (2001a). *Medicaid and Managed Care.* Washington, D.C.: The Henry J. Kaiser Family Foundation.

Kaiser Commission on Medicaid and the Uninsured (2001b). *The Medicaid Program at a Glance.* Washington, D.C.: The Henry J. Kaiser Family Foundation.

Kaiser Commission on Medicaid and the Uninsured (2002a). *Health Coverage for Low-Income Children.* Washington, D.C.: The Henry J. Kaiser Family Foundation.

Kaiser Commission on Medicaid and the Uninsured (2002b). *Health Insurance Coverage in America*: 2000 Data Update. Washington, D.C.: The Henry J. Kaiser Family Foundation.

Kaiser Commission on Medicaid and the Uninsured (2002c). *The Medicaid Resource Book.* Washington, D.C.: The Henry J. Kaiser Family Foundation.

Kaiser Commission on Medicaid and the Uninsured (2002d). *Underinsured in America: Is Health Coverage Adequate.* Washington, D.C.: The Henry J. Kaiser Family Foundation.

Kaiser Family Foundation (2001). *Medicare at a Glance.* Washington, D.C.: The Henry J. Kaiser Family Foundation.

Kaiser Family Foundation (2002). *Medicare + Choice.* Washington, D.C.: The Henry J. Kaiser Family Foundation.

Kaiser Family Foundation and Health Research and Educational Trust (2002). *Employer Health Benefits: 2002 Annual Survey.* Menlo Park, CA: The Henry J. Kaiser Family Foundation.

Meyer, J. and Stepnick, L. (2002). *Portability of Coverage: HIPAA and COBRA.* New York: The Commonwealth Fund.

Mills, R.J. (2002). *Health Insurance Coverage: 2001.* Washington, D.C.: U.S. Census Bureau.

PricewaterhouseCoopers LLP (2001). *HCFA Study of the Pharmaceutical Benefit Management Industry.* Washington, D.C.: Centers for Medicare and Medicaid. Available at www.cms.hhs.gov/researchers/reports/2001/CMS.pdf.

Rosenbaum, S. (2002). Medicaid. *New Engl. J. Med.* 346: 635-640.

Sroka, C. (2000). *CRS Report for Congress: Pharmacy Benefit Managers.* Washington, D.C.: Library of Congress Congressional Research Service.

Starr, P. (1982). *The Social Transformation of American Medicine.* New York: Basic Books.

Swartz, K., Ed. (2000). Special Conference Issue: Strategies to Expand Health Insurance for Working Americans — Strategies to Expand Health Insurance for Working Americans. *Inquiry* 38(2). Conference sponsored by Commonwealth Fund Task Force on the Future of Health Insurance.

Woolhandler, S. and Himmelstein, D.U. (2002). Paying for national health insurance-and not getting it. *Hlth. Aff.* 21(4): 88–98.

U.S. General Accounting Office (2003). *Federal Employees' Health Benefits: Effects of Using Pharmacy Benefit Managers on Health Plans, Enrollees, and Pharmacies.* Washington, D.C.: U.S. GAO.

chapter nineteen

Managed care and the pharmacy benefit

F. Randy Vogenberg

Contents

Managing pharmacy benefits

In the U.S., more than two thirds of workers and their dependents, retired workers, and family members receive health care coverage through employers. Although this represents virtually no change in the employer-covered

0-8493-1446-1/04/$0.00+$1.50
© 2004 by CRC Press LLC

population over several years,[1] several factors affect employer coverage of health care, such as cost trend increases in health benefits, arrival of techno-logical innovations, and shifting marketplace dynamics for all players in the health care system changing the nature of job-based health coverage.

It is hard to recall that just a few decades ago the typical health insurance policy did not include coverage for prescription medications. For a variety of insurance coverage, pricing, and medical–political reasons, medications were considered peripheral parts of treating an illness or injury and not integral components in the treatment continuum. Late in the 20th century, labor unions in the U.S. demanded the inclusion of drug benefits as part of health insurance coverage and employers were forced to comply.

The earliest drug benefit was a component of the major medical policy with coverage effective after an annual deductible had been met. To receive reimbursement, a plan member submitted receipts from the pharmacy for the charges incurred. The contract usually required that the U.S. Food and Drug Administration (FDA) approve the drug, that it be available by pre-scription only, and that a physician or other approved professional prescribe it for treating a medical condition.

In the 1980s, with the availability of more sophisticated, real-time com-puter networks, online access to information made it possible for pharma-cists to check a patient's eligibility for benefits at the point of sale. Pharma-cists could also verify product cost and copayment information. By this time, prescription drug benefits had tripled from 2–3% to 7–10% of the health care benefit dollar, at which point employers were becoming concerned about benefit cost.[2] Interestingly, the amount of money spent on drugs is one area in which the U.S. compares favorably with other nations. Per capita costs for pharmaceuticals are higher in England, Japan, Germany, France, Canada, and Australia than in the U.S.

In the U.S., a variety of individuals or groups purchase and pay for health service, including employers. By definition, the payer is the government, employer, or individual who pays the health care provider for providing health care services. Payers in the private sector include the following:[3]

1. Self-funded employers (large employers who provide their own funding for health care costs)
2. Groups of employers (employer coalitions)
3. Groups of employees (unions)
4. Individual patients who buy private insurance or pay for health care out of pocket.

Increasing drug costs and the affordability of health care continue to be important issues to employers and consumers. Drugs and prescription drug benefits have come a long way. At present, almost everyone recognizes that the appropriate selection and use of pharmaceuticals as part of the overall health care of individuals is an important component of the health care delivery system in the U.S.

Buyer of drugs

Since the inception of medication insurance coverage, there have been major changes in the way prescription drugs are purchased. During that time, payment for prescription medications moved from a consumer-dominant and customer-sensitive environment to a marketplace controlled by a complex process of third-party communications and payments for prescription-medication-related products and services. The direct relationship between the patient and the retail pharmacist has been replaced with a system in which the patient deals with several organizations (e.g., PBM, Health Plan, and the Employer as Plan Sponsor). These organizations frequently focus on population management, pricing formulas, and various global assumptions rather than on actual individual patient care and total benefit cost. The dynamic change in process and funding has resulted in the replacement of the retail-based consumer marketplace with a marketplace that has virtually removed consumers from the purchase decision.

Patients' direct payment for prescriptions has been replaced with third-party purchasers, who are agents for the ultimate payers, the health benefit sponsors (employers). Thus, patients have little knowledge of the total costs of the prescribed medications. As a result, the costs of the medications are hidden from patients because of fixed small dollar copayments or limited coinsurance costs at the point of service.

So who is the buyer of pharmacy services? The buyer has evolved into a combination of the patient, payer (employer or government), and third-party prescription benefit administrator.

Patients, as all consumers, want to receive the most value in products or services for the dollars they spend. Within a prescription drug benefit program, patients, as consumers, want to receive a convenient and effective treatment for the lowest out-of-pocket cost. In addition, they and their physicians expect little hindrance in providing and receiving prescribed treatments. Not encumbered by price they look for the most value, which frequently translates into the latest medication with its perceived greater value. They also want the largest quantity possible and the most medication for each plan copayment or coinsurance cost at the pharmacy.

The benefit plan sponsor, also as a consumer, wants to maintain a healthy workforce without being required to handle time-consuming employee complaints from a benefit program for a reasonable and budget-predictable cost. With all health benefits, when there are two parties who perceive themselves as consumers, there are occasional disagreements as to the best value and right cost for a product or service. Health care is a very personal matter, and with a traditional copayment arrangement there is a large difference in a patient's share of the cost vs. the sponsor's share of the cost. Similarly, there are significant differences between the two consumers in their perception of the value of drug benefit cost vs. its expense.

Seller of drugs

On the other side of the marketplace equation is the seller: the pharmacy, drug wholesaler, or prescription drug manufacturer. Drug manufacturers desire to provide FDA-approved (safe and effective) products developed and manufactured at the lowest possible cost and sell them through the distribution channel at a price that allows for maximum profit. They must sell a product that has a perceived market value equal to or greater than the costs of production, promotion, plus the projected dollars the product makes to the company's anticipated profit.

In the prescription drug marketplace, drug manufacturers have traditionally ignored the traditional consumers of the product and instead focused on the patient's health provider, intermediary, the prescribing physician or clinician in accordance with the need for a prescription under federal law. Physicians and other prescribers are effective agents for the drug manufacturer, because they are more focused on the product's perceived value than the product's cost. Physicians are unaware of the product's cost. Additionally, they are allowed to totally discount the cost since they are provided a supply of "free" samples to give out to their patients so physicians have an added reason to focus on value over cost since they went to provide a patient the best-perceived value available. This dynamic of perspectives allows the manufacturer to effectively remove the drug product cost from the perceived value in the patient decision-making process. This scenario leaves a plan sponsor as the primary payer and the only party with concerns about the actual cost of the products. In other words, the plan sponsor is required to pay the majority of resulting drug product cost without directly being involved, early on, in product value determination.

Other health-benefit-related organizations

Traditionally, the other key players in the prescription drug delivery marketplace have been the prescription claims administrators or pharmacy benefit managers, whose main purpose is to maximize the value of their pharmacy networks as components of drug benefit cost. The pharmacy network contract price, mail order pharmacy contract price, and so on can be negotiated at a more favorable cost along with the relatively inexpensive claim adjudication and detailed and timely drug claim data reporting. This assists plan sponsors with cost management, but still does not address their product value concerns. Because plan sponsors were placed in this reactive market position regarding product value determination, prescription claims administrators began to utilize claims adjudication edits. An example of this type of edit is to confirm that the recipient is eligible for coverage, as well as the formulary status of the prescription drug. These edits were intended to help assure plan sponsors that certain logic-based decisions were made before paying for the covered products, based on their intended plan of coverage. As a result, the cottage industry of prescription claims administrators evolved into the highly profitable pharmacy benefits management (PBM) industry of today.

PBM companies have used the purchasing power of the unsophisticated plan sponsor to negotiate preferred financial arrangements with drug manufacturers and pharmacy providers, and have now refocused the services intended to provide certain value decisions before paying for the products to actually promoting the products more profitable to the PBM.

There are more than 81 national PBM companies. They range in size from industry giants who cover 56 million lives and handle 350 million prescriptions a year to small, specialized PBMs who handle 7000 lives and 80,000 prescriptions per year and might operate on more local or regional levels.

At present, PBMs wield significant influence in the managed prescription drug benefits arena. They are not new, but many people think they are because they have become much more numerous and visible in the last few years.

About pharmacy benefit management firms (PBMs)

A PBM company is an organization that applies managed care principles and procedures to pharmacy benefits to contain costs and improve quality. PBMs vary in size, scope, and sophistication, but perform the same tasks. They might serve as third-party administrators solely for processing claims for payment or they might work with other clients, such as health maintenance organizations (HMOs), preferred provider organizations (PPOs), government agencies, or other third-party administrators (TPAs), as subcontractors to handle more sophisticated claim communications, e.g., drug utilization review online.

PBMs offer and can provide the following services to their various clients:

1. General support and consultative services
2. Claims processing services (including online adjudication, check writing procedures, and overpayment protection procedures)
3. Network support and development (including online access to Internet pharmacies and mail order services)
4. Formulary design, development, implementation, and maintenance
5. Rebate programs
6. Communication support
7. Clinical services
8. Report generation
9. Information services (e.g., eligibility verification, group enrollment processes, provider files)
10. Performance standards

Although PBMs vary in their capabilities and strategic focus, they all use similar techniques to manage prescription drug costs:[4]

- Discounts from the average wholesale price (AWP) and dispensing fees by pharmacies participating in the PBM network. PBMs negotiate discounts averaging 10 to 15% below AWP and dispensing fees from $1.50 to $4.00, regardless of prescription cost (the average dispensing fee is around $2.50).
- Formularies that promote the use of cost-effective drugs without diminishing quality of care.
- Rebates from drug manufacturers whose products are on the PBM's formulary. Rebates are issued based on volume of drugs sold through PBM networks. The percentage of rebate passed along to the employer depends on the number of employees covered or the type of coverage. Not all PBMs offer the same level of rebate savings. The savings range is from 0 to 100%.
- Generic substitution for brand name drugs with generic equivalents. A client can save as much as 20% of the cost of the brand name drug by using generic equivalents.
- Benefit design expertise. PBMs can deliver significant cost savings with the proper plan design. Clients still using an indemnity program can save up to 30% through a well-designed PBM program that mirrors the plan design while adding price discounts and clinical programs to manage program costs and quality. Clients with a PBM program already in place can also save money by refining their program (formulary, quantity limits), updating the plan design (multiple-tier copay), and implementing clinical programs (drug utilization review, DUR, health management).

Simply put, PBMs traditionally control costs by managing the drug's price per unit and the number of units consumed. PBMs offer their services as an inclusive package, on a menu basis, or as a combination customized for a particular client.

PBMs are also characterized by a series of relationships among many stakeholders: payers, providers, consumers, and pharmaceutical companies. Payers include employers, employer coalitions, insurers, managed care organizations, Medicare, and Medicaid. Typically, they pay the net prescription cost and a per claim or transaction fee to the PBM for claim processing. Money and information flow back to the payers in the form of rebates and a variety of utilization reports.

Providers are the pharmacists and physicians. PBMs contract with retail pharmacies to reimburse for drug costs at negotiated discount rates. Claims data — prescription number, date, drug name, quantity dispensed, physician name, and cost — flow back to the PBM. Concurrent drug utilization alerts, such as potential drug interactions or duplicate therapy, are transmitted back to the pharmacy before the prescription is dispensed. Once reviewed by the pharmacist, the claim is then adjudicated and the pharmacist learns from the PBM the amount paid and what copay to collect.

Each person with a prescription drug benefit is a consumer. The PBM maintains an eligibility file and a plan benefit design file against which claims are compared. This allows for the accurate adjudication of the claim according to the benefit and corresponding copayment. Consumers also benefit from the concurrent drug utilization program, which helps prevent drug misadventures.

Pharmaceutical companies provide per prescription rebates on their selective products that are included on the PBMs formulary or preferred drug list. In return, the pharmaceutical companies receive information on the volume of their prescriptions dispensed through the PBM pharmacy network.

Although PBMs perform many of the same claims procedures and price-oriented administrative functions as TPAs, their involvement in the clinical aspects of prescription drug management sets them apart.

Thus, PBM functions can be categorized as either administrative functions or drug use control functions.

The administrative functions include:

1. Establishing and maintaining a network of pharmacy providers
2. Processing claims
3. Designing the pharmacy plan benefit

The drug use control functions are:

1. Developing and maintaining the formulary
2. Performing DURs
3. Providing academic detailing to physicians

PBM service contracting

PBMs typically contract with employers or health plans under one of three contractual models: fee for service, capitation, or shared risk.

Under fee for service, the most common model, a PBM creates a retail pharmacy network and receives a fee for each claim processed, resulting in an average savings of 10 to 15% compared with an unmanaged benefit.

Under capitation, a fixed amount is paid to the PBM in advance (e.g., per member per month), based on past prescription utilization patterns, demographics, and other factors that attempt to balance risk and reward for both the payer and the PBM.

In a shared risk arrangement, both the employer and PBM share the risk as well as the savings. For example, if the cost exceeds the target, the PBM shares the overrun; conversely, if the cost is less than the target, the PBM shares the savings.

How pharmacy benefits are managed as part of a total health care benefit package is explained by a carve-in or carve-out model. The terms *carve-in* and *unified* are applied when prescription drug benefits are part of the general health care package. This reflects the prescription benefits' integration with other health care benefits, as opposed to them being designed and administered separately. Health insurers, such as an HMO or Blue Cross/ Blue Shield, manage the carved-in benefits and are responsible for processing the prescription drug claims. Insurers may choose to handle the claims through their own systems or subcontract that function to a PBM. The lack of flexibility and cost controls in unified programs far outweigh the advantages, particularly in traditional major medical health plans. Because of several factors, drug benefit costs in a traditional major medical environment might be substantially higher than in a separately managed plan. Furthermore, many employers with managed care benefit plans that included prescription drugs have been faced with double-digit premium increases on renewal.[5] Prescription drug costs were cited as the primary reason, along with demand for greater access, benefit mandates, increased use of medical care by an aging population, and continuing efforts by managed care companies to regain profitability.[5] Consequently, many employers choose to separate or "carve out" their prescription benefits in order to better analyze and control expenses in this increasingly complex arena.

The term *carve-out* indicates that administration and management are handled by a specialized PBM company, traditional insurer, or TPA. Carved-out pharmacy benefits provide flexibility, control, and an array of management options to help contain costs and improve quality.

Carve-out programs offer several advantages:[6]

1. It is possible to access point-of-service (POS) benefit validation, eligibility verification, and pricing information and claims submission data when drug benefits are separate.
2. A mail order program can be integrated with retail pharmacy services so that such issues as employee communications and utilization and cost reporting are coordinated.
3. Various plan member cost-sharing arrangements are possible.
4. There is flexibility in terms of payment to the pharmacy. For example, members required to pay the full cost of the drug to their pharmacy and submit paper claims for reimbursement receive the benefit of the contracted pharmacy's discounted rate, or, conversely, pay a $5 co-payment per prescription, with the pharmacy's POS system handling claims processing automatically.

There are two major disadvantages to carve-out programs:

1. In cases where prescription costs are part of the major medical deductible, an employer must pay two administrative service fees: one to the PBM for claims adjudication and another to the medical carrier for claims reimbursement and reporting.

2. A carve-out plan typically pays all pharmaceutical claims because they are filed electronically. A traditional major medical paper-based plan might incur higher costs as a result of the shoebox effect. This is a result of patients paying for prescription drugs, saving and then submitting their receipts for reimbursement at a later date, usually all at the same time and near the end of the year.

Evaluating the pharmacy benefit: auditing performance of PBMs

There are a variety of audits or reviews of services delivered and paid for by the PBM, including the following.[6]

Comprehensive audits measure overall PBM performance over a 1-year period. Retrospective in nature, all prescription claims are audited to determine whether the product dispensed was covered under the plan design, the person was eligible to receive services at the time of sale, the discounts were applied according to contract, dispensing fees were accurate, copays were applied correctly, and so on. PBM clinical services and rebates may also be included in the scope of a comprehensive audit.

Retail network audits are typically conducted on an ongoing basis by the PBM, managed care organization, or a large employer group that contracts directly with chain and independent pharmacies. These audits ensure the validity of prescription claims and curb attempts of fraud and abuse at the pharmacy level.

Repricing audits measure adherence to the contract's financial terms. They require limited data and use an independent source to confirm average wholesale price on the date of service. Discounts are recalculated and compared with the contracted rates, and dispensing fees and copayments are verified on a sample set of claims. Compliance with plan design may also be included in the scope of the audit.

Rebate audits measure the ability of the PBM to obtain and recover rebate amounts and to pass the appropriate portion back to the client according to contract terms.

Performance guarantee audits measure the extent to which the PBM has complied with any performance guarantees included as part of the contract, such as ID card production turnaround time, mail service turnaround time, dispensing accuracy, customer service response time, and member satisfaction.

Operational audits are performed onsite at the PBM and verify that the operational and clinical procedures are in place and being performed as stated. They also verify any operational procedures specific to plan administration.

PBM plan design

The management of prescription medication benefits has evolved with the overall health benefits structure. The processes of medication coverage have similarly evolved to a primarily automated activity via computer systems that has incorporated increasingly sophisticated utilization management capabilities.

Medication therapy costs continue to rise as a percentage vs. prior year(s) and have risen slightly as the total percentage of health care spending overall to 13% of GDP.[7] New drug therapy products continue to enter the marketplace just as other improvements have occurred in the health care delivery system. The resulting changes in care impact the relative component costs of treatment, such as medication therapy.

Managing pharmacy benefits

For cost, quality, and accessibility reasons, pharmacy benefits, like all other employee benefits, are managed. PBM may be defined as a range of organizational activities designed to influence the behavior of prescribers, pharmacists, and patients, with the goal of impacting the cost and use of prescription drug coverage. Drug therapy has become costly, complex, and important enough to justify this organizational oversight, management, and intervention in the drug use process. A number of interrelated parties are involved and affected by the process of PBM:

- Patients (subscribers/enrollees)
- Pharmacies
- Pharmacists
- Prescribers (physicians and others)
- Manufacturers
- Private or public sector (self-funded employers, insurance companies or health plans, and Medicare or Medicaid programs)
- Third-party or PBM organizations

Pharmacy benefit plan design

Benefit plan design refers to the agreement between the employer/payer or the designated plan administrator/manager and the individual enrollees, also referred to as members, subscribers, or patients. Benefit design basics include such issues as what drugs the plan covers (and does not cover), in what quantities, from which pharmacies or other drug sources, and at what out-of-pocket cost to members. Plan design also involves such operational issues as pharmacy reimbursement, claims processing, and utilization review.[8]

The importance of the basic plan design itself cannot be overemphasized. It does not matter whether one is creating a new pharmacy benefits plan, improving an existing one, or preparing to work with a PBM company. If the basic plan is not well thought out and tailored to a company's own needs and circumstances, it will make little difference how effective the other components of benefits management are. All the parts of PBM are interrelated, but the long-term quality and effectiveness of an overall plan begins with how well the benefits are designed.

The ideal pharmacy benefits plan

According to the *National Pharmaceutical Council Prescription Medicine Benefit Program Checklist*,[9] benefits managers and the companies they represent want a pharmacy benefit plan that:

1. Covers medications that are effective in treating patients as well as reducing overall medical costs
2. Allows prescribers the flexibility to select medications that meet the needs of individual patients
3. Gives plan members the freedom to choose a pharmacy that is readily accessible to them
4. Encourages written instruction sheets, medications monitoring, and personalized counseling by the pharmacist
5. Monitors patient compliance with drug therapy
6. Maintains and utilizes patient medication records to prevent unnecessary and potentially harmful drug interactions and other problems (called medication misadventures)
7. Employs strict quality assessment standards
8. Conducts appropriate review of drug utilization
9. Promotes prudent patient utilization of benefits by plan members with strategies that include copayments or plan limitations

Basic plan elements include the following:

1. Member cost share
2. Pharmacy reimbursement
3. Plan limitations, restrictions, and exclusions
4. Provider network
5. Claim processing and administration
6. Data collection and reporting
7. DUR
8. Communication

Characteristics of an effective pharmacy benefit

The overall goal is to create pharmacy benefits that meet employees' needs at a reasonable cost. An effective pharmacy benefit promotes the following features: quality, accessibility, member satisfaction, and efficiency.[9]

Quality involves excellence and meeting expectations. It can be defined in terms of its structure, process, and the outcomes of care. For example, the structure of pharmacy care deals with the adequacy of the personnel, facilities, and technology that provide pharmacy services.

Accessibility refers to minimizing barriers to receiving pharmacy benefits. Other barriers might be issues of transportation or geography.

Efficiency is whether available resources are used wisely; for example, drug therapy is inefficient if unnecessary drugs are prescribed or if only expensive drugs are prescribed.

Member satisfaction involves interpersonal as well as technical aspects of care. Do plan members feel that their drug benefits are of high quality? Are they convenient to access and pay for? Do participating pharmacists treat patients courteously and adequately explain the drugs being dispensed?

Basic plan elements

Cost share

Copayments at the point of service are the most common form of cost sharing. One advantage of copayments is that covered plan members know what their out-of-pocket expenses will be when they pick up their prescriptions, and these amounts are deducted from what the PBM or insurer pays to the pharmacy. For example, if a prescription has a retail price of $50 and the copayment is $15, the pharmacy collects $15 from the member and the remaining $35 from the PBM. Recently, efforts to contain costs and still meet employee expectations for choice have led to the introduction and widespread use of copayment tiers. Copayment tiers offer different levels of cost share for various drug categories. For example, in a classic two-tier copay design, a lower copay such as $5 applies to generic drugs, and a higher copay such as $15 applies to brand-name drugs. This type of arrangement (1) incents members to use generic drugs through use of a lower cost share and (2) helps reduce the cost burden to employers by passing on some of the higher cost of brand name drugs to members. A variation on this is to apply the lower cost share to formulary drugs, both brand and generic, and the higher cost share to nonformulary drugs. The savings to the employer are less, but it lays the foundation for formulary utilization. It also opens the door for rebates as it promotes the use of preferred drugs on the formulary. Rebates are offered by pharmaceutical manufacturers to offset the cost of some single-source brand-name drugs.[8]

The trend currently, however, is the multiple or the most common three-tier copay structure. This approach offers the lowest tier for generics, middle tier for preferred or formulary brand-name drugs, and highest tier for nonpreferred or nonformulary drugs. Used in combination with a formulary, this arrangement helps lower the drug cost for employers while maximizing the member's choice. Another advantage is that drug manufacturers offer a larger rebate when a three-tier copay system is part of the benefit design. At least one plan offers a fourth tier to this type of arrangement for lifestyle or life-enhancing drugs and the more expensive self-injectable bioengineered drugs. Often, the fourth tier uses coinsurance rather than a fixed copayment amount.[1]

Coinsurance maintains the member's portion of the drug cost as a constant percentage. For example, the member will always pay 20% of the prescription drug costs. The payment to the pharmacy for the prescription will vary based on the allowable retail cost for the prescription. The same prescription might have a different cost each time a member purchases it because of price changes (increases or decreases) from the drug manufacturer. Employers look to coinsurance as a means to moderate their increasing drug benefit costs and as a hedge against drug product cost inflation.

Cost sharing affects the total cost of prescription drug benefits in two ways: It affects the amount paid for each prescription, and it also affects utilization. According to the law of demand in economics, as price increases, demand tends to decrease. In the case of drug prescriptions, price is the member's out-of-pocket expense. As cost-sharing (i.e., out-of-pocket expense) increases, utilization decreases.

Cost sharing can also be set up to reward desired behaviors. This is the case with incentives to use generic products, which are usually less expensive than brand-name drugs. Generic products are chemically equivalent to the brand-name (also called the originator or innovator) products, which are protected under patent for, approximately, their first 7 years on the market.

In every state, drug product selection laws and regulations specify means by which the prescriber can mandate the use of a branded product (dispense as written rule, DAW). When the prescriber insists on a brand-name drug, is the patient responsible for paying the price difference between the brand name and the generic drug? The answer depends on the benefit design. Some designs do not hold the patient responsible for a prescriber's decision and do not require that the difference be paid. On the other hand, for plans in which the goal is to encourage the use of generic products, patients might be required to pay the price difference, even though the decision to go with the brand name drug was not theirs. This gives patients plenty of incentive to request that their doctors prescribe generics whenever possible.

Plan limitations, restrictions, and exclusions

Plan limitations, restrictions, and exclusions typically are major cost-containment elements of pharmacy benefits plan designs. Examples include a cap or limit on outpatient drug benefits (usually $2000 a year per member), the formulary or preferred drug list, and a limit on the quantity of drugs dispensed per prescription (the plan pays for only a limited supply of medication at one time). The most common scenario is that the plan pays for a 30- to 34-day supply of a prescribed drug at a pharmacy.

Select drugs or categories, such as those used to treat migraines or male erectile dysfunction, may be subject to quantity limits based on FDA or manufacturer recommendations. For example, Viagra® may be limited to 8 tablets per 30 days.

One alternative to all these limitations is to allow larger quantities, such as a 3- to 6-month supply, to be purchased for chronic conditions, such as diabetes or cardiovascular disease, through a mail order provider. Although a larger supply of medication increases convenience for the patient and reduces the number of dispensing fees paid, there are fewer chances to intervene on drug misadventures. The advantages of a smaller supply include reduced product waste if a prescription is discontinued, more member cost sharing, and frequent monitoring for compliance with the patient's drug therapy.

The category of coverage limitations (which drugs are covered and which are not) is often important in plan limits. Typically, drugs that are FDA approved and available only by prescription are covered when authorized by a professional for the treatment of a medical condition or are medically necessary. Typically, over-the-counter (OTC) or nonprescription drugs are not covered by insurance, although insulin for diabetes is traditionally exempt from this rule. The rationale is that most OTC products are affordable to patients without the use of insurance, and insurance coverage could easily be abused by plan members, thus increasing cost to the payer. Interestingly, as prescription drugs receive FDA approval to move from prescription to nonprescription status (e.g., Lotrimin®, Zantac®, and hydrocortisone), some experts feel that coverage of selected prescribed OTC products should be allowed if they are prescribed by authorized providers because it might lower costs and consequently improve clinical and financial outcomes in the pharmacy and medical benefit.

A second category of drugs that many plans traditionally do not cover is referred to as drug efficacy study implementation (DESI) drugs. These drugs were reclassified by the FDA in 1962 as safe, but they have not been proven fully effective under current regulations. Examples of DESI drugs (brand and generic forms) include triple sulfa vaginal cream (Sultrin®), Tedral®, promethazine cough and cold combinations, and pentaerythritol. Coverage is selectively extended to certain categories of DESI drugs that have been tested for efficacy.

Third, experimental drugs are usually excluded from coverage, just as health insurance policies do not cover experimental therapies or procedures. Deciding whether a drug is experimental is easier than deciding whether a type of surgery, for instance, is experimental because the safety and efficacy of a drug must be demonstrated in large clinical trials before the FDA allows it on the market. Because approval by the FDA is typically granted by Medicaid indication, a related issue is the use of FDA-approved drugs for unapproved or off-label indications (non-FDA-approved use of an approved drug). Once a drug is on the market, though, it is often used for additional purposes. However, these new indications have not been subject to the rigorous scientific study involved in FDA approval. The question of whether off-label use constitutes experimental use remains hotly contested, but the current trend is to cover approved drugs for off-label indications when sufficient peer-reviewed published literature supports the treatment.

Other prescription drugs commonly excluded from coverage include injectables administered by a clinician, anorexiants (appetite suppressants), smoking cessation products, fertility drugs, oral contraceptives, vitamins, prescriptions used for cosmetic purposes, allergy and biological sera, dental fluorides, and therapeutic or medical devices.

A different but common type of plan limitation involves a prior authorization (PA) program. This occurs when the drug has to be approved by the plan administrator or benefits manager on a case-by-case basis before it is covered. Typically, a PA program applies to targeted drugs that are expensive, require monitoring to reduce the risk of serious side effects, or whose effectiveness is limited. PAs can be inconvenient at the very least because of the time the approval process might take and the delay in getting a needed prescription filled. However, many plan administrators have implemented programs in which a 42- to 72-hour supply can be dispensed until the authorization can be received. The member does not go without medication and there is time enough for the PA process to be completed.

Pharmacy networks

Pharmacies as a provider network

A provider network is a group of pharmacies that a health plan has contracted and from which members must choose when they have prescriptions filled. PBMs, insurers, and pharmacies themselves accomplish establishing and maintaining a network of pharmacy providers. For example, PBMs recruit pharmacies into a group, negotiate payment terms, and monitor and audit network performance.

As with physician networks, pharmacies might be in a preferred, standard, or secondary network position. The network type can limit access by patients to select pharmacies who are not part of a particular network. In addition, through designing the pharmacy plan benefit, PBMs can offer varied coverage positions, including copayment arrangements, mail order, and promotion of generic or formulary drugs, or both, through the types of networks.

Contracting

Pharmacy reimbursement consists of a variety of factors, but the basic components are as follows:

1. A dispensing fee (a set amount paid to a pharmacist by the plan administrator per prescription order filled) that is added to the ingredient cost of the medication. This fee covers preparation and labor costs.
2. Ingredient cost of the drug, which can be based on an average wholesale price (AWP), maximum allowable cost (MAC), estimated

acquisition cost (EAC), wholesale acquisition cost (WAC), or actual acquisition cost (AAC).

3. Any applicable sales tax.

Claims processing at present is handled through electronic switch companies that PBMs and others use to provide electronic online claims adjudication for eligibility or payment, reports to clients on benefit utilization, and payments made to providers.

Claims processing and administration are fundamental elements of a PBM. Three methods are typically utilized in handling a prescription claim for payment:

1. *Direct claim.* The plan member pays for the prescription at the pharmacy, then submits a claim form for reimbursement. This was the most common method before the use of electronic claim submissions.

2. *Discount prescription card system.* Plan members are issued a card or coverage document to be presented at the pharmacy when a prescription is filled. The member pays 100% of the negotiated discounted cost of the prescription. This method has become more popular with Medicare eligible patients who do not currently have prescription drug coverage, but join or purchase a card program from a third-party organization such as AARP or the manufacturer.

3. *Point of service (POS):* An electronic system is used for exchanging information that can handle plan design elements, such as eligibility for product coverage, plan limits, member cost-share amounts, and product information, between the pharmacy and the claims administrator in real time as the pharmacist dispenses the prescription.

Purchasing

Pharmacies purchase their medication inventories through traditional supply chains that include drug wholesalers and manufacturers. Third parties or PBMs do not purchase medications in the traditional sense of physical ownership. Instead, they authorize payment for medications and related pharmaceutical services as part of the claim processing function.

Quality management, drug utilization review, and data collection

Data collection, in general, includes gathering information required for quality review, DUR, and outcomes research. Like community pharmacies, insurers and PBMs employ concurrent (at point of sale), retrospective (over time), and prospective (before dispensing) drug utilization strategies. Based on the information generated for DUR and claims processing, robust pharmacy databases are created, which can be used for a variety of management and outcomes improvement initiatives by those organizations. Performing and understanding details about DUR is covered in Chapter 13.

One application of this information is to provide academic detailing to physicians and other prescribers in the PBM network. This detailing or in-person educational session is similar to activities performed by pharmaceutical manufacturers' representatives. Physicians are profiled and selected for face-to-face visits with PBM pharmacists, who review the physicians' actual prescribing patterns against expected peer comparison profiles within selected drug categories within the same geographic region.

Another application relates to the auditing function (described earlier in the section "Evaluating the pharmacy benefit") as well as initiatives designed to improve compliance with prescribed therapies, warnings, or reminders to clinicians (pharmacists and physicians), and patient information that might improve their clinical outcomes of pharmaceutical care.

Future ideas

Although managed care has proven to be cost effective for employers, they are now balancing cost containment objectives against the need to maintain employee satisfaction for retention or recruitment. As a result, employers have begun to open up restricted managed care networks and formularies and are using different cost management strategies in the current decade. By shifting from limiting health benefits, employers are moving to employee-specific interventions, employee contribution risk sharing, and establishing more explicit performance standards with their health care providers. They are also rapidly moving into real-time information and access through the Internet, call centers, and other employee self-service applications. Another trend emerging is to combine the principles of managed competition with other business tactics or value purchasing. This strategy integrates health benefits into the corporate business plan.

The following are examples of trends that can impact prescription drug benefits over the next few years:

- Genomic-related drug development will become more established, resulting in both diagnostic and drug therapy advances heretofore unknown.
- Mergers, alliances, and other partnerships among health care providers and related businesses will strain ethical and moral boundaries for health care professionals, such as pharmacists
- Clinical drug therapy management will play an increasingly important role in overall health care as evidence continues to accumulate that drug therapy itself is often the least expensive component of health care. As a result, pharmacists will be paid for and recognized as consultants to other clinicians and to patients.
- As the population ages and chronic diseases become more crucial to health care cost assessment, increasingly expensive but more effective prescription medications will be used.

- Preventative care will have a renewed presence in the marketplace through initiatives such as employee wellness and health management programs aimed at reducing incidence of chronic diseases that can help keep health care costs in check for all payers.

It is both an exciting and perilous time for pharmacists involved in the clinical care of patients. Creative ways of thinking and incorporating evolving technologies into pharmaceutical care delivery make possible advances that people in the last century could barely consider. Pharmacists with clinical and financial expertise will be required to better manage the cost, quality, and accessibility of health care and prescription drugs. Prepare now for a positive, exciting future as a pharmacist who will be engaged in managing pharmaceutical care.

References

1. The Takeda and Lilly Prescription Drug Benefit Cost and Plan Design Survey Report, 2001 ed. Kikaku Publishing, Washington, D.C., October 2002.
2. Report on health in America. *Business and Health*, 8(4), Supplement A: 1990, 6–7.
3. *International Health Systems: A Chartbook Perspective*, 2nd ed. American Medical Association, Chicago, 1995.
4. Sica JM. Managing prescription drug costs. Presented at the International Foundation of Employee Benefit Plans, June 24–26, 2000, Lake Tahoe, NV.
5. Healthcare premiums to rise 11%–12%, *Richmond Times-Dispatch*, August 21, 2000.
6. Vogenberg, FR, and Sica, JM. Evaluating and selecting a pharmacy benefits management company. In *Managing Prescription Drug Benefits*. Vogenberg, FR and Sica, JM, Eds. International Foundation of Employee Benefits Plans, Brookfield, WI, 2001, chapter 8.
7. CMS. Office of Actuary, May 2, 2000.
8. Vogenberg, FR and Sica, JM. Pharmacy benefit plan design. In *Managing Pharmacy Benefits*. Vogenberg, FR, and Sica, JM, Eds. International Foundation of Employee Benefit Plans, Brookfield, WI, 2001, chapter 3.
9. National Pharmaceutical Prescription Medicine Benefit Program Checklist. National Pharmaceutical Council, Reston, VA, 1990.

chapter twenty

Pharmacy practice and health policy within the U.S.: An introduction and overview

Jennifer H. Lofland* and Alan Lyles

Contents

* Dr. Lofland's time was sponsored by the Agency for Health Care Research and Quality K-08 00005 Mentored Clinical Scientist Award and a PhRMA Foundation grant.

Introduction

In the U.S., there has been considerable change in the practice of pharmacy during the 20th century. At many points throughout history, seminal events in health care policy and the health care system have brought about changes in pharmacy practice. This chapter provides an overview of these seminal events and discusses the context in which these events have impacted pharmacy practice in the U.S. (See Table 20.1 at the end of the chapter for a list of these seminal events and their impacts.) By using the five stages of major change in pharmacy practice presented by Holland and Nimmo,[1] the key health care policy issues and events within the last 150 years are discussed. In addition, the impact and influence of these events on pharmacy practice, either as imposed, mandated policy actions or as initiatives from within the profession, are examined.

Pharmacy practice begins with manufacturing

In its first stage in the 19th century, pharmacy practice was primarily a cottage industry (Figure 20.1).[1] Because the country's population was so scattered and medical knowledge was rudimentary at this time, large-scale manufacturing of pharmaceuticals was not only impractical but impossible.[2] Pharmacists created, prescribed, and dispensed medications from their own apothecaries. The manufacturing of pharmaceuticals was generally limited to a specific population within a given geographic area. In general, pharmacists created compounded medications for physicians practicing within the local area.[2]

Rise of pharmaceutical industry: pharmacists as compounders

During the second phase of pharmacy practice, health care within the U.S. experienced changes in capabilities, regulations, and financing, from the development of the pharmaceutical industry and the establishment of the Food and Drug Administration (FDA) to the creation of the first health maintenance organization (HMO).

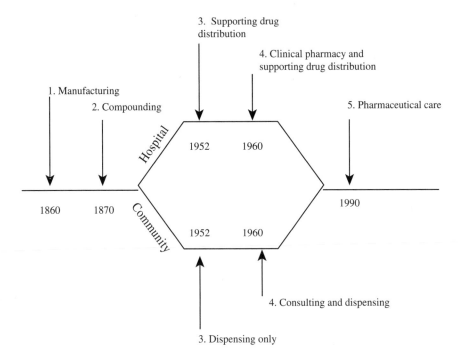

Figure 20.1 Five stages of major change in pharmacy practice. (Adapted from Holland R, Nimmo C. *Am. J. Hlth.-Syst. Pharm.* 1999; 56: 1758–1764.)

With the development of large-scale pharmaceutical manufacturers, pharmacy practice evolved from principally manufacturing to principally compounding and dispensing. Three factors coalesced to permit the rise of the U.S. pharmaceutical manufacturing industry: (1) the need for pure and standardized products, (2) the creation of a national distribution system for products (i.e., railroads), and (3) the growing U.S. population.[2]

During the 19th century, the population of the U.S. expanded. In the 1820s and 1830s, the country's first railroads were under construction. By 1869, when the transcontinental railroad was completed, the country's population was more than 23 million.[2] The ever-increasing population supplied a market for medications, and the completion of the railroad provided a system for transporting products across the country.

As the population increased, the use of patent medicines increased as well. During the late 1800s, few scientifically trained physicians were available, their fees were relatively expensive, and there was a general distrust of their curative procedures (e.g., bloodletting).[2] However, patent products were readily available inexpensive and claimed to be panaceas for many ailments. Unfortunately, the ingredients in these products were not disclosed and many of the products were simply alcohol, water, or flavoring.[2]

Together, these conditions provided the setting for the development of the pharmaceutical industry. Frederick Stearns & Company, the first U.S. pharmaceutical company, was founded in 1855.[2] Before 1900, there were 21 established firms, including the predecessors of some of today's largest research-intensive pharmaceutical companies, such as Sharp & Dohme, Eli Lilly and Company, and Johnson & Johnson.[2] With the rise of the pharmaceutical industry, more pharmacists discontinued manufacturing drugs in their apothecaries and began to compound medications. This fundamental shift in professional functions is notable because it was a reaction to external forces rather than the result of initiatives from within the profession of pharmacy.

U.S. Food and Drug Administration

As the use of patented medicines grew, so did the concern that products could easily be adulterated and misbranded. In 1862, President Lincoln addressed this concern by appointing Charles M. Wetherill, M.D., to serve in the newly created Department of Agriculture.[3] With Dr. Wetherill's appointment, the Bureau of Chemistry, the predecessor of the FDA, was created within the Department of Agriculture. The Bureau of Chemistry, beginning in 1867, conducted studies to investigate the adulteration of food products.

It was not until 1883, however, with the appointment of Dr. Wetherill as chief chemist, that these investigations were greatly expanded. Under Dr. Wetherill's leadership, the Bureau of Chemistry completed a widely publicized study analyzing the effects of food additives. However, it was ultimately a novel, rather than scientific evidence, that galvanized public attention. In 1906, Upton Sinclair published *The Jungle*, a candid depiction of the filthy conditions in the U.S. meat-packing industry.[3]

These events collectively led to the passage of the 1906 Federal Food and Drug Act. This act, administered by the Bureau of Chemistry, stated that drugs could not be sold unless they met the specifications of strength, quality, and purity defined by the U.S. Pharmacopoeia and National Formulary.[3] This marked the beginning of the modern era of the FDA. In 1930, the name of the federal agency was shortened to its present name. The agency has been under several different administrations since then and is currently under the Department of Health and Human Services.[3]

The passage of the 1906 Federal Food and Drug Act illustrates a key principle and theme throughout health policy changes in the U.S.; rarely does health policy change because of proactive involvement and pressure from interested parties. Rather, agendas for health policy change are often dictated by seminal, typically tragic, events. Kingdon posits a framework of agenda setting within the federal government that consists of three families of processes: problems, policies, and politics. Each family develops and functions independently. However, when a window of opportunity opens, the three families may unite and policy change can occur.[4]

For the 1906 act, the Bureau of Chemistry had been proactively investigating the adulteration of food products. However, it was not until a window of opportunity was opened, with the publication of *The Jungle*, that the public became enraged with such conditions and legislation could finally be passed prohibiting the interstate commerce of misbranded medications.

The 1938 Food, Drug, and Cosmetic Act

With Dr. Wetherill's departure in 1912, the Bureau of Chemistry began to concentrate its efforts on examining drug regulation and patent medications. Based on its findings, there was growing concern within the bureau over both the misbranding of medications and pharmaceutical manufacturers' use of false therapeutic claims. To address these concerns, unsuccessful proactive attempts were made by the bureau to amend the 1906 Federal Food and Drug Act.[3]

However, in 1937, a national pharmaceutical tragedy focused the nation's attention on the safety of pharmaceutical products. A pharmaceutical manufacturer created an elixir of sulfanilamide, a new dosage form of the antibiotic. However, the solvent of this product was a highly toxic analog of antifreeze.[3] Use of this new formulation resulted in over 100 deaths, many of them children. This tragedy created a health policy window of opportunity. The public outrage surrounding this incident resulted in the passage of the Food, Drug, and Cosmetic Act of 1938. With this act, manufacturers were required to demonstrate that all new drug entities were safe before receiving marketing approval. In addition, the Food, Drug, and Cosmetic Act of 1938 marked a change in regulatory focus by prohibiting false therapeutic claims for medications.[3]

The National Institutes of Health

In addition to changes in the nation's health policy to address the safe handling of pharmaceuticals, there were developments to increase the scientific understanding and determine the etiology of disease. In 1887, Dr. Joseph J. Kinyoun established the Laboratory of Hygiene on Staten Island, NY, an entity that was to become the National Institutes of Health (NIH).[5] As the first federal research institution established to identify and develop cures for infectious diseases, the laboratory represented a new direction for medical policy in the U.S.

Over time, the Laboratory of Hygiene was relocated to Washington, D.C., and renamed the Hygienic Laboratory.[5] In the early 1900s, the laboratory began the first long-term epidemiological study of a chronic disease, pellagra, which was then an epidemic in the southern U.S. With the laboratory's successes in fighting pellagra, Senator Joseph E. Ransdell sponsored the Ransdell Act in 1930 to reorganize the laboratory and rename it the National Institute of Health.[5]

After World War II (WWII), the National Institute of Health broadened its research scope to include chronic diseases such as cancer and mental illness. In 1948, the institute was expanded and the name was changed to the National Institutes of Health (NIH). At present, the NIH consists of 17 institutes and is an agency within the U.S. Public Health Service, Department of Health and Human Services.[5] Its budget in 1999 was U.S.$15.6 billion.[6] The establishment and subsequent growth of the NIH reflects the emerging priority placed on scientific inquiry and treatments based on understanding pathologic processes at a fundamental level. This trend continues currently as evidence-based medical practice.

The first health maintenance organization (HMO)

In the early part of the 20th century, both the practice of pharmacy and the medical profession were cottage industries. The majority of physicians worked alone or in small group practices, delivering medical care on a fee-for-service (FFS) basis.[7] Although most physicians were not hospital employees, they were members of a hospital's medical staff in order to have hospital-admitting privileges.[7] However, by the 1930s, a new model for medical care delivery, known as the prepaid group practice, was emerging. This new model would challenge the traditional FFS system and serve as the basis for the development of today's health maintenance organizations (HMOs).[7]

One of the most successful prepaid group practices was the Kaiser Health Plan. In 1938, Sidney Garfield, M.D., began to provide prepaid health care services to the employees of Henry J. Kaiser,[7] who were working at the Grand Coulee Dam in Washington State. Instead of receiving a salary, Dr. Garfield was paid a fixed fee for each employee (i.e., capitation) for whom he was responsible. Over time, this concept of physician prepayment based on a person's enrollment status rather than the actual services received spread across the U.S. It was not until the 1970s that Dr. Paul Ellwood, an advisor to President Richard Nixon, suggested that prepaid group practices be renamed health maintenance organizations.[7,8]

Hill–Burton Act

The 1940s witnessed further changes in the structure of the U.S. health care system, not only for physicians but for hospitals as well. The 1946 Hill–Burton Hospital Construction Act allocated almost U.S.$4 million from 1946 to 1971 for the expansion of hospitals and hospital services within the U.S.[7] This act was one of the federal government's first investments in health care.[7] By funding the construction of hospitals throughout most communities after WWII, the Hill–Burton Act created new opportunities, positions, and technical challenges for pharmacists.

Pharmacists as dispensers

WWII stimulated advances in the pharmaceutical manufacturing industry and science. The conclusion of WWII marked the beginning of the third phase of pharmacy practice — pharmacists as medical product dispensers. Pharmaceutical manufacturers began incorporating more sophisticated technologies into the production and manufacturing of pharmaceutical products.[9] For example, in the 1930s approximately 75% of prescriptions required some compounding, whereas by 1950 the need for prescription compounding had decreased to only 25%.[9] Fundamental changes within the pharmacy profession were dictated by external events. Increased capabilities within the pharmaceutical manufacturing industry shifted the roles of pharmacists, from compounders to dispensers of medication.

Durham–Humphrey Act of 1951

With the passage of the Food, Drug, and Cosmetic Act of 1938, the FDA began to identify drugs (e.g., sulfanilamide) that were potentially dangerous for patients and could not be labeled for safe use.[9] Because of these growing concerns, in 1951, Carl Durham and Hubert Humphrey, a pharmacist, proposed an amendment to the Food, Drug, and Cosmetic Act of 1938. The amendment created and defined the two classes of medications that we have at present: (1) legend drugs, which require a prescription from a legally recognized prescriber, and (2) over-the-counter medications, which can be obtained without a prescription.[9]

With passage of the Durham–Humphrey Act of 1951, the pharmacy profession was subject to regulatory restrictions that marked a significant change in the practice of pharmacy within the U.S. This amendment removed the professional autonomy and discretion that a pharmacist practicing in the first half of the 20th century had over dispensing and selling medications. [9] The extent of these new restrictions on pharmacy practice is exemplified in the American Pharmaceutical Association's (APhA) Code of Ethics of 1952:

> The primary obligation of pharmacy is the service it can render to the public in safeguarding the preparation, compounding, and dispensing of drugs and the storage and handling of drugs and medical supplies ... The pharmacist does not discuss the therapeutic effects or composition of a prescription with a patient. When such questions are asked, he suggests that the qualified practitioner is the proper person with whom such matters should be discussed.[10]

With the decreased need for compounded medications and the passage of the Durham–Humphrey Act of 1951, the practice of pharmacy had entered the era of "count, pour, lick, and stick." This caused many to question the future of pharmacy as a profession.

Development of hospital pharmacists

The Hill–Burton Act of 1946 and concurrent changes within the pharmaceutical industry resulted in new positions and professional opportunities for hospital pharmacists. During the third stage of the profession, the primary professional functions of pharmacists began to differentiate by the pharmacists' practice setting, community vs. hospital.[1] Within a hospital, the pharmacist's day-to-day responsibilities varied, and included participating on pharmacy and therapeutics committees, compounding, managing, educating nurses, and distributing products.[1] However, similar to the community pharmacy, emphasis was still on product and not on cognitive services or processes of care.

During the 1950s, there was explosive growth in the number of new pharmaceutical products available.[9] However, many of these products were for the same chemical entities. For financial reasons as well as a means to improve the quality of patient care, hospitals and hospital pharmacists began to develop medication formularies, create pharmacy and therapeutics (P&T) committees, and establish systems for generic drug substitution and selection.[9] These hospital-based activities were a departure from previous fundamental changes in pharmacy practice — they arose from within the profession. These services were increasingly dependent on expertise and professional judgment, which helped to move the product-focused practice of pharmacy toward the delivery of clinical services.

Clinical services and dispensing

The 1960s were a time of significant change not only for pharmacy practice but for national health policy as well. The fourth stage of pharmacy practice marks the emergence of clinical pharmacy. Pharmacists who were practicing within hospitals were the major force behind this development.[9] The diffusion of clinical pharmacy faced cultural and financial hurdles, requiring changes in how pharmacists interacted with other health care professionals and in the services for which they received compensation.

With the establishment of P&T committees in the 1950s, hospital pharmacists acquired more influence over the use of pharmaceuticals within their institutions. Pharmacists now had the opportunity to demonstrate the value of their expertise through advice and guidance in therapeutic decisions.[9] Within hospitals, pharmacists had direct access to patient-specific clinical data, medical literature, and clinicians, which allowed them to provide therapeutic advice to physicians.[1] Hospital pharmacists began to demonstrate their value as medical information resources — a resources that could lead to the delivery of better patient care.

The APhA Code of Ethics of 1969 best shows how the practice of pharmacy changed its restrictive nature in the 1950s to become a proactive profession whose members saw themselves as part of the health care team: "A pharmacist should . . . render to each patient the full measure of his ability as an essential health practitioner."[9]

The emergence of clinical services during this phase of pharmacy practice is exemplified by the development of clinical pharmacy services in the U.S. Indian Health Service (IHS). The IHS provides health care services for 1.4 million American Indians and Alaska Natives.[11] The IHS's health care facilities are in rural areas near or on Indian reservations in 34 states, mainly in the western part of the U.S. and Alaska.[11] In the 1960s, pharmacists within the IHS began to provide services that were the predecessors for current models of patient care. Pharmacists working within the IHS provided primary care to patients with minor conditions, monitored them for adverse drug reactions, provided patient education, and developed disease prevention programs.[11]

At present, pharmacists within the IHS have even more professional authority and latitude to provide patient care. Pharmacists provide primary care for patients beyond treating minor illnesses: they can initiate medication orders, and, under medical staff protocols, diagnose, manage, and monitor patients with chronic diseases.[11] The care delivered by pharmacists in this unique setting continues to serve as an exemplary model of the capabilities and impact of the pharmacy profession on direct patient care.

Kefauver–Harris Amendments

As pharmacy practice was experiencing internal changes in the 1960s, modifications to health policy at a national level were impacting the profession. First was the passage of the Kefauver–Harris Amendments to the Food, Drug, and Cosmetic Act of 1938, requiring manufacturers to demonstrate a drug's efficacy. As with the 1938 act, the impetus for these amendments was a medical tragedy.

Thalidomide, a new sedative, was associated with birth defects in thousands of newborns throughout Europe.[3] Fortunately, the medication had not been approved for use within the U.S. In 1962, with the support of Senator Estes Kefauver, another health policy window was opened; the amendments were passed to ensure that medications were both safe and efficacious.[3] With the Kefauver–Harris Amendments, the effectiveness of a medication has to be proven by "substantial evidence" which includes "adequate and well-controlled trials."[12] For the first time, pharmaceutical manufacturers had to demonstrate a product's efficacy to the FDA. The Kefauver–Harris Amendments led the way for randomized clinical trials and the FDA drug approval process.

Creation of Medicare and Medicaid

The second major change in the nation's health policy during this fourth phase in the evolution of pharmacy practice was the establishment of the Medicare and Medicaid programs in 1965, as amendments to the Social Security Act.

Medicare

Medicare is a federal health care program, and its recipients include people over the age of 65, the disabled, and those with end-stage renal disease.[13] Medicare is administered by the Centers for Medicare and Medicaid Services (CMS), formerly known as the Health Care Financing Administration. The Medicare program consists of two parts (parts A and B), but is funded by four different sources: (1) general tax revenues, (2) beneficiaries' premiums, (3) mandatory contributions from employers and employees, and (4) deductibles and copayments paid by patients.[13]

With Medicare's Hospital Insurance Trust Fund, also known as Medicare Part A, workers make required contributions to the fund while they are employed. Upon retirement, workers receive health care benefits.[13] By law, employers and their employees are required to pay equal portions of a payroll tax, which totals 2.9% of earned income.[13] In 1997, almost 90% of the trust fund's income was from payroll taxes. The remaining income was generated from the interest earned from the trust fund.[13] A beneficiary's Medicare Part A insurance is limited to only those hospitals accredited by the Joint Commission on Accreditation for Healthcare Organizations (JCAHO). The JCAHO accreditation standards include explicit and extensive professional pharmacy activities, indirectly supporting professional trends for clinical practice (see Chapter 18).

Medicare Part B pays for physician and outpatient services, diagnostic tools, and home health services. The majority of the funds for Part B are provided by the general tax revenues, which have been appropriated by Congress. Beneficiaries enrolled in Part B are required to pay an annual deductible ($100 for 2002) and a monthly premium ($50 for 2002). Because payments to beneficiaries represent 99% and 98% of the expenditures for Medicare Part A and Part B, respectively, the administrative costs associated with Medicare are quite low.[13]

Medicaid

Medicaid is a federal–state entitlement program for low-income Americans who meet certain criteria.[14] Even though Medicaid is administered by CMS as well, it has very little in common with the U.S. Medicare program. Medicaid primarily covers three groups of individuals: the elderly, the disabled, and parents and their dependent children.[14]

In 1998, Medicaid provided services for approximately 40.6 million people,[15] of which 10.6 million (26%) were elderly, blind, or disabled; 18.3 million

(53%) were children; and 7.9 million (19%) were adults in families with dependent children.[15] Even though 47% of Medicaid beneficiaries are children, minors account for only 16% of Medicaid's payments for health care services.[15] The elderly, blind, and disabled represent 26% of the Medicaid beneficiaries but account for 71% of the costs.[15]

State participation in the Medicaid program is voluntary; however, since 1982, all states participate in the program.[14] For each state, the federal government funds at least 50% and up to 83% of the costs of Medicaid, depending on the state's per capita income.[14] States that agree to participate in Medicaid must provide its beneficiaries a minimum set of health care resources, which include the following:[14]

- Hospital care
- Nursing home care
- Physician services
- Laboratory and x-ray services
- Immunizations and other periodic screenings
- Family-planning services
- Health center and rural health clinic services
- Nurse midwife and nurse practitioner services

However, a state may cover additional health care benefits for its beneficiaries. Therefore, the Medicaid benefit packages vary greatly from state to state. States that include additional health care benefits receive matching funds from the federal government for those services. The additional services may include, but are not limited to, the following:

- Prescription medications
- Institutional care for individuals with mental retardation
- Dental and vision care
- Personal care and services for people with disabilities
- Home- and community-based care for the elderly

The Medicare and Medicaid programs have had a significant impact on the practice of pharmacy. The Medicare program stimulated the growth of the hospital pharmacy profession. Only those hospitals with a pharmacy department that was directed by a pharmacist and met a minimum set of federal standards could receive federal funding for Medicare reimbursement.[9,10]

For community pharmacists, the new Medicaid program had a tremendous impact on the pharmacy profession, which is still seen in today's community pharmacies. The establishment of Medicaid created millions of new prescriptions that needed to be filled in a beneficiary's local pharmacy and for which the pharmacy would be reimbursed. With the increased number of prescriptions, however, came many additional administrative tasks. These tasks included negotiating pharmacist reimbursement levels; staying current with and following regulations regarding proper prescription documentation; and selecting, installing, and operating third-party prescription payment systems.[9,10] With the creation of third-party payment systems within the Medicaid program, the unmet pharmaceutical needs of beneficiaries were addressed, which resulted in substantial cost increases. As the costs continued to exceed forecasts, the federal government began to consider ways to decrease health care costs.

HMO Act of 1973

In the early 1970s, the Medicare program was less than 10 years old, but it was generating health care costs for the federal government considerably beyond what was anticipated. The CMS spent U.S.$7.4 billion on health care resources for its beneficiaries in 1966 and $17.6 billion in 1970.[16] Fee-for-service payments were seen as providing incentives to health care providers to expand the number of patient services with little thought of the actual need for these services and their associated costs. One potential solution to restrain health care costs was to change the financial incentives for health care providers. The main approach relied on shifting health care coverage from indemnity to prepaid health care, as seen in the Kaiser Health Plan.[8]

Based on the counsel of his advisors, President Richard Nixon believed that the Kaiser Health Plan could be replicated at a national level as a means to control health care costs. Because many of President Nixon's advisees were Californians, they were familiar with the Kaiser health system, the home of some of Mr. Kaiser's first prepaid health plans.[8] They knew that HMOs at the time offered numerous possible advantages to the traditional health care system. These HMOs (1) were cost effective, (2) provided quality care, (3) decreased administrative waste, (4) instituted health care utilization controls, and (5) demonstrated a high degree of patient satisfaction.[8]

In addition to these possible advantages, President Nixon and his advisors felt that the introduction of HMOs would increase competition among health care providers within the existing health care system, potentially leading to decreased health care costs.[8] Based on the potential of HMOs to decrease costs and provide quality care, the Nixon administration proposed legislation for the encouragement and growth of managed care and HMOs.

Despite opposition by the American Medical Association (AMA) and others over the course of 3 years, Congress passed the HMO Act of 1973. Certain restrictive features of the HMO Act of 1973 limited its immediate impact on the U.S. health care system. The original legislation defined federally qualified HMOs, required annual open enrollment periods, assured quality standards, required that certain employers offer indemnity as well as HMO insurance, mandated equal employer contributions to indemnity and HMO insurance coverage, and provided grants to initiate the creation of new HMOs.[17] However, it created the environment within the U.S. for the health care changes yet to come.[8] Even though the growth of HMOs was slow at first, at present HMOs and managed care organizations are a dominant method of health care financing and delivery in the country.[18]

FDA Modernization Act of 1997

As mentioned, external forces have influenced the practice of pharmacy. FDA regulations in particular have had a substantial impact. In 1997, Congress enacted the Food and Drug Administration Modernization Act (FDAMA), which resulted in changes to the Kefauver–Harris Amendments of 1962 and key FDA reforms.[12] With the changes in the Kefauver–Harris Amendments, pharmaceuticals are now subject to the FDA drug review and approval process. Since its inception, the approval process has been the center of much congressional discussion regarding FDA reform.[12] The greatest criticism of the FDA by Congress and the public was that the approval process was too lengthy, thereby delaying patient access to new and effective medications.[12] One possible solution to this concern was FDA reform.

The principal concern and part of the stimulus for the development of the FDAMA was the length of the FDA's medication review process. Congressional FDA reformers wanted to construct the FDA similar to the regulatory systems of Europe, which they argued were faster than those of the U.S.[21] One of the first steps toward reforming the FDA's review process was the Prescription Drug User Fee Act (PDUFA) of 1992. This act authorized the agency to charge the pharmaceutical manufacturers a fee for reviewing their medications. This fee, $88 million in 1997 alone, has been used to train and hire approximately 600 reviewers.[22]

According to the FDA Commissioner at the time, David Kessler, the increased money resulted in faster drug application reviews. The General Accounting Office (GAO) reported that the average approval times for new drug applications (NDAs) submitted to the FDA in 1987 and 1992 were 33 and 19 months, respectively.[23] As Dr. Kessler states:

These improved approval times have been made possible by shortening the time for completion of most first reviews to only 12 months. For the drugs submitted to the FDA in fiscal year 1994, we reviewed and acted upon 96 percent of them on time. In addition the GAO found that by 1994, FDA review and approval times were faster than those in the United Kingdom. [23]

The pharmaceutical industry supported this act based on the demonstrated improvement in review times. Both industry and the FDA wanted to ensure that the PDUFA was not allowed to expire at the end of its 5-year authorization.

In the 105th Congress in 1997, the legislation that was to become the FDAMA was drafted. The 1997 bill:

1. Allowed third-party review for the less crucial medical devices

2. Codified programs the FDA created to give patients experimental drugs pending approval
3. Gave the FDA more discretion over how many clinical trials manufacturers must conduct on new drugs to prove their effectiveness
4. Loosened restrictions on health claims companies can make
5. Gave companies greater latitude to make economic claims for their drugs
6. Allowed companies to disseminate information on unapproved uses of their medications
7. Gave companies incentives to test for and establish the pediatric doses of pharmaceuticals [22]

A window of opportunity provided the catalyst for FDAMA's passage. The 1997 bill came when a critical deadline was approaching: the PDUFA has a 5-year life span and was due for reauthorization or expiration. By allowing the FDA to collect user fees with the PDUFA, the approval time for NDAs was greatly reduced.[12] Without the reauthorization of PDUFA, FDA reviewers added under PDUFA funds would lose their jobs on September 30, 1997. "We're down to crunch time," said Carl Feldbaum, executive director of the Biotechnology Industry Association. "All the gains of the last five years are at stake."[22]

Following enactment of the FDAMA, the pharmaceutical industry had guidelines under which it could disseminate economic information as well as data on the unapproved indications (off-label) of medications. With data now available on pediatric dosing for medications, pharmacists would have critical additional information to use in their professional practices. Finally, linking PDUFA funding with the passage of FDAMA assured that there will be a debate concerning the agency and FDA reform on the congressional calendar every 5 years.

Guidance on direct-to-consumer advertising (DTCA) issued

Dr. David Kessler's departure from the FDA removed a major barrier to expanding DTCA in the U.S. Under Dr. Kessler's FDA tenure, pharmaceutical firms were able to sponsor advertisements in which the pharmaceutical name (reminder advertisement), the disease that it treated (help-seeking advertisement), or both (product-claim advertisement) could be mentioned. The communication had to present the brief summary information from the approved labeling, providing a fair balance of gains and risks associated with the product. The format for broadcast communications is brief; consequently, the extensive medical warnings that were required under these guidelines made direct-to-consumer television and radio advertisements relatively unattractive.[24]

With the growing use of help-seeking and reminder advertisements and with the limited information they provide to consumers, there was growing pressure to revisit the guidelines for broadcast advertisements.[24] However, Dr. Kessler was opposed to increasing these advertisements. Therefore, his departure from the FDA was the impetus for modifications to DTCA.

In 1997, the FDA's Draft Guidance on direct-to-consumer broadcast advertisements allowed radio, television, and telephone communications to discuss the risks associated with medications differently than in reminder and help-seeking advertisements.[24] The audio or the audio–visual components of the advertisement had to contain a major statement of the most important risks, and adequate provisions had to be made for four additional sources for the full label information (brief summary).[24]

These changes made broadcast communication directly to the patient more attractive to the pharmaceutical industry and its use underwent explosive growth from $790 million in 1996 to $2.9 billion in 2000. The increased public awareness of specific, often newer medications provides an opportunity for the pharmacist to provide guidance and patient counseling. However, because of the continued link between product and payment, limited compensation from health care providers is offered for delivering these services.

Pharmaceutical care as the new paradigm

The 1990s marked the beginning of the fifth stage of pharmacy practice and a new paradigm, *pharmaceutical care*, "the responsible provision of drug therapy for the purpose of achieving definite outcomes that improve the patient's quality of life."[1] For the first time, the profession made a fundamental shift away from the product (i.e., medication) toward the cognitive aspects of medical care.

In pharmaceutical care, pharmacists' knowledge, skills, and capabilities are the same as in clinical pharmacy; however, their attitudes and values differ. The shift from clinical pharmacy to pharmaceutical care focuses more attention on the profession, and pharmacists begin to assume responsibility for the outcome of medication therapy.[1]

The Omnibus Budget Reconciliation Act of 1990 (OBRA 90) includes aspects of pharmaceutical care that "recognized pharmacists as professionals whose expertise can be effectively utilized to ... promote rational outcomes from drug therapy."[9] OBRA 90 requires mandatory drug utilization review and that pharmacists offer medication counseling for Medicaid beneficiaries.[9] Although this legislation recognized an enhanced professional role for community pharmacists, requiring that they offer to provide medication counseling and answer any questions that patients might have regarding their prescribed medications, it did not change the reimbursement structure. External forces dictated the content of professional practice, with no regard for a pharmacist's compensation.

Pharmacy Technician Certification Board established

The establishment of the Pharmacy Technician Certification Board (PTCB) in 1995 supported the implementation the pharmaceutical care paradigm.[19] Consistent with the professional model of pharmaceutical care, more pharmacists are beginning to provide direct patient care and counsel patients on the appropriate uses of pharmaceuticals. As pharmacists devote more time to services involving direct patient contact, they need to rely on pharmacy technicians as extenders to obtain patient data, enter patient and prescription information into computer systems, and compile patients' prescriptions.[19]

When the PTCB began, there were 7,000 applicants for certification. At present, the program continues to grow and has certified over 104,000 pharmacy technicians.[19] For the future, the PTCB is seeking ways to promote the role of pharmacy technicians as a profession and to better serve pharmacists and patients in the delivery of quality health care.

The Fleetwood Project

With the change in professional pharmacy practice to the pharmaceutical care model, pharmacists and pharmacy organizations realized the importance of acquiring evidence of the impacts these services have on patient care. The American Society of Consultant Pharmacists Research and Education Foundation began a research program, the Fleetwood Project, to demonstrate the impacts of consultant pharmacy services on patient outcomes and health care costs.[20] The Fleetwood Project is an initiative that arose from within the profession to support change in professional practice in contrast to the practice responding to the next external mandate.

The Fleetwood Project consisted of three phases of research. The first phase quantified the cost of medication-related problems in nursing facilities and estimated the value of consultant pharmacists in these settings. This phase determined that drug regimen review conducted by consultant pharmacists improved patients' outcomes by 43% and saved $3.6 billion a year by avoiding medication-related problems.[20]

The goal of the second research phase was to transition consultant pharmacists from performing retrospective chart reviews to performing prospective evaluations in which the pharmacists intervene in the delivery of care. The settings in which the Fleetwood Project model was implemented increased clinical pharmacist decision making, increased pharmacists' interactions with patients and families, and improved communication among patients' health care team members.[20]

Incorporating findings from the first and second phases, the third phase aimed to identify pharmacist-sensitive outcomes. During this phase, patient outcomes most sensitive to pharmacist interventions were identified and quantified. Once these were identified, the Fleetwood Project model was modified to highlight these specific conditions and processes associated with pharmacist-sensitive outcomes.[20] Projects such as this can establish evidence of pharmaceutical care. For a program to be implemented successfully, pharmacists will need to routinely document their services so that their impacts on patient outcomes can be evaluated. The Fleetwood Project demonstrates professional initiated change and serves as a model for the profession and pharmaceutical care.

Institute of Medicine's To Err Is Human *and* Crossing the Quality Chasm

In the late 1990s, quality of health care became a major issue for health care policy in the U.S. Repeatedly, research produced evidence of small area clinical variations in preventing and treating various diseases across the country. Kresowski et al.[25] conducted a study to describe the variation in the utilization, health care processes, and outcomes for carotid endarterectomy (CEA) procedures in 10 states. The utilization rates of CEA, mortality 30 days after CEA, stroke 30 days after CEA, and warfarin therapy use for Medicare patients between June 1, 1995, and May 31, 1996, were evaluated. Utilization rates of CEA varied from 25.7 to 38.4 procedures per 10,000 Medicare beneficiaries in the 10 states. This suggests that there is a need for improvement in the utilization, processes of care, and outcomes of CEA.[25]

In addition to regional variations for treating and preventing stroke, there is variation surrounding the care for patients with breast cancer. In 2001, Stephens et al.[26] performed an evaluation comparing the performance of West Virginia physicians and hospitals to those in other states. The research used a set of 22 quality indicators for 6 health conditions (breast cancer, acute myocardial infarction, diabetes, heart failure, pneumonia, and stroke) that had been targeted by Medicare's Health Care Quality Improvement Program (HCQIP) and presumed to represent national priorities.

Of the 19 states evaluated, West Virginia ranked below the 50th percentile on 19 of the 22 quality indicators. For the breast cancer quality indicator, only 44% of female beneficiaries had a medical claim for a mammogram within the past 2 years.[26] The lowest rates of mammography screening were seen in the southwestern part of the state. In addition, physician-specific rates varied from less than 10%, with the highest rate of greater than 90% seen in obstetrician–gynecologists.[26]

In addition to evidence of regional variation, health services research had demonstrated decreased rates of adherence to accepted evidence-based therapeutic guidelines. Despite widely known professional guidelines (i.e., sixth report of the Joint National Committee, JNC-VI), medical consensus on the health benefits of blood pressure control, and availability of effective mediations, blood pressure is poorly controlled in the U.S.[27] Data from a national research study found that only 68% of patients with hypertension are aware of their condition, and of those treated, only 27% have their blood pressures controlled.[27]

With the growing evidence of regional variation in the delivery of health care and the low adherence to established therapeutic guidelines, the Committee on the Quality of Health Care in America was formed in 1998. The committee's charge was to create a plan to improve the quality of health care within the U.S. over the following 10 years. Its first report, *To Err Is Human: Building a Safer Health System*, reported that thousands of Americans die each year from medical errors.[28] In the U.S., more people die each year from medical errors than from motor vehicle accidents, breast cancer, or AIDS.[28] The data used within this report had been available and known for some time; however, with the presentation and endorsement by the well-respected Institute of Medicine (IOM), the data gained increased significance and served as the evidence for making quality health care in the U.S. a national priority.

To Err Is Human contains a four-part plan for decreasing the number of medical errors, and each part has implications for the pharmacy profession. To provide leadership and a research focus for patient safety, Part one recommends the creation of a center for patient safety within the Agency for Healthcare Research and Quality (AHRQ). Pharmacy organizations and pharmacists have the opportunity to contribute by including the study of medical errors in their applied research agendas. Using their expertise, pharmacists can provide input to the national goals, their content, and professional responsibilities for medication safety.[29]

Part two of the plan calls for establishing an error-reporting system. The report suggests a two-prong approach in which a national program is first implemented at the state level to detect the most serious errors. Then, a voluntary, confidential system is established to encourage individuals to report near misses.[29] Pharmacists can participate in both activities to provide their expertise and help create such systems in their institutions.

Part three involves creating safety-related performance standards. In terms of health professionals, the report asks licensing organizations to examine how they identify unsafe practitioners. In addition, professional organizations should address patient safety in national conferences, journals, and training programs (e.g., residencies).[29]

The last part of the strategic plan is to ensure that health care organizations implement patient safety improvement initiatives within their organizations. Similar to the aviation industry, health care organizations need to establish a culture of patient safety.[29] Instead of waiting for imposed mandates, pharmacists can work within their organizations to develop systems and a culture of safety. Pharmacists understand a unique aspect of medical care delivery; with this knowledge, they can contribute to the design and help lead the way for improvements in safe health care delivery.

Safety is only one aspect of the quality of health care in the U.S. The committee's second report, *Crossing the Quality Chasm: A New System for the 21st Century*, states that fundamental changes are needed to achieve an expected level of quality in health care services within the U.S. In *Crossing the Quality Chasm*, the IOM posits 13 recommendations to health care providers, decision-makers, purchasers, and stakeholders on how to transform the health care delivery system. For example, under Recommendation 5, the IOM suggests that as one of the first steps to change, the system should place greater emphasis on prevalent conditions. By focusing attention on widespread diseases, considerable improvements can be made in the quality of the care that patients receive.[6] Pharmacists can play a vital role in this effort by identifying opportunities for improved medication use by this subset of patients.

These IOM reports can serve as stimuli for the pharmacy profession to initiate improvements in the quality of care delivered to patients and to reduce the extent and severity of medical errors within the U.S. This is an opportunity for pharmacists to institute improvements from within the profession, instead of waiting for imposed changes from other health professions, industries, or regulatory bodies. Pharmacists are trained with a unique set of skills and expertise regarding medication use. Working as part of a team of health care professionals, these skills can be used to better serve the public, lead to improvements in the quality of care, and enhance the professional aspects of pharmacy practice.

Future health policy

As we enter the 21st century, many health policy concerns face the U.S.: the uninsured, an aging population, rising health care costs, barriers to access to health care services, and bioterrorism. With the unfolding of these issues, there will surely be changes in the practice of pharmacy, yet it is essential that the profession be proactive rather than reactive. Over the last 150 years, many of the changes within the profession have been due to mandates imposed on the practice of pharmacy as opposed to initiatives from within the profession. Now, pharmacists may begin to change this historical paradigm within the profession and institute modifications to the practice of pharmacy.

For the future, one of the greatest concerns for the nation, and always up for debate, is the structure and financing of the Medicare program.

Restructuring and refinancing Medicare

Restructuring the Medicare program's financing is a continuing debate. Since its inception in 1965, the Medicare program has become a health care program for individuals with chronic diseases. However, the program was designed and structured primarily to provide insurance for acute health care episodes (i.e., hospitalizations), as evidenced by the lack of specific health care insurance benefits covered through the Medicare program. Neither Part A nor Part B of the Medicare program offers the following services: outpatient prescription medications, routine physical examinations, complete long-term care services, vision care, eyeglasses, or preventive services.[30]

Despite measures to control the health care expenditures via adjustments to reimbursements, Medicare health care costs continue to rise. The cohort of U.S. baby boomers is aging and will soon be eligible for Medicare benefits. With their eligibility will also come increased demand, use, and costs of health care services. As currently financed, the Medicare trust funds might not continue to be solvent and might not be able to provide adequate coverage for beneficiaries in the future. The latest report predicts that Medicare Part A, the hospital trust fund, should be solvent until 2029.[31] However, this estimate can fluctuate greatly, given both modeling assumptions and the current economic conditions of the U.S. Therefore, there is still a need to consider modifications to the financing mechanisms for the Medicare program to maintain its viability.

Quality-based Medicare provider payment

As concerns over the costs and the quality of the health care for Medicare beneficiaries grew, in 1992, the CMS developed a new program for assessing quality, the Health Care Quality Improvement Program (HCQIP).[32,33] The HCQIP's aims are to:

1. Develop scientifically based quality indicators.
2. Identify opportunities to improve the care provided to Medicare beneficiaries by examining patterns of care.
3. Communicate the patterns of care with health care professionals and providers.
4. Promote quality improvement via system enhancements.
5. Evaluate programs.[34]

The HCQIP concentrates on six clinical areas of national priority: acute myocardial infarction, breast cancer, diabetes, heart failure, pneumonia, and stroke. The CMS selected these specific areas based on their public health importance as well as the feasibility of their measurement and quality improvement.[34]

With the HCQIP, there is an opportunity to restructure provider payments under the current Medicare program to emphasize the quality of care that beneficiaries receive. Medicare, as the purchaser of health care for over 39 million individuals in the U.S., has an opportunity to demand quality health care services. Quality indicators for HCQIP's six clinical areas have been developed; these could serve as an early implementation phase of a new reimbursement program.

However, only determining a provider's adherence to a set of quality indicators for a population with a particular clinical condition is not sufficient. Within a disease category, there are levels of severity and associated morbidity. It is presumed that the sicker the patients, the less likely they might be to exhibit improvements, and therefore less likely to have positive outcomes due to clinical care received. To ensure equitable payment based on the quality of care provided, the severity of illness of a provider's Medicare patient population needs to be considered explicitly in the payment structure.

Pharmacists as Medicare health care providers

As of this writing, legislation is before the U.S. Congress proposing reimbursement of pharmacists' services delivered to Medicare beneficiaries. Currently, pharmacists receive Medicare reimbursement for providing education to patients with diabetes. To illustrate how this legislation could build on the experience with pharmacists in disease and drug therapy management (collective drug therapy management, CDTM) to improve the quality of care delivered in the U.S., issues surrounding atrial fibrillation and stroke will be discussed.

In various settings such as Veterans Administration outpatient clinics, Kaiser Permanente outpatient services, hospital-based outpatient clinics, physician offices, and community pharmacies, pharmacists have been successfully managing patients' warfarin therapy.[35–40] Research demonstrates the positive outcomes associated with, and the cost-effectiveness of, pharmacist-run warfarin clinics.[41,42] In addition, with over 60,000 pharmacies across the U.S., pharmacists are readily available within most communities.[43]

In the future, the CMS could mandate that in order to receive reimbursement, a pharmacist needs to be certified in anticoagulation management. Currently, the American College of Clinical Pharmacy, through selected training sites, offers anticoagulation certification across the country.[44] Medicare could then reimburse pharmacists for the management of warfarin therapy for patients with atrial fibrillation. As Medicare providers, pharmacists would be held to the same standards and provisions for reimbursement as other providers. By utilizing ubiquitous community-based health care professionals such as pharmacists as a means for primary stroke prevention, the quality of care for Medicare beneficiaries will improve (see Chapter 18).

Pharmacogenetics and pharmacogenomics

Pharmacogenetics and pharmacogenomics are emerging health care issues that will increasingly affect the profession of pharmacy. Since 1990, the Human Genome Project has been working to complete the mapping of human genetic information. Because of improvements in the sequencing technology, the complete DNA sequence should be completed 2 years ahead of schedule, in 2003.[45]

Pharmacogenetics is the study of the variability in medication response and toxicity due to an individual's genetic factors. Pharmacogenomics is the field in which the data gained through pharmacogenetics are used to develop and prescribe medications. A clear implication is that a pharmacist may be able to use a patient's genetic information to select the most appropriate medication for therapeutic response with the least risk of side effects. For example, mutations in patients' CYP450 enzymes may result in differences in metabolism of medications and therefore differences in responses to and adverse effects of a given medication.[45]

With genetic information, pharmacists can begin to counsel patients on their genetic information and why that determines their specific medications.[45] However, knowledge of a patient's genetic information has ethical, legal, and social implications. How will this data be used? What additional privacy protections are needed? Who will pay for this information and decide which drugs are most appropriate? Such questions need to be resolved before the wealth of information gained from the Human Genome Project can be effectively and appropriately used to select medications for individuals.

Internet and e-prescriptions

With the advent of the Internet, pharmacy practice has changed considerably (see Chapter 24). Pharmacists practicing in the 1940s would probably have never imagined the technological capabilities of present times. Not only are almost all prescriptions filled with the use of computers, but patients now get online, gain information about medications, order prescriptions, and come to the pharmacy with probing questions based on the information they obtain from the Internet.

With the Internet, e-prescriptions have emerged. Physicians can now transmit electronic prescriptions directly into managed care pharmacy networks and pharmacy benefit management systems.[46] In addition, physicians can send prescriptions to online pharmacies (e.g., www.CVS.com) via their office computers or personal digital assistants (e.g., Palm™ Pilot).[46] This technology is revolutionary and may change the current U.S. health care system. In light of the recent IOM reports[6,28] discussed earlier, this technology has the potential to decrease medical errors and increase the quality of health care. With e-prescriptions, pharmacists do not have to decipher a physician's handwriting to determine the name, dose, and strength of a prescribed medication. In addition, e-prescriptions can potentially increase the productivity of pharmacists as well as prescribers with the associated decrease in telephone time. By using their unique knowledge of medical information and delivery, pharmacists can become involved in developing the decision rules, software, and technology for e-prescriptions. However, the exact roles that pharmacists will perform in this new arena and the impacts of e-prescriptions on the daily activities of pharmacists are still developing.

Conclusion

In the U.S., there has been considerable change in the practice of pharmacy over the last 150 years. At key points during the profession, seminal events within health care policy and the U.S. health care system forced change within the field of pharmacy practice. However, few of these instances for change were initiated from within the profession. The pharmacy profession has seen an amazing evolution from the passage of legislation to ensure safe and effective medication use to the recent emergence of pharmacogenomics and the potential for the selection of high-tech medications in the 21st century.

Health care policy in the U.S. is sure to change over the next century. Individual pharmacists and those in positions of leadership have the opportunity to participate in formulating the emerging health care policies and developing initiatives to enhance the profession. It is up to pharmacists, as members of the health care team, to ensure that these changes lead to improved quality of care for Americans.

Pharmacists must continue to differentiate the services that they deliver from the pharmaceutical product, i.e., pharmaceutical care, and demonstrate the impact of their professional training on patient care. Pharmacists need to be proactive, which requires sacrificing time and committing to long-term goals. Remaining reactive to external pressures may mean the marginalization of the profession.

Table 20.1 Seminal Health Policy Events

Year	Event	Implication or Impact for Pharmacy Practice
1855	Establishment of pharmaceutical industry	• Moved pharmacists manufacturing to dispensing activities
1860s 1906	Creation of the Food and Drug Administration (FDA) Passage of Federal Food and Drug Act	• Required medications to meet specifications for strength, quality, and purity
1938	Food, Drug, and Cosmetic Act of 1938	• Required medications to demonstrate they are safe • Prohibited pharmaceutical industry from making false therapeutic claims
1930s–1940s	Creation of first Health Maintenance Organization	• Created a new system for the organization and reimbursement of health care services
1940s	Creation of National Institutes of Health	• Increased research initiatives to determine the etiology of diseases
1946	Hill–Burton Hospital Construction Act	• Allocated monies for the construction of hospital across the country • Helped create hospital pharmacy positions
1951	Durham–Humphrey Act of 1951	• Created two classes of medications: legend and over-the-counter medications • Placed greater restrictions on pharmacists • Helped create the era of "count, pour, lick, and stick"

Table 20.1 Seminal Health Policy Events (continued)

Year	Event	Implication or Impact for Pharmacy Practice
1962	Kefauver–Harris Amendments to the Food, Drug, and Cosmetic Act of 1938	• Required medications to demonstrate their safety and effectiveness • Created the FDA drug approval process • Required randomized clinical trials for medications
1965	Creation of U.S. Medicare and Medicaid Programs	Medicare • Stimulated the growth of hospital pharmacy positions Medicaid • Created demand for millions of prescriptions • Created administrative issues • Created prepaid third-party prescription payment systems
1973	HMO Act of 1973	• Created the environment for HMO expansion in the future
1995	Pharmacy Technician Certification Board established	• Created a credentialing body for pharmacy technician practices • Allowed pharmacists to engage in pharmaceutical care more readily
1997	FDA Modernization Act of 1997	• Created FDA reform • Allowed the pharmaceutical industry to disseminate economic information and unapproved indications for medications • Increased information (e.g., pediatric dosing) for pharmacists
1997	Draft Guidance for Industry on DTCA	• Allowed broadcast advertisements to contain limited risk and benefit information • Required adequate provision for alternative sources of complete labeling information
1998–2000	Creation of Committee on the Quality of Health Care in America • *To Err Is Human: Building a Safer Health System* • *Crossing the Quality Chasm: A New System for the 21st Century*	• Created opportunities for pharmacists to provide guidance on system to decrease medical errors • Created opportunities for pharmacy organizations to include medical errors on research agendas

References

1. Holland R, Nimmo C. Transitions, Part I: Beyond pharmaceutical care. *Am. J. Hlth.-Syst. Pharm.* 1999; 56: 1758–1764.
2. Worthen D. The pharmaceutical industry: 1852-1902. *J. Am. Pharm. Assoc.* 2000; 40: 589–591.
3. Swann, JP. *History of the FDA*, 2001, pp. 1–7. www.fda.gov/oc/history/historyoffda/fulltext.html, accessed December 29, 2003.
4. Kingdon JW. *Agendas, Alternatives and Public Policy*, 2nd ed. New York: Addison-Wesley, 1995.
5. National Institutes of Health. History of NIH. www.training.nih.gov/catalog/nihhistory.html, pp. 1–3, accessed July 1, 2002.
6. Institute of Medicine. *Crossing the Quality Chasm: A New Health System for the 21st Century*, executive summary. Washington, D.C.: National Academy of Sciences. 2000, pp. 1–22.
7. Bodenheimer TS, Grumbach K. How healthcare is organized: II. In: Bodenheimer TS, Grumbach K, Eds, *Understanding Health Policy: A Clinical Approach*, 2nd ed. New York: Mange Medical Books/McGraw-Hill, 1998, pp. 97–113.
8. Doherty J. Evolution of the contemporary health care delivery system. In: Wertheimer AI, Navarro RP, Eds., *Managed Care Pharmacy.* 1st ed. Binghamton, NY: Pharmaceutical Products Press, 1999, pp. 1–14.
9. Higby GJ. The continuing evolution of American pharmacy practice. *J. Am. Pharm. Assoc.* 2002; 42: 12–15.
10. Higby GJ. American pharmacy in the twentieth century. *Am. J. Hlth.-Syst. Pharm.* 1997; 54: 1833–1836.
11. Paavola FG, Dermanoski KR, Pittman RE. Pharmaceutical services in the United States Public Health Service. *Am. J. Hlth.-Syst. Pharm.* 1997; 54: 766–772.
12. Merrill RA. Modernizing the FDA: an incremental revolution. *Hlth. Aff. (Millwood)* 1999; 18: 96–111.
13. Iglehart JK. The American health care system: expenditures. *N. Engl. J. Med.* 1999; 340: 70–76.
14. The Henry J. Kaiser Family Foundation. *Medicaid: A Primer.* Washington, D.C.: The Henry J. Kaiser Foundation, 1999, pp. 1–10.
15. The Centers for Medicare and Medicaid Services. Medicaid beneficiaries, and vendor payments by basis of eligibility. www.hcfa.gov/medicaid/msis/2082-3.htm, accessed July 3, 2002.
16. The Centers for Medicare and Medicaid Services. National health expenditures aggregate, per capita, percent distribution, and annual percent change by source of funds: calendar years 1960-00. www.hcfa.gov/stats/nhe-oact/, accessed July 12, 2002.
17. Mitka M. A quarter century of health maintenance. *JAMA* 1998; 280: 2059–2060.
18. Lyles A, Palumbo FB. The effect of managed care on prescription drug costs and benefits. *Pharmacoeconomics* 1999; 15: 129–140.
19. Murer MM. A pharmacy success story: 104,644 pharmacy technicians certified nationwide. *J. Am. Pharm. Assoc.* 2002; 42: 158–159.
20. American Society of Consultant Pharmacists, Research and Education Foundation. The Fleetwood project research initiative. www.ascpfoundation.org/programs/prog_fleetwood.htm, accessed July 12, 2002.

21. Schwartz J. FDA reforms have momentum as hearings open; at least three measures under consideration, including one that allows private review of drugs. *The Washington Post* May 1, 1996, p.8.
22. Schwartz J. Another shot at FDA "modernization"; bill to revamp food and drug agency draws less controversy than predecessor. *The Washington Post* July 22, 1997, p.13.
23. Food and Drug Administration Department of Health and Human Services. Senate Labor Changes in FDA, S1477, February 21, 1996. Labor and Human Resources.
24. Lyles A. Direct marketing of pharmaceuticals to consumers. *Annu. Rev. Pub. Hlth.* 2002; 23: 73–91.
25. Kresowik TF, Bratzler D, Karp HR, Hemann RA, Hendel ME, Grund SL et al. Multistate utilization, processes, and outcomes of carotid endarterectomy. *J. Vasc. Surg.* 2001; 33: 227–234.
26. Stephens MK, Cochran RF, Schade CP. Improving medical care for West Virginia seniors. *W. Va. Med J.* 2001; 97: 188–193.
27. Sheps SG, Dart RA. New guidelines for prevention, detection, evaluation, and treatment of hypertension: Joint National Committee VI. *Chest* 1998; 113: 263–265.
28. Institute of Medicine. *To Err Is Human: Building A Safer Health System*, executive summary. www.nap.com, accessed July 7, 2002, pp. 1–16.
29. Kohn L. The Institute of Medicine report on medical error: overview and implications for pharmacy. *Am. J. Hlth.-Syst. Pharm.* 2001; 58: 63–66.
30. Shi L. Health services financing. In: Shi Leiyu, Ed., *Delivering Health Care in America*, 1st ed. Gaithersburg, MD: Dow Jones & Company, 1996, pp. 171–211.
31. Wilensky GR. Medicare reform: now is the time. *N. Engl. J. Med.* 2001; 345: 458–462.
32. Cleves MA, Weiner JP, Cohen W, Athon C, Banks N, Boress L et al. Assessing HCFA's health care quality improvement program. *Jt. Comm. J. Qual. Improv.* 1997; 23: 550–560.
33. Jencks SF, Cuerdon T, Burwen DR, Fleming B, Houck PM, Kussmaul AE et al. Quality of medical care delivered to Medicare beneficiaries: a profile at state and national levels. *JAMA* 2000; 284: 1670–1676.
34. Health Care Financing Administration. Medicare priorities. 10156 Baltimore, MD: U.S. Department of Health and Human Services, pp. 22–29, 2000.
35. Kroner BA. Anticoagulation clinic in the VA Pittsburgh healthcare system. *Pharm. Pract. Manag. Q.* 1998; 18: 17–33.
36. Conte RR, Kehoe WA, Nielson N, Lodhia H. Nine-year experience with a pharmacist-managed anticoagulation clinic. *Am. J. Hosp. Pharm.* 1986; 43: 2460–2464.
37. Norton JL, Gibson DL. Establishing an outpatient anticoagulation clinic in a community hospital. *Am. J. Hlth.-Syst. Pharm.* 1996; 53: 1151–1157.
38. Knowlton CH, Thomas OV, Williamson A, Gammaitoni AR, Kirchain WR, Buttaro ML et al. Establishing community pharmacy-based anticoagulation education and monitoring programs. *J. Am. Pharm. Assoc. (Wash.)* 1999; 39: 368–374.
39. Dager WE, Branch JM, King JH, White RH, Quan RS, Musallam NA et al. Optimization of inpatient warfarin therapy: impact of daily consultation by a pharmacist-managed anticoagulation service. *Ann. Pharmacother.* 2000; 34: 567–572.

40. Dedden P, Chang B, Nagel D. Pharmacy-managed program for home treatment of deep vein thrombosis with enoxaparin. *Am. J. Hlth.-Syst. Pharm.* 1997; 54: 1968–1972.

41. Mamdani MM, Racine E, McCreadie S, Zimmerman C, O'Sullivan TL, Jensen G et al. Clinical and economic effectiveness of an inpatient anticoagulation service. *Pharmacotherapy* 1999; 19: 1064–1074.

42. Wilt VM, Gums JG, Ahmed OI, Moore LM. Outcome analysis of a pharmacist-managed anticoagulation service. *Pharmacotherapy* 1995; 15: 732–739.

43. National Association of Chain Drug Stores. Total Retail Sales 2001. www.nacds.org/wmspage.cfm?parm1 = 507, accessed May 11, 2002.

44. American College of Clinical Pharmacy. Anticoagulation training program. www.accp.com/ClinNet/ri02anti.pdf, accessed May 11, 2002.

45. Carrico JM. Human genome project and pharmacogenomics: implications for pharmacy. *J. Am. Pharm. Assoc. (Wash.)* 2000; 40: 115–116.

46. Pankaskie M, Sullivan J. New players, new services: e-scripts revisited. *J. Am. Pharm. Assoc. (Wash.)* 2000; 40: 566.

chapter twenty-one

Pharmacist credentials and accreditation of pharmacy programs

Steven L. Sheaffer

Contents

0-8493-1446-1/04/$0.00+$1.50
© 2004 by CRC Press LLC

Regardless of one's accomplishments or the recognition one receives for such laudable programs and activities, professional excellence ultimately implies more. I believe such accomplishments, while recognized as milestones of excellence, are only byproducts of the consistent day-to-day journey toward such worthy goals. In other words, professional excellence is more than any destination or achievement, it includes the journey itself. [1]

Billy W. Woodward

Introduction

The U.S. health care system is a unique integration of private and public organizations that regulate, provide, and pay for health care services. In most other countries, national governments exert much more control over how health care is provided, funding for their nations' health services, and defining the roles and training of health professionals. The result is that national authorities, such as the ministry of health, are able to exert significant and central authority over health care, how and to whom it is delivered, and the qualifications and practice expectations of health professionals. In the U.S., the state-based regulation of pharmacy and pharmacists by boards of pharmacy, payers of health care and pharmacist services that include employer sponsored insurance programs, state-controlled Medicaid programs, and federally funded Medicare, along with a myriad of nongovernmental national standard setting and assessment organizations, meet the need of pharmacy to pharmacy practice. Over the past two decades, the increased focus on pharmacist-provided patient care services and increased specialization within pharmacy has lead to the creation of new standard-setting organizations and new practice credentials, with the ultimate goal to define, validate, and advance pharmacist patient care responsibilities and capabilities.

Defining standards for pharmacists, pharmacy practice, and pharmacy education and assessing whether these standards are achieved meets various needs of the profession, the public, state, and federal governments, and funding organizations. The standards may apply to entry-level education and training programs for pharmacists and pharmacy technicians or to individual pharmacists and pharmacy technicians seeking to demonstrate achievement of entry-level or advanced practice abilities. Pharmacies, or patient care organizations such as hospitals that provide pharmacy services, also seek to demonstrate their adherence to program standards that impact pharmacist roles and the effectiveness of pharmacy services and how medications are used. This chapter reviews such programs and the outcomes that each seeks to achieve.

Overview of pharmacy licensure, accreditation of organizations, and credentialing of practitioners

When pharmacists obtain the authority to practice the profession by passing the pharmacy licensure examination and obtaining their state pharmacist license, they have demonstrated their ability to meet the minimum standards required to practice as a pharmacist. To reach this point, they have either graduated from an accredited college of pharmacy or passed an equivalency evaluation of their pharmacy education obtained from a foreign college of pharmacy. They have also passed a state board examination that assesses the broad-based knowledge and skills learned during the didactic and experiential education in pharmacy school.

It becomes quickly apparent to pharmacy students considering employment that they must choose from a wide range of practice settings and types of pharmacy practice that demand ongoing commitment to education to further develop, achieve, and sustain a baseline level of specialty knowledge to meet effectively the unique expectations of their chosen area of pharmacy practice. Although the pharmacy profession in the U.S. currently does not, by law, require any periodic reassessment of a pharmacist's competency, practicing pharmacists are confronted with a wide range of credentials that allow them or an organization (employer, privileging body, accrediting body, etc.) to verify that they have achieved unique or advanced levels of knowledge and skill. To guide the profession and pharmacists pursue such credentials, 11 pharmacy organizations joined together to form the Council on Credentialing in Pharmacy (CCP) in 1998. In 2000, this council published a white paper entitled "Credentialing in Pharmacy,"[2] which has provided guidance to the profession. A very useful component of the white paper is the definition section describing and defining credentialing programs (Table 21.1). The entire white paper can be found on CCP's Web site at www.pharmacycredentialing.org. The process, scope, and value of technician education and certification face similar issues and are also addressed in this chapter.

Organizations that educate or employ pharmacists are subject to standards that assure the quality of their graduates or that the services they provide to patients meet established standards. Although such accreditation is often described as voluntary and conducted by nongovernmental organizations established and controlled by professionals, government requirements or reimbursement criteria usually necessitate organizations to become accredited. For example, all U.S. pharmacy colleges seek American Council for Pharmaceutical Education (ACPE) accreditation because a condition of

Table 21.1 Definitions

Accreditation: The process whereby an association or agency grants public recognition to an organization that meets certain established qualifications or standards, as determined through initial and periodic evaluations.

Certificate training program: A structured, systematic postgraduate education and continuing education experience for pharmacists that is generally smaller in magnitude and shorter in duration than a degree program. Certificate programs are designed to instill, expand, or enhance practice competencies through the systematic acquisition of specific knowledge, skills, attitudes, and performance behaviors.

Certificate: A document issued to a pharmacist on successful completion of the predetermined level of performance of a certificate training program or of a pharmacy residency or fellowship.

Certification: The voluntary process by which a nongovernmental agency or association formally grants recognition to a pharmacist who has met certain predetermined qualifications specified by the organization. This recognition designates to the public that the holder has attained the requisite level of knowledge, skill, or experience in a well-defined, often specialized, area of the total discipline. Certification entails assessment, including testing, an evaluation of the candidate's education and experience, or both. Periodic recertification is usually required to retain the credential.

Competence: The ability to perform one's duties accurately, make correct judgments, and interact appropriately with patients and with colleagues. Professional competence is characterized by good problem-solving and decision-making abilities, a strong knowledge base, and the ability to apply knowledge and experience to diverse patient-care situations.

Competency: A distinct skill, ability, or attitude that is essential to the practice of a profession. Individual competencies for pharmacists include, for example, mastery of aseptic technique and achievement of a thought process that enables one to identify therapeutic duplications. Pharmacists must master a variety of competencies in order to gain competence in their profession.

Continuing education: Organized learning experiences and activities in which pharmacists engage after they have completed their entry-level academic education and training. These experiences are designed to promote the continuous development of the skills, attitudes, and knowledge needed to maintain proficiency, provide quality service or products, respond to patient needs, and keep abreast of change.

Credential: Documented evidence of professional qualifications. For pharmacists, academic degrees, state licensure, and board certification are examples of credentials.

Credentialing: (1) The process by which an organization or institution obtains, verifies, and assesses a pharmacist's qualifications to provide patient care services. (2) The process of granting a credential (a designation that indicates qualifications in a subject or an area).

Fellowship: A directed, highly individualized postgraduate program designed to prepare a pharmacist to become an independent researcher.

License: A credential issued by a state or federal body that indicates that the holder is in compliance with minimum mandatory governmental requirements necessary to practice in a particular profession or occupation.

Table 21.1 Definitions (continued)

Licensure: The process of granting a license.

Pharmacy technician: An individual who, under the supervision of a licensed pharmacist, assists in pharmacy activities not requiring the professional judgment of the pharmacist.

Privileging: The process by which a health care organization, having reviewed an individual health care provider's credentials and performance and found them satisfactory, authorizes the individual to perform a specific scope of patient care services within the organization.

Residency: An organized, directed, postgraduate training program in a defined area of pharmacy practice.

Traineeship: A short, intensive, clinical and didactic postgraduate educational program intended to provide the pharmacist with knowledge and skills needed to provide a high level of care to patients with specific diseases or conditions.

Source: From CCP, White paper: credentialing in pharmacy (September 2000).

their graduates taking state board examinations is that their college has been accredited by the ACPE. Although the profession, through the ACPE, defines the standards for how a pharmacy student is educated, a state's requirements provide little alternative to colleges other than to assure that they meet ACPE requirements. Likewise, the JCAHO accreditation of hospitals is linked to eligibility for Medicare payments; therefore, pharmacists practicing in hospitals and other types of health care facilities are impacted by the pharmacy and medication use standards defined by JCAHO and other accrediting organizations.

The continued evolution of drug knowledge and medication systems, the growing number and complexity of medications, and the public's heightened expectations of quality heath care and safe use of medications have created new opportunities and challenges for pharmacists. These developments have brought about the need for pharmacists to demonstrate continued advancement of baseline and specialized knowledge and competency to meet patient care needs. Increasingly, pharmacists are achieving advanced training and practice credentials beyond their initial, entry-level licenses. Each pharmacy student, and especially pharmacists early in their professional practices, should understand the options, requirements, and implications of pursuing such credentials and the associated organizations and requirements.

Improving and assuring quality of practitioners' pharmacist education

The ACPE was formed in 1932 by the American Association of Colleges of Pharmacy (AACP), the American Pharmaceutical Association, and the National Association of Boards of Pharmacy (NABP) for the accreditation of preservice education. At present, graduation from an ACPE-accredited college of pharmacy is required by most U.S. state boards of pharmacy in order to take pharmacy licensure exams. The U.S. Department of Education also recognizes the ACPE accreditation of the professional degree program in pharmacy. Whereas the three founding organizations and the American Council on Education recommend appointees to its board, the ACPE functions as an autonomous and independent agency. ACPE standards define the educational, scientific, and professional principles and expectations of both didactic and experiential pharmacy education.[3]

The ACPE continues to assess its standards as a means of advancing the profession and in response to changes in pharmacy practice and in the field of education both domestically and internationally. One of the most significant changes in pharmacy education resulted from the 1999 decision by the ACPE to recognize the Doctor of Pharmacy degree as the only accredited pharmacy degree program, effective with all 2005 graduating classes. As a result, all U.S. colleges of pharmacy have transitioned from the Bachelor of Science in pharmacy for all incoming students. In 2005, the ACPE will discontinue its accreditation standard for the B.S. in pharmacy. In 2002, the ACPE also accredited the Beirut College of Pharmacy in Lebanon. Although the Beirut program is unique to international pharmacy education because it is similar to U.S. pharmacy education, it reflects the change in international pharmacy education to include an increased patient focus. The ACPE is also taking initiatives to recognize the equivalency of graduates of Canadian colleges of pharmacy that meet Canadian accreditation standards.

Pharmacist licensure

State boards of pharmacy are responsible for the licensure of pharmacists and pharmacies. Although most boards of pharmacy are primarily comprised of practicing pharmacists, their primary purpose is to assure public safety through regulation of pharmacy practice in their states. In most states, an internship requirement traditionally requires a pharmacy student to work in a licensed pharmacy under the supervision of a board-registered pharmacist preceptor. With the evolution of experiential education in colleges of pharmacy, many state boards of pharmacy have accepted college-coordinated clerkships as equivalent to (or as a significant portion of) state-mandated internships. Given the wide variability from state to state in this requirement and related registration procedures for hours to qualify, pharmacy students should anticipate where they hope to become licensed and gain the experience and documentation to meet intern requirements.

Graduates of foreign colleges of pharmacy must document that they have education and experience equivalent to their U.S.-trained colleagues. They must also pass the Foreign Pharmacy Graduate Equivalency Examination (FPGEE), the Test of English as a Foreign Language (TOEFL), and the Test of Spoken English (TSE). Once these requirements are met, they receive the Foreign Pharmacy Graduate Examination Committee's (FPGEC) certificate.[4]

Upon meeting training prerequisites as an intern and graduating from an ACPE-accredited college, or obtaining the FPGEC certificate, an individual may apply to take board examinations in one or more states. The NAPLEX (National Association of Boards of Pharmacy Licensing Examination) is used by all states except California, which administers its own exam. The exam is taken in one state, but the scores can be reported to other NAPLEX states where licensure is being pursued. In addition to NAPLEX, all states administer a law exam, with some states administering a practical lab exam or additional testing. For the law examination, many states participate in the Multistate Pharmacy Jurisprudence Examination (MPJE). This exam, taken at the same time as the NAPLEX, is a combination of federal law questions common to all participants, with a segment devoted to laws specific to the state where licensure is being pursued.[4]

Continuing education requirements

In most states, continued licensure requires pharmacists to complete a specified number of continuing education (CE) credit hours each year from providers accredited by the ACPE. Although there is a growing interest and perceived need for career-long assessment of pharmacist competency, there is disagreement on whether this should be the responsibility of the state boards or a nongovernmental professional-based group. The growing specialization of pharmacist practice further complicates ongoing competency assessment. Currently, in most states, as long as pharmacists achieve state CE requirements and do not violate pharmacy laws, they can renew their pharmacy licenses even if they do not actively practice pharmacy.

The ACPE has established accreditation standards for organizations that approve the content and conduct of pharmacy education programs that meet ACPE criteria. The majority of ACPE-approved providers are professional pharmacy organizations, colleges of pharmacy, and pharmaceutical companies. Each program is reviewed every 6 years by the ACPE. Boards of pharmacy in 48 states accept CE credit from ACPE provider organizations to meet their CE requirements for license renewal.[3]

Pharmacy technicians

Pharmacy technicians are an increasingly important component of the pharmacy workforce. A pharmacy technician has been defined as "an individual working in a pharmacy (setting) who, under the supervision of a licensed pharmacist, assists in pharmacy activities that do not require the professional judgment of a pharmacist."[5] The training of pharmacy technicians varies widely from on-the-job training to graduates of American Society of Health-System Pharmacists (ASHP)-accredited technician training programs. Formal training programs can range from a hospital- or trade-school-based program that typically provides student didactic and experiential education to 2-year associates degree programs offered by community colleges. The ACPE initiated a process in 2003 to develop a profession-wide consensus on technician education and training needs and determine whether there is a need for a national standard for pharmacy technician education. In anticipation of this discussion, the CCP published the document "White Paper on Pharmacy Technicians 2002: Needed Changes Can No Longer Wait." [6] This document provides a history and evolution of technicians; an overview of current technician roles; and related issues, including competency assessment and education. It challenges the profession to address critical issues in the partnership between pharmacists and pharmacy technicians.

Although there is no standardized national approach to educating and training pharmacy technicians, the pharmacy profession, and, increasingly, state boards of pharmacy are addressing the competency of the pharmacy technician workforce. The Pharmacy Technician Certification Board (PTCB) was founded by the American Pharmaceutical Association, the ASHP, the Illinois Council of Health System Pharmacists, and the Michigan Pharmacists Association. In 2002, the NABP also became a partner in the governance of PTCB. Since administering its first technician certification examination in 1995, almost 150,000 pharmacy technicians have earned the designation of certified pharmacy technician (CPhT). The exam is broad based and applies to all pharmacy practice settings.[7]

The PTCB exam is used and endorsed by many national pharmacy chains, many independent community and hospital pharmacies, and the U.S. military. Employers use the exam as a condition of employment as a requirement to perform selected functions, to justify career or salary advancement, and so forth. To create a minimum standard for pharmacy technician capabilities, a growing number of state boards of pharmacy require technicians to be PTCB certified. In addition, many state boards of pharmacy have developed processes for technicians to register with the state. This process allows pharmacy boards to identify individuals currently employed as technicians in their states. Most professional pharmacy organizations and state boards of pharmacy oppose licensure of pharmacy technicians. As the roles of pharmacy technicians continue to evolve and the public becomes more aware of their contributions, the profession will need to provide the required training and competencies to assure the public that the technicians are able to fulfill their vital roles in pharmacy.

Postgraduate training programs

Pharmacy residency programs

A residency program is defined as "an organized, directed, postgraduate training in a defined area of pharmacy practice." Most residency programs last 12 months. The ASHP Commission on Credentialing accredits pharmacy residency programs in the U.S. The commission started accrediting hospital pharmacy residency programs in 1952. Since then, significant changes in the levels and diversity of residency training have occurred. The intent of a residency program is to "provide the knowledge and experience that pharmacy practitioners need to face challenges of today's complex health care systems, while also providing essential skills to meet the practice demands of the future."[8] As pharmacy practice in hospitals and health systems evolved, residency training expanded to include ambulatory care and advanced specialty practice. Table 21.2 lists the types of residency programs currently accredited by the ASHP Commission on Credentialing. All ASHP residency accreditation standards and currently accredited programs with detailed, updated information can be found on the ASHP Web site (www.ashp.org). The American College of Clinical Pharmacy (ACCP) also publishes a list of pharmacy practice and specialty practices residency programs (accredited and unaccredited) offered by its members. Compliance with the residency accreditation standard also reflects positively on the quality of the pharmacy practice at the residency practice site. An added incentive to seek pharmacy residency accreditation is that it qualifies a hospital to receive Medicare funding for the residency program.

A recent advance in pharmacy residency training is expansion of residency accreditation to include community and managed care pharmacy residencies. In partnership with the APhA for community pharmacy and the AMCP for managed care, the ASHP has established residency standards and reviews of these programs. In addition, expansion of community pharmacy residency programs has also been supported by the NACDS and

Table 21.2 Residency Programs Accredited by ASHP Commission on Credentialing

Pharmacy practice
Pharmacy practice residency (traditionally conducted in health systems)
Pharmacy practice with emphasis on community pharmacy
Pharmacy practice with an emphasis on managed care
Pharmacy practice with emphasis on home care
Pharmacy practice with emphasis on long-term care
Specialized Residencies
Cardiology
Clinical pharmacokinetics
Critical care
Drug information
Emergency medicine
Geriatrics
Infectious diseases
Internal medicine
Managed care pharmacy systems
Nuclear pharmacy
Nutrition support
Oncology
Pediatrics
Pharmacotherapy
Pharmacy practice management
Primary care
Psychiatric

NCPA, including development of the NACDS/NCPA community pharmacy residency guidelines.[9] The Institute for the Advancement of Community Pharmacy, an organization founded by the NACDS and NCPA, has provided grants to encourage schools of pharmacy and community pharmacies to develop additional community pharmacy residency programs nationwide.

Fellowship training

Unlike a residency, which focuses on developing practice knowledge and skills, a pharmacy fellowship is defined as "a directed, highly individualized, postgraduate program designed to prepare the participant to become an independent researcher."[10] Although no formal accreditation process exists, the ACCP has developed guidelines for the conduct of clinical fellowships. To improve consistency in the quantity and quality of the research experience, the ACCP has implemented a process for peer review of pharmacy fellowship training programs. If the preceptor qualifications and the training program meet the guidelines based on a review by the ACCP Fellowship Review Committee, they are recognized and the program and preceptor are listed on the ACCP Web site.[10]

Certificate programs and traineeships

For practitioners to acquire new capabilities without enrolling in an academic degree program, a wide variety of certificate programs (see definitions in Table 21.1) evolved. These programs can vary considerably in rigor and the amount, if any, of didactic education and structured experiential training required. Such programs, however, assist pharmacists in developing knowledge and skills in a specific area, with the value of such programs depending on individuals' goals or in instances when an employer or regulatory body recognizes the importance of the certificate. Examples are state boards of pharmacy that allow pharmacists to administer vaccines provided they have completed a certificate program in vaccine administration that was developed and administered by the American Pharmacists Association. In 1999, the ACPE published the "Standards and Quality Assurance Procedure for ACPE-Approved Providers of Continuing Pharmaceutical Education Offering Certificate Programs in Pharmacy." This document defines certificate programs in pharmacy as forms of accredited CE that involve "in-depth commitment on the part of learners" with approval of such programs by existing ACPE-approved providers. Several attributes that differentiate a certificate program from a CE program include the "instructional design to include (a) practice experiences, (b) simulations, and/or (c) other activities so as to assure demonstration of the application of the stated professional competencies." It is also "expected that this will *generally* require a minimum program of 15 contact hours or 1.5 CEUs."[3]

Traineeships allow practicing pharmacists to receive abbreviated clinical training experience under the supervision of a pharmacist practicing in a given specialty. Most traineeships define expected outcomes achieved by a combination of self-study and didactic instruction that supports an intense clinical training experience usually conducted at the practice site of the preceptor. Examples of such programs are anticoagulation management, critical care pharmacy, and diabetes management. These programs are commonly offered through the foundations of professional organizations such as the ACCP, American Society of Consultant Pharmacists (ASCP), and ASHP and are often supported by grants from the pharmaceutical industry.

Individual pharmacist advanced practice credentials

Entry into the profession requires graduation from an ACPE-accredited college of pharmacy and passing the state licensure examination. There is a growing number of means by which individual pharmacists can obtain credentials to differentiate themselves in specialized areas of practice. These can range from an employer-based certificate program to develop and assess the competency of pharmacists to board certification in nuclear pharmacy as a requirement to practice in this specialty area. In addition to credentials specific to pharmacy, there are also opportunities for pharmacists to be recognized through programs that assess different types of health care providers with a common area of practice.

Specialty certification (BPS)

A specialty practice credential granted by the Board of Pharmaceutical Specialties (BPS) is highly regarded in the profession, based on the rigorous practice experience and testing requirements for pharmacists to be BPS certified. According to BPS, its mission "is to improve public health through recognition and promotion of specialized training, knowledge, and skills in pharmacy, and certification of pharmacist specialists."[11] BPS was formed in 1976 as an independent agency of APhA. The first five specialty areas of practice to be recognized were nuclear pharmacy (1978), followed by nutrition support pharmacy (1988), pharmacotherapy (1988), psychiatric pharmacy (1992), and oncology pharmacy (1996). As BPS states, "new specialties are considered for recognition upon the submission of a petition to BPS from a group of interested pharmacists." BPS uses seven criteria to evaluate the request, which range from having a reasonable number of pharmacists practicing in the specialty to requiring specialized knowledge and performance of specialized functions that are "acquired through education and training beyond the basic level attained by licensed pharmacists."

Once a specialty has been recognized, a number of actions are required before a certification exam can be implemented. This relatively intensive and costly process includes conducting "a role delineation study to analyze the specialty practice area, which results in a comprehensive list of knowledge, skills and functions."[11] From this, an examination content outline; a bank of test questions; criteria for candidates, including education, training and practice experience; and a process for recertification are established before testing is initiated. Each exam is administered annually, with recertification required every 7 years. An ongoing evaluation and updating process is in place for each specialty area. The number of BPS-certified pharmacists has increased from 951 in 1993 to 3400 in 2001. The largest number is in pharmacotherapy, with 1843 pharmacists in 2001.

In 1997, BPS implemented an added-qualifications program to recognize focused practice areas within the currently recognized specialties. The added-qualifications designation may be granted to a BPS-certified pharmacist specialist who can document a level of focused training and experience in an area. Candidates for added qualifications submit a structured portfolio, which is assessed relative to published standards. Infectious diseases and cardiology are currently approved added qualifications within pharmacotherapy.[11]

Disease management certification

The National Institute for Standards in Pharmacist Credentialing (NISPC) was formed in 1998 by the APhA, NABP, NACDS, and NCPA "to create a consolidated, nationally recognized, credential for pharmacists seeking certification in a variety of disease states."[12] The primary motivation to develop DSM credentials for pharmacists is that state Medicaid programs will compensate DSM-credentialed pharmacists to provide advanced pharmacy services. NISPC offers certification in asthma, diabetes, dyslipidemia, and anticoagulation. To be certified by the NISPC, a pharmacist must pass an examination with questions that are specific to the specialty area, developed by experts, and designed to address four different areas of competency expected of all pharmacists who provide disease state management services to patients. There are no practice experience or clinical training requirements in the specialty area. After passing the exam, pharmacists may use the designation of certified disease manager (CDM) and are listed on the NISPC Web site (www.nispcnet.org). Recertification is required every 3 years and is based on completion of 30 hours of CE in the specific disease state.[12]

Certified geriatric pharmacist

The Commission for Certification in Geriatric Pharmacy (CCGP) is an independent credentialing organization founded by the ASCP. ASCP's membership is composed primarily of pharmacists with practices involving nursing facilities, subacute care and assisted living facilities, and other settings where the challenges and complexities of drug therapy in geriatric patients create numerous opportunities for pharmacist involvement. The Certified Geriatric Pharmacist (CGP) exam was first administered in 1997.[13] Federal laws require nursing facilities to have a pharmacist conduct drug regimen reviews on every resident in the facility at least monthly, along with other specified duties. Pharmacists who have CGP credentials are able to provide additional assurances to employers and nursing homes that contract for their consultant pharmacist services that they are capable of achieving the outcomes expected.

Pharmacist certification by multiprofessional organizations

Pharmacists patient care management and education services provided to specific types of patients often require similar postgraduate training, experience, and expertise as those required of other health professionals. Several national specialty organizations have developed criteria for multiple health care disciplines, including pharmacy, to become credentialed.

Certified diabetic educator (CDE)

The longest standing (since 1986) multidisciplinary certification program involving pharmacists is for those with expertise and a practice in diabetic education. Becoming a certified diabetic educator is open to numerous licensed health professionals, including registered nurses, physicians, physician assistants, registered dieticians, and pharmacists. Diabetic educator certification is managed by the National Certification Board for Diabetic Educators (NCDME). The primary intent of this credential is to recognize professionals who have advanced knowledge and experience in diabetic education and consistent practice in the area. Before applying for the certification exam, three experiential requirements must be met: (1) a minimum of 2 years professional practice experience in diabetes self-management, (2) a minimum of 1000 hours of diabetes self-management education experience in the last 5 years, and (3) current employment in a primary role as a diabetes educator for a minimum of 4 hours per week at the time of applying. Upon passing the 200-question examination, the successful candidate may use the designation CDE. Renewal of the CDE credential is required every 5 years and requires reexamination.[14] A new credential in advanced clinical diabetes management is being developed by the American Association of Diabetes Educators and the American Nurses Credentialing Center. It is expected that, unlike the CDE, a separate examination will be offered for resident nurses (RNs), registered dieticians, and pharmacists. The focus of this process will be on clinical practice with "a core of knowledge for all advanced practitioners, but specific and unique content for each discipline."[15] The APhA is collaborating to develop this certification process.

Asthma educator-certified (AE-C)

The first examination for asthma educators, including pharmacists, to achieve the designation AE-C was administered in September 2002. The exam is available to candidates who are licensed or credentialed health care professionals, health educators, or persons with at least 1000 hours of asthma education experience. The mission of the National Asthma Educator Certification board is "to promote optimal asthma management and quality of life among individuals with asthma, their families and communities by advancing excellence in asthma education through the Certified Asthma Educator process." One of the seven areas of expertise that an asthma educator must achieve is to teach "the best use of medications and delivery devices, explaining technical concepts in understandable terms." The other areas reflect a need to have a broad-based knowledge of asthma and the ability to work closely with patients and families to define and achieve broad-based patient care needs of asthmatics.

Certified anticoagulation care provider

The National Certification Board for Anticoagulation Providers established a certification program for registered nurses, advanced practice nurses, pharmacists, physician assistants, and physicians in 1998. This "certification process is designed and intended for practitioners whose primary role as an anticoagulation provider includes systematic, organized, and on-going patient education and drug therapy management"[17] in patients requiring anticoagulation. To take the exam, practitioners "must submit substantial evidence of their practice experience." Practitioners who meet practice requirements and pass the examination may use the designation of certified anticoagulation care provider or CACP.

Assuring quality of pharmacy practice sites in health systems

The Joint Commission on Accreditation of Healthcare Organizations (JCAHO)

Pharmacy practice, especially in hospitals, has been evaluated during accreditation visits by the JCAHO. The JCAHO's development and evolution of standards for hospital pharmacy practice has had a marked impact on the level and scope of pharmacy services provided. From the implementation of unit dose systems and IV admixture programs in the 1970s and 1980s to the current focus on the entire medication use process and medication safety, the role of the pharmacist has been a focal point of developing JCAHO standards and during visits by JCAHO surveyors to sites seeking accreditation. At present, JCAHO's focus is increasingly on a multidisciplinary outcomes-focused review process. Although this has reduced the focus on the pharmacy per se, it has created greater opportunities and responsibilities for the pharmacist during the entire medication use process (prescribing, dispensing, and administering the medication). The outcomes of how drugs are used, e.g., impacting and assessing prescribing practices relative to nationally defined best practices as well as the clinical management, reporting, and prevention of medication errors and adverse drug events, are increasingly the focus of how pharmacy services are assessed.

The JCAHO review process for hospitals (and other JCAHO-accredited programs) is evolving from an onsite review process, which normally occurs every 3 years, to a process of continuous assessment of quality and patient outcomes. It is a major challenge for hospitals and pharmacy managers to keep up with new initiatives, changing areas of focus, and procedural changes in the review process.[18]

One advantage of JCAHO accreditation for hospitals is that it may make them eligible for Medicare and Medicaid payment without needing to undergo routine government review of their services. Even with JCAHO accreditation, hospitals may be reviewed by the Center for Medicare and Medicaid Services (CMS). Such reviews are based on CMS's conditions for participation criteria, using a process similar to JCAHO onsite reviews. These reviews can result from a complaint regarding the quality of care at an institution or as part of a random review by CMS to validate JCAHO findings.[19]

Over the past two decades, the Joint Commission on Accreditation of Hospitals has evolved from comprising only acute care hospitals to including other health system practice settings, as reflected in its name change. Of the eight practice settings where JCAHO has developed accreditation standards, hospitals and home care and long-term-care settings focus heavily on pharmacy and medication use practices. The home care accreditation process specifically provides for accreditation of pharmacy programs in clinical/consultant pharmacy services, long-term-care pharmacy services, pharmacy dispensing services, and pharmacy services (i.e., combined clinical and despensing services). Other areas of home care, including hospice, home health services, and freestanding ambulatory care services, may survey pharmacy services as part of their accreditation visits.[20]

The following are specific areas of focus for the JCAHO that are important to pharmacists practicing in hospitals. Many of these activities have similar applications and expectations as the JCAHO-accredited programs noted previously.

Medication management chapter

Before moving from discipline-specific standards to a review process that focuses on a multidisciplinary and systems-based approach to care, medication standards were in department-specific chapters, such as pharmacy, nursing, and medical staff, with the latter centered around the Pharmacy and Therapeutics committee, the formulary and adverse drug reaction reporting. Over time, the pharmacy standard disappeared and was integrated into the overall patient care chapters. For the 2004 standards, the JCAHO has published a new chapter entitled "Medication Management," which reflects increased focus on medication systems and safety.[21] This chapter divides the medication process into six segments:

1. Selection and procurement
2. Storage
3. Ordering and transcribing
4. Preparing and dispensing
5. Administration
6. Monitoring

The following are the proposed JCAHO expectations and intended outcomes when medication systems are designed and implemented in hospitals:

1. Reducing practice variation, errors, and misuse
2. Monitoring medication management processes as regards efficiency, quality, and safety
3. Standardizing equipment and processes across the organization to improve the medication management system
4. Using evidence-based good practices to develop medication management processes
5. Managing critical processes associated with medication management to promote safe medication management throughout the organization
6. Handling all medications in the same manner, including sample medications

Of note is the broad definition that the JCAHO draft uses to define medications. It may include medications that pharmacy departments do not provide, such as those brought into institutions by patients or purchased and used independent of pharmacy departments. According to the definition:

> *Medication includes prescription medications, sample medications, herbal remedies, vitamins, neutraceuticals, over-the-counter drugs, vaccines, diagnostic and contrast agents used on or administered to diagnose, treat, or prevent disease or other abnormal conditions; radioactive medications; respiratory therapy treatments; parenteral nutrition; blood derivatives; intravenous solutions (plain, with electrolytes and/or drugs); and any product designated by the FDA as a drug.*[21]

Such a broad definition and the expectation regarding consistency in the way all medications are used in organizations necessitates that pharmacies approach medication systems in a multidisciplinary and integrated manner.

The details of hospital medication management standards and the resulting expectations of pharmacy service and on pharmacist responsibilities are beyond the range of this chapter. The following are examples of how the standards impact pharmacy practices:

1. The organization must define what minimum patient information must be available for health professionals, including pharmacists, to fulfil their responsibilities. This includes, at minimum, a patient's relevant laboratory values, diagnosis, allergies, and past sensitivities, and, as appropriate, height and weight. For the pharmacy to properly assess medication orders and monitor a patient's drug therapy, including pediatric and chemotherapy patients, it is critical for the pharmacy to have routine access to this information.

2. The proposed standard requires all medication storage areas to be periodically inspected according to the organization's policy to ensure that medications are stored properly. This statement reflects much weaker prescriptive language than for previous standards. Although the specifics of what, how often, and by who are not specified, the outcomes of assuring proper security, consistent temperatures in refrigerators, where medications are stored, and the presence of authorized or absence of unauthorized medications still needs to be documented.

3. Examples of specific types of medications and standards regarding their availability or use include emergency medications, investigational drugs, floor stock medications, intravenous compounded medications, recalled or discontinued medications, medications unavailable due to a shortage, investigational drugs, medications brought to the hospital by patients or that are self-administered, and high-risk medications. The last is a focus of the JCAHO patient safety goals as noted later.

4. A more detailed requirement for how medication orders are to be written is included in the new draft standards. Again, the focus is on the institution needing to develop its own written policy that addresses such areas as defining which abbreviations are unacceptable (such as U for units); when the indication for use must be required as part of an order; and what actions are to be taken with incomplete, illegible, or unclear orders. Where permitted, organizations must also develop procedures for order types, such as hold orders, automatic stop orders, titrating orders, taper orders, for which there is increased potential for misinterpretation and error.

5. Expectations for hospitals that do not have 24-hour pharmacy service are required, including how medication orders are to be processed and medications accessed when the pharmacy is closed.

6. There is continued focus on adverse drug events and medication errors. Processes must respond to actual or potential adverse drug events and medication errors and properly report them internally and externally (e.g., to the FDA, ISMP, or USP). Other standards address how adverse drug events and medication errors should be addressed to improve systems, support staff education and training, and minimize the risk of medication-related errors and adverse events.

Sentinel event reporting and patient safety goals

The JCAHO initiated a sentinel event reporting expectation by health care organizations and began tracking sentinel events in 1996. The JCAHO defines a sentinel event as "an unexpected occurrence involving death or serious physical or psychological injury, or the risk thereof. Serious injury specifically includes the loss of limb or function. The phrase *or the risk thereof* includes any process variation for which a recurrence would carry a significant chance of a serious adverse outcome. Such events are called 'sentinel' because they signal the need for immediate investigation and response." When an accredited organization experiences a sentinel event, it is expected that reporting, evaluation, and response processes will occur that minimize the potential of the event reoccurring. A key component of the review process is the conduct of a root cause analysis, which by design is intended to identify the underlying causes and contributing factors that contributed to the sentinel event. According to the JCAHO:

> *The product of a root cause analysis is an action plan that identifies the strategies an organization intends to implement to reduce the risk of similar events occurring in the future. The plan should address responsibility for implementation, oversight, pilot testing as appropriate, time lines, and strategies for measuring the effectiveness of the actions. During a survey process, compliance to this expectation is through document review, interviews with the organization's leaders and staff, and review of an example of the organization's response to a sentinel event within the previous year.[22]*

The sentinel event reports submitted to the JCAHO are reviewed and cataloged for error type and underlying causes. Medication errors are one of the most common types of sentinel events reported to the JCAHO. When a trend of similar errors is identified, the JCAHO issues a sentinel event alert, which alerts others of the risk and recommends actions to minimize risk in organizations. The first alert issued in 1998 focused on deaths due to the inadvertent IV push administration of IV potassium chloride (KCl). Awareness of these events and actions by pharmacists to remove concentrated KCl from patient unit floor stocks has markedly reduced reports of this type of error. Of the 27 subsequent alerts issued in January 2003, seven focus on different types of medication errors and prevention strategies.

In 2002, a sentinel event advisory committee was established to review JCAHO initiatives regarding sentinel events. A charge of this group is to annually recommend to the JCAHO a set of no more than six national patient safety goals and associated recommendations. During the survey process, each organization is evaluated on implementation of the recommendations, or acceptable alternatives, as a condition of accreditation. Two of the initial six goals relate to medications: the need to improve the safety of high-alert medications and to improve the safety of using infusion pumps. The six goals are evaluated annually; some may continue for multiple years, while others are replaced because of new areas of priority. The new goals are announced by July 1 each year and are surveyed during the following calendar year.[22]

Survey methodology

Traditionally, teams of surveyors trained and employed by the JCAHO were scheduled to visit facilities pursuing accreditation. Hospital surveys scheduled for every 3 years often prompted a flurry of activities in anticipation of the visit. Questions about the level of ongoing compliance with the standards have led the JCAHO to announce new processes and move to unannounced surveys. By 2006, it is expected that all routine surveys will be unannounced, and accredited sites are expected to conduct an online self-assessment regarding their compliance with published standards. A new tracer methodology, wherein surveyors follow the care of selected patients, will be used to evaluate patient care practices vs. the accreditation standards.[18]

ORYX indicators

A related initiative to provide ongoing measurement of the quality of care provided by health systems are the ORYX indicators. ORYX is intended "to integrate the use of outcomes and other performance measurement data into the accreditation process."[23] Performance measures are expected to be applicable across the accredited health care organizations with the evolution of core performance measures applicable to each accreditation program. The initial four core measurement areas will be for hospitals and will focus on acute myocardial infarction, heart failure, community-acquired pneumonia, and pregnancy and related conditions. Hospitals are expected to collect data that will allow assessment of patient care based on the standards. The ORYX standards for acute myocardial infarction in Table 21.3 reflect the focus on medications and how pharmacists can impact their organizations' performance.[23]

The only thing certain about the survey process is that the methods and areas surveyed will continue to change to reflect current standards of care in order to assure quality and safety of patient care provided by accredited organizations. Pharmacists can expect that the JCAHO views them as critical members of the patient care team and integral to ensuring safe and effective

Table 21.3 JCAHO ORYX Acute Myocardial Infarction Performance Measures for Hospitals

Measure ID No.	Measure Name
AMI-1	Aspirin received[a] within 24 h of admission
AMI-2	Aspirin prescribed[a] at discharge
AMI-3	Angiotensin converting enzyme inhibitor prescribed[a] for left ventricular systolic dysfunction (LVSD)
AMI-4	Adult smoking cessation advice or counseling provided
AMI-5	Beta blocker prescribed[a] within 24 h of admission
AMI-6	Beta blocker prescribed[a] at discharge
AMI-7	Time to thrombolysis (future measure is receipt within 30 min from arrival)
AMI-8	Time to PTCA (future measure is receipt within 90 min from arrival)
AMI-9	Inpatient mortality rate

[a] Unless contraindicated.

medication use and that related systems that support prescribing, dispensing, drug administration, and evaluating patient outcomes meet current standards of care.   •

Managed care organizations

Pharmacy department performance and compliance with medication use processes that are impacted by pharmacists are often used to evaluate quality of health care providers. Managed care organizations are accredited by the National Committee for Quality Assurance (NCQA). The NCQA collects quality indicator information, including medication utilization that can be impacted by pharmacists within and by those contracting with the MCO. The program used by the NCQA is the Health Plan Employer Data and Information Set (HEDIS). HEDIS is a set of standardized performance measures designed to ensure that purchasers and consumers have the information they need to compare reliably the performance of managed health care plans. Example HEDIS medication-use measures include rates of flu vaccine administration, use of beta blockers after heart attacks, and appropriate use of medications by asthma patients.[24]

Community pharmacy

At present, no distinct accreditation programs for community pharmacies exist. The only community pharmacies involved in accreditation processes are those that have implemented accredited community pharmacy residency programs or those participating in the JCAHO home care accreditation program.

State boards of pharmacy are responsible for licensing pharmacies and how pharmacy services are provided in these locations. This is accomplished by an initial and then ongoing board-authorized inspections to assure that pharmacies meet the minimal standards for providing pharmacy services as defined by state pharmacy acts and regulations. Violations found during routine reviews or in response to a complaint may lead to fines or revocation of a pharmacy license. Pharmacy boards are increasingly challenged by the growing diversity of pharmacy practices and the licensure requirements for specialty pharmacies that have evolved. Examples include nuclear pharmacies and pharmacies providing home infusion or IV compounding services.

Online pharmacy

The Verified Internet Pharmacy Practice Site (VIPPS) program is a voluntary certification program for online pharmacies and is sponsored by the NABP. This program, initiated in 1999, provides a means for online pharmacies to demonstrate compliance with VIPPS criteria "including patient rights to privacy, authentication and security of prescription orders, adherence to a recognized quality assurance policy, and provision of meaningful consultation between patients and pharmacists."[25] Patients can determine whether an online pharmacy is VIPPS certified by looking for the VIPPS hyperlink seal on the pharmacy's Web site or by going to the NABP Web site (www.nabp.net) and viewing the list of VIPPS-certified pharmacies.

Other standard-setting organizations impacting pharmacy practice

Many organizations, both pharmacy and nonpharmacy, develop standards that impact pharmacists and pharmacy practice. These standards may be used by accrediting organizations, the federal government (e.g., the FDA), or state boards of pharmacy when creating their own standards or laws. Pharmacists also look to such standards to provide guidance when establishing new programs or creating policies and procedures. The following are examples of such organizations and how they impact pharmacy.

United States Pharmacopeia (USP)

The USP is a nongovernment organization that "promotes the public health by establishing state-of-the-art standards to ensure the quality of medicines and other health care technologies."[26] It is traditionally known for publishing the USP-NF that establishes standards for prescription and nonprescription drugs. The USP also develops practice standards, such as its document "Sterile Products for Home Use." The USP also operates two medication error reporting, tracking, and analysis programs. The medication error reporting program, operating in collaboration with the Institute for Safe Medication Practices (ISMP), receives voluntarily submitted medication error reports. Their evaluation and trending allows them to identify problems and recommend corrective actions. The USP MEDMARx program in an Internet-based system for hospitals to report and track their own medication errors. This information is anonymously entered into a larger database, permitting broad-based trending of hospital-based errors and underlying causes. Both of these USP systems assist others, such as the JCAHO, professional organizations, and individual practitioners in medication safety initiatives.

National Quality Forum (NQF)

The NQF is a "not-for-profit membership organization that was created to develop and implement a national strategy for health care quality measurement and reporting."[27] Its membership has broad participation by organizations representing all parts of the health system, including consumers; public and private purchasers; employers; and health care professionals, such as pharmacists, labor unions, and supporting industries. The goal is to work together to "promote a common approach to measuring health care quality and fostering system-wide capacity for quality improvement." Their focus is on quality centers on errors, overtreatment, and undertreatment; which all lead to undesirable patient outcomes and unnecessary costs.

Of particular interest to pharmacists is the NQF report entitled "Safe Practices for Better Healthcare."[28] This report "details 30 healthcare practices that should be universally utilized in applicable clinical care settings to reduce the risk of harm to patients." Eleven of the thirty endorsed practices deal specifically with or are relevant to medication practices. Of particular interest to pharmacists is the fifth practice, which states:

> *Pharmacists should actively participate in the medication-use process, including, at a minimum, being available for consultation with prescribers on medication ordering, interpretation, and review of medication orders, preparation of medications, dispensing of medications, and administration and monitoring of medications.*

This statement strongly advocates for active involvement of pharmacists in all phases of medication use. Other standards, such as number 18, which advocates for use of "dedicated anti-thrombotic (anti-coagulation) services that facilitate coordinated care management" supports those pharmacists who have developed anticoagulation expertise and services. The broad-based support of these standards is a strong statement of the value that pharmacists provide to patients and other members of the health care team.

The Leapfrog Group

This unique group that focuses on health care quality is composed of over 140 public and private organizations that provide health care benefits. Its goal is to use its purchasing power to drive changes in the way health care is delivered by directing the patients it serves to hospitals meeting their standards. By working with medical experts to identify problems and propose solutions, Leapfrog believes it can improve hospital systems. It has initially identified three areas of focus. The first, of greatest interest to pharmacists, is to implement computerized prescriber order entry (CPOE) for medications. The other two are to develop surgery data for hospitals that allow comparison of death and complication rates for high-risk treatments and procedures, and to ensure that hospital ICU care be managed or comanaged by a physician certified (or eligible for certification) in critical care medicine. Hospital pharmacists are already aware of how Leapfrog's focus on CPOE for medication use has stimulated senior hospital management interest in moving forward with such systems. The short- and long-term impacts are very significant for pharmacy. Given the national focus on medication safety, it is likely that future areas of Leapfrog's focus will impact pharmacists.[29]

Pharmacy professional organizations

Many of pharmacy's national professional organizations develop professional practice standards to support their members' needs and to foster improvements in pharmacy practice and patient care. Many of these standards are developed by appointed groups of members and then approved by the organizations' house of delegates, reflecting broad-based input and support by the membership. An example of this is the APhA. The ASHP has the most extensive list of documents, referred to as "Best Practices in Health-System Pharmacy," which is published in hard copy and available on its Web site. This list is a combination of professional policies approved by the ASHP house of delegates and more detailed guidance documents approved by the ASHP board of directors. Other specialty organizations, such as ASCP for long-term-care pharmacy and AMCP for managed care pharmacy practice, develop policies specific to their areas of practice that reflect the values and priorities of their members. Readers are referred to Chapter 22 for more detailed comments and contact information for professional organizations.

What is the value and who benefits?

The issues and opportunities currently evolving in the medication use and the roles of pharmacists create an exciting and bright future for the pharmacy profession. The transition of pharmacy education and pharmacy practice from a product-based profession to one that increasingly focuses on patients and pharmacist contributions to improving patient medication use have created new challenges for the profession, employers of pharmacists, and individual pharmacists. Assuring the capabilities and qualities of both pharmacy services and pharmacists providing such services is and will become an increasingly important focus of the profession and the public. Although the pharmacy license is currently the only credential essential to enter and practice pharmacy, pharmacists seeking to differentiate themselves and assure continued engagement and growth in an increasingly diverse and specialized profession must understand the process and the value of pharmacist credentials.

As Billy Woodward notes in the quote at the beginning of the chapter, pharmacists should not focus too heavily on credentials they need to achieve their career goals. Rather, they should continue to grow and develop their capabilities and knowledge each day. By enjoying and realizing the benefits of each day in their professional journeys in pharmacy, pharmacists will view credentials as outcomes of their experience, and not as endpoints. This approach will help ensure that organizations where pharmacists work meet the standards they are held to, assure payers that the quality of drug therapy they are reimbursing for is provided, and, most importantly, that the patients they serve realize their goals to minimize risk and improve their health through the benefits of the medications they use.

Appendix

Accrediting, Credentialing, and Standard-Setting Organizations

Accrediting Organizations	Credentialing Organizations (continued)
American Council on Pharmaceutical Education (ACPE) 20 North Clark Street Suite 2500 Chicago, IL 60602-5109 www.acpe-accredit.org	National Certification Board for Diabetes Educators (NCBDE) 330 East Algonquin Road, Suite 4 Arlington Heights, IL 60005 www.ncbde.org
ASHP Commission on Credentialing American Society of Health-System Pharmacists (ASHP) 7272 Wisconsin Ave. Bethesda, MD 20814 www.ashp.org	National Institute for Standards in Pharmacist Credentialing (NISPC) 205 Daingerfield Road Alexandria, VA 22314 www.nispcnet.org
Joint Commission on Accreditation of Healthcare Organizations (JCAHO) One Renaissance Blvd. Oakbrook Terrace, IL 60181 www.jcaho.org	The Pharmacy Technician Certification Board (PTCB) 2215 Constitution Avenue, NW Washington, D.C. 20037-2985 www.ptcb.org
Credentialing Organizations	**Standard-Setting Organizations**
	Center for Medicare and Medicaid Services (CMS) Department of Health and Human Services http://hhs.cms.gov
Board of Pharmaceutical Specialties (BPS) 2215 Constitution Ave. NW Washington, D.C. 20037-2985 www.bpsweb.org	Council on Credentialing in Pharmacy (CCP) www.pharmacycredentialing.org
Commission for Certification in Geriatric Pharmacy (CCGP) 1321 Duke St Alexandria, VA 22314 www.ccgp.org	The Leapfrog Group www.leapfroggroup.org The National Association of Boards of Pharmacy (NABP) 700 Busse Highway Park Ridge, IL 60068 www.nabp.net
National Asthma Educator Certification Board (NAECB) 1150 18th St. NW, Ste. 900 Washington, D.C. 20036 www.naecb.org	The National Quality Forum (NQF) 601 Thirteenth Street, NW Suite 500 North Washington, D.C. 20005 www.qualityforum.org
National Certification Board for Anticoagulation Providers C/O Anticoagulation Forum Boston University Medical Center, Room E-113 www.carsgroup.org	United States Pharmacopeia 12601 Twinbrook Parkway Rockville, MD 20852 www.usp.org

References

1. Woodward, B. The journey to professional excellence: a matter of priorities. *AJHP* 1998; 55: 782.
2. Council on Credentialing in Pharmacy. White paper: credentialing in pharmacy. http://www.pharmacycredentialing.org, accessed October 22, 2002.
3. The American Council on Pharmaceutical Education. Who we are. http://www.acpe-accredit.org/, accessed January 6, 2003.
4. National Association of Boards of Pharmacy. http://www.nabp.net, accessed June 24, 2003.
5. American Society of Hospital Pharmacists. ASHP outcome competencies for institutional pharmacy technician training programs (with training guidelines). *Am. J. Hosp. Pharm.* 1982; 39: 317–320.
6. Council on Credentialing in Pharmacy. White paper on pharmacy technicians 2002: needed changes can no longer wait. *AJHP* 2003; 60: 37.
7. Pharmacy Technician Certification Board. http://www.ptcb.org, accessed June 25, 2003.
8. American Society of Health-System Pharmacists. Pharmacy residencies. http://ashp.org/rtp/Starting/definitions.cfm, accessed January 6, 2003.
9. National Community Pharmacists Association. NCPA/NACDS community pharmacy practice residency guidelines. http://66.113.233.142/management/guidelines.shtml, accessed June 25, 2003.
10. American College of Clinical Pharmacy. Residencies and fellowships. http://www.accp.com/resandfel/?page=definition, accessed January 7, 2003.
11. Board of Pharmaceutical Specialities. http://www.bpsweb.org, accessed January 7, 2003.
12. National Institute for Standards in Pharmacist Credentialing. http://www.nispcnet.org, accessed January 6, 2003.
13. Commission for Certification in Geriatric Pharmacy. http://ccgp.org, accessed June 19, 2003.
14. National Certification Board for Diabetes Educators. About NCBDE certification. http://ncbde.org/, accessed January 8, 2003.
15. American Nurses Association. Advanced practice programs; advanced diabetes management exams. http://www.ana.org/ancc/CERTIFY/cert/exams03.htm#ADMP, accessed June 26, 2003.
16. National Asthma Educator Certification Board. http://naecb.org, accessed June 19, 2003.
17. National Certification Board for Anticoagulation Providers. http://www.carsgroup.org/certified.htm, accessed January 8, 2003.
18. Gannon, K. JCAHO plans major change for hospital surveys in 2004. *Drugtopics.com* February 17, 2003.
19. Centers for Medicare & Medicaid Services. Conditions of participation and conditions of coverage. http://cms.hhs.gov/cop/, accessed June 20, 2003.
20. Joint Commission on Accreditation of Healthcare Organizations. Facts about the Joint Commission on Accreditation of Healthcare Organizations. http://www.jcaho.org/about+us/index.htm, accessed June 7, 2003.
21. ———. Medication management. http://www.jcaho.org/accredited+organizations/hospitals/standards/new+standards/, accessed June 20, 2003.
22. ———. Sentinel event policy and procedure. http://www.jcaho.org/accredited+organizations/hospitals/sentinel+events/se_pp.htm, accessed June 20, 2003.

23. ———. Information on final specifications for national implementation of hospital core measures as of 05/20/03. http://www.jcaho.org/accredited+organizations/hospitals/oryx/core+measures/information+on+final+specifications.htm, accessed June 25, 2003.
24. National Committee for Quality Assurance. NCQA report cards. http://hprc.ncqa.org/menu.asp, accessed June 25, 2003.
25. National Association of Boards of Pharmacy. Internet pharmacy and online pharmacies verification; VIPPS. http://www.nabp.net/vipps/intor.asp, accessed June 23, 2003.
26. United States Pharmacopeia. About USP. http://www.usp.org/aboutusp/index.htm, accessed June 23, 2003.
27. National Quality Forum. Welcome to the National Quality Forum. http://qualityforum.org/, accessed June 23, 2003.
28. ———. Safe practices for better healthcare, executive summary. http://www.qualityforum.org/txsafeexecsumm+order6-8-03PUBLIC.pdf, June 23, 2003.
29. The Leapfrog Group. http://leapfroggroup.org, accessed June 23, 2003.

chapter twenty-two

The role of professional organizations and pharmacy practices

Victoria E. Elliott

Contents

0-8493-1446-1/04/$0.00+$1.50
© 2004 by CRC Press LLC

The leader of the future ... will be one who creates a culture or a value system centered upon principles. Creating such a culture in a business, government, school, hospital, nonprofit organization, family, or other organization will be a tremendous and exciting challenge in this new era and will only be achieved by leaders, be they emerging or seasoned, who have the vision, courage, and humility to constantly learn and grow.[1]

Stephen R. Covey

Introduction

The nearly 1 million nonprofit organizations currently active in the U.S. provide excellent opportunities to learn about leadership. Of all the nonprofits, trade and professional associations constitute a large portion and are a pervasive force in society. There are more than 23,000 national and over 140,000 state and local associations in the U.S., making it the only country with such an active and fully developed association sector.[2]

Most people join at least one voluntary association at some time. According to statistics gathered by the American Society of Association Executives (ASAE) in 1995, 7 out of 10 American adults belong to 1 association, and 1 out of 4 belong to 4 or more associations. As the largest providers of adult education services in the U.S., associations contribute nearly $100 billion each year to the economy and employ nearly as many people as the computer or airline industries.[2]

What does it mean to belong to an association? What is the overall purpose of a professional association? How can membership in a professional association impact one's professional and personal development?

This chapter explores the answers to these and other questions regarding associations, in particular professional pharmacy associations. The purpose of this chapter is twofold. First, it imparts to students of pharmacy the value of membership and active involvement in professional associations. Second, it provides an understanding of the importance of professional associations to the advancement of pharmacy practice in the U.S. At the conclusion of the chapter, students should be able to:

- Define associations and describe how they impact pharmacy practice, legislation, and regulation.
- List the benefits of membership in an association.
- State how individual involvement in an association can stimulate personal professional development and foster increased career satisfaction.

History of modern associations

Many modern associations are classified by the IRS as not-for-profit under Section 501(c) of the U.S. Tax Code. Most business-related organizations are classified in the 501(c)3 category, meaning that their missions are largely supported through dues income or revenue generated through organizational activities related to the purpose of the organizations. Some professional societies opt for 501(c)4 status as charitable organizations that focus on activities such as direct mail fundraising, development of major gifts, service delivery, and research support. Beyond that, however, it is often hard to distinguish between associations and charitable organizations.

It is believed that associations existed in ancient Egypt and China. The apprentice training agreements and protective regulations maintained in Roman times are also seen as precursors to the modern association. By the 16th century, merchants and artisans throughout western Europe formed guilds that governed production, monitored sales, managed apprentice programs, oversaw wages and hours, and inspected finished products.[2]

In the U.S., guilds of the colonial period became unpopular because of their price fixing and regulatory practices that ran counter to the entrepreneurial spirit of the time. They were replaced by other types of trade associations — organizations in which companies or businesses hold memberships. The first trade association still in existence is the Chamber of Commerce of New York, which was formed by 20 merchants in 1768. The New York Stock Exchange, formed in 1792, is the second-oldest continuing association.

Trade associations continued to develop throughout the 19th century, by the end of which they were serving several purposes, including lobbying, quality control, credit improvement, industrial standardization, and a social function. They, however, also exhibited many of the same traits as those of the guilds they sought to replace. Associations engaged in price fixing, production controls, and distribution management to help business owners maintain monopolies. In the early 1900s, associations formed in order to provide price and sales data to their members. This information exchange was eventually limited by the U.S. Supreme Court in 1925, when it ruled that an association could provide price information but only on past transactions and that members could make no agreements to maintain prices based on such information. This information had to be made available to nonmembers, banks, and the U.S. Department of Commerce.

Throughout World War I and into the early part of World War II, associations transitioned into professional societies through the hiring of staff members and the formation of the American Trade Association Executives, now known as the American Society of Association Executives (ASAE).

The establishment of professional societies — organizations in which individuals hold membership — dates back to the 1500s, with the formation of the first scientific society, the Academia Secretorum Naturae of Naples, in 1560. Professional societies flourished in the 18th century as the divisions between labor and scholarly specialization became more evident. Developing bodies of knowledge were systematically collected and documented in order to preserve them for future generations, resulting in the modern development of professionalism. With the advent of economic printing and communication technologies brought about by urbanization and industrialization in the post–Civil War era, professional societies provided arenas for the establishment of specialties and expanding bodies of knowledge. Their meetings and publications provided a forum for the exchange of ideas and techniques, presentations, discussions, and airing of professional controversies. Societies served to disseminate the new information, maintain standards of professionalism, and consult governments and universities on the needs, desires, and ideals of their members.

Ernstthal and Jones categorize professional societies as follows:[2]

> *Scientific, engineering, or learned.* The purpose is to advance the body of knowledge in the field and keep members updated on trends and developments in the respective profession or trade. Examples are the American Pharmacist Association (APhA) or the Academy of Managed Care Pharmacy.
>
> *Affinity groups.* They are made up of people with nonemployment-related common interests, e.g., the National Rifle Association or the American Painted Horse Association.
>
> *Religious, charitable, public service, or fraternal organizations.* Central to these organizations is a cause or belief that brings members and supporters together. Examples include the American Cancer Society or the National Wildlife Foundation.

The unique social structure of associations

Associations and other not-for-profits can be differentiated from for-profit businesses in a number of ways. A comparison of associations and businesses can help clarify their roles. Table 22.1 illustrates differences between associations and businesses based on organizational infrastructure. Table 22.2 focuses on the leadership function in for-profit vs. member-based organizations such as associations.

Both for-profits and associations function as systems in achieving their mission, each component dependent on the other to accomplish this mission. For-profit systems are dependent on the economic relationship between the buyer and seller, and therefore work to build a customer base that will purchase their goods and services over a lifetime. Successful businesses

Table 22.1 Association Infrastructure Compared to that of For-Profit Entities

Businesses	Associations
Size and Revenue	
Large, medium, small (less than $50 million revenue annually).	Most considered small. Only 5 of the 50 largest report revenues of more than $50 million (principles of association management).
Mission	
Profitability.	Tax-exempt purposes, including research, public service and education, representation of private interests to government. About member's personal and professional development.
Structure	
Pyramid-shaped hierarchy for ease of assigning authority and decision-making responsibility. Requires understanding future of own business environment.	Combination of staff (which might be a typical business organization chart) and any of one of several volunteer governance structures. Requires balancing future of own organization with future of the trade or profession the organization represents.
Market	
No limits. The work of a for-profit organization benefits shareholders.	Defined by primary membership that pays dues in exchange for services and information. The work of an association benefits its members.

Source: Adapted from Ernstthal, H. and Jones, B., *Principles of Association Management.* 3rd ed., American Society of Association Executives, Washington, D.C., 1996, chap. 3.

obtain the necessary customer base and show their appreciation, but the relationship is always based on profit and value.

Associations are dependent on the mutual gain between the organization and its members. Leaders identify the tasks necessary to accomplish the mission and goals, based on members' perspectives, and then match these to members' interests, talents, and skills. Members' active involvement in the organization results in valuable information, contacts, and techniques that further their personal and professional goals. Successful associations maximize and appreciate the full potential of members to achieve positive changes for the trade, profession, or cause they represent.[3] Figure 22.1 illustrates the complex social system of an association.

The organization — the governing body, staff, and volunteers — is but one component of this system. The organization's operating and support systems produce the programs and services that are developed based on the organization's strategic plan. The plan is driven by the mission and goals of

Table 22.2 Organizational Structure: For-Profit vs. Membership-Based Organizations

For-Profit Organizations	Membership-Based Organizations
Decision Making	
Decisions are made directly or the authority is delegated to specific individuals to gather and incorporate ideas from others.	Building consensus is the goal; therefore, members need to be involved in order to gain ownership and commitment.
Team Selection	
Teams are selected by hiring, firing, and deciding who gets the job. Peer interviews can provide value.	Fellow leaders are already elected or appointed, and often suggest members and should be considered for other leadership or volunteer positions. Organizational leaders cannot be hired, fired, or threatened.
Setting Direction	
Priorities, goals, and direction are established, often with the input of others, to guide how the business or program will proceed.	Members are involved in setting direction using a team effort to ensure commitment to the goals of the organization.
Appropriating Awards	
Job satisfaction is a key to employee retention. Rewards are afforded through bonuses, benefits, and perks.	Traditional economic incentives do not exist; recognition of efforts must be continuous.
Creating the Environment	
There is an opportunity to make a direct impact on changing the company's image, realizing that others support its creation and management.	The organization's image already exists, but the influence, abilities, and support that members and leaders gain from others can change it. Volunteer leaders represent the organization, so their image is the organization's image.

Source: From Hudson, P., Making the transition. Presented at the Pennsylvania Society of Health-System Pharmacists Leadership Forum: Mysteries of Millennium Membership, Harrisburg, November 16–17, 2001. (With permission from the National Association of Home Builders.)

the organization, which are in turn established through the careful collection and evaluation of industry trends, members' needs, and the finite resources and capabilities available within the organization's infrastructure. In the not-for-profit community, the organization's leaders must focus on the common self-interests of their members.

Members have a set of self-interests that collectively comprise the common purpose for which they voluntarily chose to associate with each other

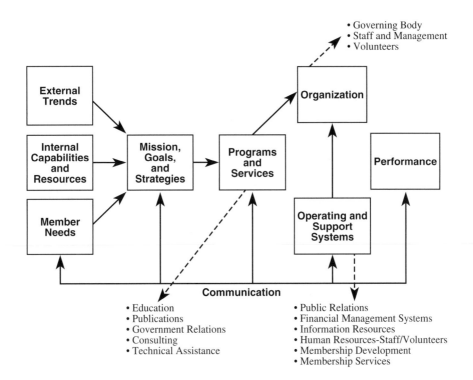

Figure 22.1 Associations as systems. (From Tecker, G., Eide, K., and Frankel, J., Building a knowledge-based culture, American Society of Association Executives, Washington, D.C., 1997. With permission.)

— hence the term *association*. The challenge to the organization and its leaders is to look beyond the limited interests of the moment into the longer-term opportunity or consequence to membership involved. In other words, what is the organization doing for its members beyond meeting their present needs? Second, leaders must consider the contribution of the organization to the community at large. In the not-for-profit sector, exemption from income tax requires a contribution to the public good. Unlike for-profits, therefore, by their definition and purpose, associations have an obligation to both members and their collective self-interests, as well as to the community at large.

The role of associations

Advocacy

Defined in the *American Heritage Dictionary* as active support of a cause, advocacy is considered by many association executives as the most important function of an association. Advocacy efforts can be legislative and professional. Every trade or profession has policy interests it would like to advance, preserve, or protect. Most associations identify representation of the interests of their members to government as the most important benefit of membership. In fact, representation on public policy issues is the primary motive for joining a trade association.[2]

Most national associations monitor legislation at both the federal and state levels. Many have full-time staff dedicated to government relations activities, including direct lobbying of regulatory or executive agencies or elected officials. Government relations activities include the following:

- Collecting and disseminating information about emerging public policy issues that may have an impact on members, and developing strategies for intervening or participating in these issues should the need arise.
- Formulating the organization's position on the issues and communicating it to members.
- Implementing a grassroots or lobbying campaign targeted to legislators or other key government decision makers to persuade them of the merits of the organization's position.

The latter, if used effectively, can be the most influential resource a volunteer-member organization has at its disposal. Although paid lobbyists can be very effective, elected representatives more likely respond to voters. Many volunteer organizations expend a lot of resources to educate key members who agree to contact their elected official and request support of the organization's position. With the advent of the Internet, e-mail, and broadcast fax, grassroots lobbying efforts have even more potential for greater influence, because associations can communicate almost immediately with members about key political issues. Unfortunately, in the U.S, there is more apathy than enthusiasm among people when it comes to interacting with elected officials about issues of importance to them or their profession.

Some associations operate a political action committee (PAC) to raise funds in support of grassroots education and political lobbying. PAC funds, which are simply pools of individual contributions, are typically used to support a candidate's election campaign. Although PACs are tightly regulated, they can facilitate the government relations initiatives of an association by providing to members a sense of being part of the political process.

Additionally, organizations form coalitions around issues of similar concern or interest. This allows the organization to pool its collective information, knowledge, and members in support of a common cause. Coalitions can be informal, forming when needed and dissolving as issues are resolved or go away, or they can be long-term relationships.

Table 22.3 provides examples of two coalitions of pharmacy organizations formed to address issues of common interest. In Pennsylvania, a coalition of pharmacy organizations was formed in 1985 in support of legislative issues of common interest. The coalition, known as the Pennsylvania Pharmacy Liaison Group, is an informal network of member and trade associa-

Table 22.3 Two Examples of National Pharmacy Coalitions

Joint Commission of Pharmacy Practitioners	Alliance for Pharmaceutical Care
Structure	
Forum on matters of common interest and concern to national organizations of pharmacy practitioners.	Consortium of national organizations.
Purpose	
Facilitate the effective representation of pharmacists on professional, educational, legislative, and regulatory issues through analysis, interpretation, and exchanges of views on relevant issues.	Educate the public, policy makers, and other key decision makers about the import role that pharmacists play in the ever-evolving health care system.
Member Organizations[a]	
AMCP, ACCP, ACA, ACCP, APhA, ASCP, ASHP, NABP, NCPA, NCSPAE	AACP, AMCP, APhA, ASCP, ASHP, Healthcare Distribution Management Association (HDMA), NACDS, NCPA, NCSPAE
Activities	
Adoption of identical policy statements by each member organization on National Health Insurance, which covers issues such as mechanisms for health care delivery, necessity of pharmacy services, reimbursement policies, role of deductibles and copayments in pharmacy services, cost control and quality assurance mechanisms. Recommendations have been made to AACP on pharmaceutical education, NABP on internships, and NABPLEX for licensing of foreign graduates.	Health care screening exhibit at annual National State Legislators Conference; compile and distribute evidence of the value of pharmacists on improved patient outcomes and health care savings to legislators.

[a] See Table 22.5 for full names of organizations.

tions, including the Pennsylvania Pharmacists Association, the Pennsylvania Society of Health-System Pharmacists, the Pennsylvania Chapter of the American Society of Consultant Pharmacists, the Pennsylvania Council of Deans, and the Pennsylvania Association of Chain Drug Stores. Initially, the coalition members gathered to craft a new pharmacy practice act, first introduced in the Senate in 1996, which served to modernize the first practice act originally written in 1961 and amended only once in the mid-1980s. Through six years of active lobbying and grassroots activities in support of the bill, five of the six coalition organizations in support of the final version were successful in ensuring passage of a bill, which now represents important amendments to the original Pennsylvania Pharmacy Practice Act. Key to these amendments are the definition of pharmacy practice as the provision of health care services, recognition of the provision of collaborative drug therapy management by a pharmacist to patients in the institutional setting as standard practice, and ability of pharmacists to administer immunizations.

In some sectors, association government relations activities are viewed as the equivalent of buying votes in support of favorable legislation. However, most 501(c)3 organizations spend less than 6% of their total income on government affairs activities.[4] Ernstthal and Jones point out that "almost all Americans are represented within the democratic process ... through their direct or indirect membership in professional societies, religious associations, employer groups, labor unions, consumer groups, hobby or affinity organizations."[2]

Professional representation

Successful advocacy efforts require representation of the members' professional ideals to organizations and groups outside the organization. In the case of legislators, this often requires educating and informing them of the standards of practice unique to the particular profession that will be impacted through a change in legislation. Sometimes legislative advocacy efforts also require organizations to represent their members to other professional organizations. In the case of pharmacy associations, outside organizations, such as the American Medical Association, the American Hospital Association, and the American Nurses Association, can be pivotal during a legislative process that requires their support or lack of opposition. Similarly, members of these organizations look to pharmacy associations to create and publish industry standards on appropriate drug use that can be used in their own training and advocacy efforts.

In early 2001, the Joint Commission on Healthcare Organizations (JCAHO) put forth proposed revisions to its standards addressing medication use. One proposed revision would have exempted hospitals with computerized physician order entry (CPOE) systems for medications and other patient therapies from the requirement that a pharmacist prospectively review the medication order. Many organizations opposed this recommendation, citing published best practice evidence in support of incorporating a pharmacist in the medication use process before medication administration. These organizations, many of which included state and national professional societies, advocated on behalf of their members that the JCAHO reconsider its position in light of their own organizations' concerns and documented evidence on the use of a pharmacist as a key component of medication review and distribution process. In July 2002, the JCAHO reversed its recommendation for pharmacist retrospective review of orders in hospitals with CPOE.

The JCAHO too can be considered an advocacy organization. In advocating for the public's safe health, the JCAHO strives to "continuously improve the safety and quality of care provided to the public through the provision of health care accreditation and related services that support performance improvement in health care organizations."[5] Some of these services are discussed in subsequent sections of this chapter.

AARP (formerly known as the American Association of Retired Persons) is a nonprofit membership organization dedicated to addressing the needs and interests of persons 50 years and older. AARP's volunteer leaders advocate on behalf of their members on important issues, such as ensuring the long-term solvency of Social Security; protecting pensions; fighting age discrimination; prescription-drug coverage in Medicare; patient protections in managed care and long-term care; antipredatory home loan lending; and other protections for older consumers. AARP advocates in the nation's capital, in state houses across the country, and in the courts on behalf of AARP members and their families (for more details see the AARP Web site, www.aarp.org).

Standard development and setting

In addition to political advocacy, industry regulation through the establishment of voluntary standards can be viewed as one of the most inherently important roles of an association. According to Ernstthal and Jones, "associations engage in standard setting activities to encourage and recognize quality."[2] Industry standards, certification, and accreditation are meant to be used as a framework for establishing the best system or practice for accomplishing an intended outcome. They do not guarantee success. Accredited and certified programs, institutions, and individuals must undertake a process of continuous quality improvement to ensure successful outcomes of their endeavors. Ernstthal and Jones categorize association voluntary standards into four categories: codes of ethics, certification, accreditation, and technical standards.

Codes of ethics

Pharmacists are health professionals who assist individuals in making the best use of medications. This Code, prepared and supported by pharmacists, is intended to state publicly the principles that form the fundamental basis of the roles and responsibilities of pharmacists. These principles, based on moral obligations and virtues, are established to guide pharmacists in relationships with patients, health professionals, and society.

APhA Code of Ethics for Pharmacists, Preamble

An association's code of ethics governs the conduct of its members. Compliance with the code varies. In many associations, it is largely ignored and not enforced; in others, compliance with the code is necessary for continued membership. In some cases, compliance with the industry code of ethics is required for continued licensure to practice. In professional health associations, compliance can be enhanced through the use of peer review to assure that members provide an appropriate standard of care.

Certification

Certification programs formally confirm that an individual has successfully met the standards set by the organization (association) for a particular practice or area of specialty. For example, the Board of Pharmaceutical Specialties (BPS)* certifies that a pharmacist has demonstrated an advanced level of education, experience, knowledge, and skills in one of five specialty areas: nuclear pharmacy, nutrition support, oncology pharmacy, pharmacotherapy, and psychiatric pharmacy.

Certification differs from licensure or registration, which are both regulatory requirements set individually by states for the practice of an individual in a particular profession. Numerous professions offer certification programs, such as accounting, association management, teaching, medical, and nursing. Like licensure, renewal requirements are often associated with certification, which may include retesting or documentation of required continuing education.

Accreditation

Accreditation is a means of certifying that an institution has successfully met a prescribed standard or set of standards. One of the most prominent examples of a health care accrediting body is the JCAHO. Hospital and other health care organizations are state licensed but seek accreditation by the JCAHO, an independent standard-setting organization. JCAHO accreditation is recognized nationwide as a symbol of quality that reflects an organization's commitment to meeting certain performance standards. To earn and maintain accreditation, an organization must undergo an onsite survey by a JCAHO survey team at least every 3 years. Laboratories must be surveyed every 2 years.

The Joint Commission's Hospital, Home Care, Laboratory, and Ambulatory Surgery Centers Accreditation Programs are recognized by the federal Health Care Financing Administration (HCFA) as meeting or exceeding the federal quality standards for these organizations. Thus, many of these organizations are able to use their Joint Commission accreditation to obtain

---

* BPS was established in 1976 by the American Pharmaceutical Association (APhA) to respond to the evolving requirements of patients and the health care system. BPS's mission is to recognize specialty practice areas, define knowledge and skill standards for recognized specialties, evaluate the knowledge and skills of individual pharmacist specialists, and serve as a source of information and coordinating agency for pharmacy specialties (see the APhA Web site, www.aphanet.org).

Medicare certification through a process known as deemed status. Similar reliance for licensure purposes exists for hospitals and other types of provider organizations in many states.

Technical standards

According to Ernstthal and Jones, technical standards are categorized as either design or performance. "Design standards outline specific materials to be used and the dimensions of the finished product. Performance standards deal with how the finished product should work, rather than how it is designed or manufactured."[2] The U.S. is unique in that many industry standards are established by associations or private organizations rather than the government. Standards are formulated by a group of knowledge volunteers and then all affected parties are provided an opportunity to comment before standards are finalized. Most organizations also arrange for an appeals process once a standard is set in the event of an affected organization disagreeing with a standard. Once the standards are published, the association is typically involved in technical support to its members to assist in assuring their compliance with the standards.

An example of a technical standard are the generally accepted accounting principles (GAAP) set by the Financial Accounting Standards Board. The NCCLS (formerly the National Committee for Clinical Laboratory Standards) is a global, interdisciplinary, nonprofit, standards-developing, and educational organization that promotes the development and use of voluntary consensus standards and guidelines within the health care community. It is recognized worldwide for the application of its unique consensus process in the development of standards and guidelines for patient testing and related health care issues (see the NCCLS Web site, www.nccls.org).

Education and meetings

Most members indicate that continuing education is one of the primary benefits they receive from their professional association. For most health professions, continuing education is required for relicensure. In addition, it is an important tool for remaining current on advancements within the profession.

Educational programming is available in numerous formats, including live programs and seminars and written home study through professional journals, e.g., Internet programs and audio conferences. Seminars and live programs have the added benefit of allowing members to network with peers to learn how the topics have affected others' practices and what they are doing to respond to necessary changes. The other live formats, e.g., audio conference and Web-based audio streaming, allow participants limited interaction with faculty and with each other, in the convenience of the participants' homes or offices. Of course, static Internet programs and home study lack the networking and peer interaction component, but can be used at a time and place most convenient for the participants.

The most successful meetings consider members' preferences for topics and speakers, location, length, time of year, and day of week. Educational programs and seminars vary in length and are often part of a large annual convention or meeting. In addition to the educational components, many associations conduct board and committee meetings, install new officers, and celebrate members' accomplishments by bestowing awards and honors. Exhibit shows are another popular component of conventions, during which members can browse displays set up by industry suppliers and vendors. In the case of pharmacy associations, the largest national exhibit show is held in conjunction with the Midyear Clinical Meeting of the American Society of Health-System Pharmacists.

Other unique components of several national and regional pharmacy association meetings are employment service and residency showcase programs. Practicing pharmacists and graduating students can select from a number of different employers, or postgraduate residency programs, and set up interviews conducted at the meeting location. In addition, many employers who provide residency programs participate as exhibitors to market their programs to pharmacists and students.

Publications and information

Associations use print publications to sustain member communication between face-to-face meetings and to provide consistent information to all members. The production and distribution of periodicals is considered by many members to be the most important benefit of membership, because it allows associations to carry out their most important function in the most efficient manner — the exchange of information among members.

Newsletters, common to most associations, allow for exchange of information among members and provide a mechanism for keeping members abreast of industry-related news, regulatory and legislative issues, association trends, organizational accomplishments, and member achievements. Many associations are moving their newsletters to electronic formats, which are more cost effective and timely. However, electronic versions compete for viewing time with the numerous other e-mails that members receive from work or other associations. Some organizations are limiting electronic newsletters to a secondary means of communication by providing a condensed, printed version of the newsletter to each member while encouraging them to log on to the Internet for further details about a particular article or subject.

Other distribution options for newsletters and magazines are e-mail and fax broadcast. Although timely, they are limited in the amount of information that can be provided without overwhelming the reader. E-mail and fax broadcasts are most effective for short messages regarding time-sensitive issues of an urgent nature, e.g., grassroots action on a key piece of legislation or a news bulletin on a current issue or important association business.

The most favored publication of professional societies is the magazine or periodical, which keeps members abreast of developments and research in their field. For many, it is also a means by which they can publish their research findings or share the discovery of a solution to a problem that many of their colleagues may also be looking to resolve. Examples in pharmacy include journals such as the *American Journal of Health-System Pharmacy* (published by the American Society of Health-System Pharmacists, ASHP), *Pharmacotherapy* (published by the American College of Clinical Pharmacy, ACCP), and the *Journal of Managed Care Pharmacy* (published by the Academy of Managed Care Pharmacy, AMCP). Other association publications might include reference texts for use in practice settings. Such publications can also provide a source of nondues-related revenue to the association, which helps support the costs to sustain member services.

Standard-setting organizations also publish texts for use by individuals or organizations seeking compliance with a particular set of industry standards or best practices. For example, the JCAHO publishes an annual accreditation manual for several health care settings, including hospitals, laboratories, and long-term care, ambulatory care, home care, and behavioral health care facilities. The ASHP publishes its positions and best practices in the "Best Practices for Health-System Pharmacy: Positions and Practice Standards of ASHP."

The Internet is fast becoming a cost-effective and efficient means of housing association and other industry information and publications. Often, this information is limited to dues-paying members who view the information in a members-only section of the association's Web site. Associations also make the same information available in electronic format, e.g., on CD-ROM or floppy disks, to others who wish to purchase the products.

Research and statistics

According to Ernsttahl and Jones, two thirds of associations conduct research or gather data on their members' profession or industry.[2] The information, which can be economic, demographic, social, or industrial, is used by businesses and government and is often less expensive to obtain than that produced by for-profit consulting and research firms. Associations also use the information and data they collect to provide value to members as a way to retain their membership.

Salary surveys, industry-specific studies, and benchmarking studies are just some examples of studies undertaken by pharmacy and related associations. Salary surveys enable employers to compare their staff salaries with others in the same region or state, or with national averages. The ASHP conducts a national survey of pharmacy practice in hospital settings, and each year focuses on a different issue. For example, in 2001, the survey questions centered on prescribing and transcribing, and in 2000 the focus was on monitoring, patient education, and wellness. The survey allows pharmacy managers to benchmark their pharmacy services with others across the country for the purposes of justifying new programs or policy changes.

Leadership development

In the *Gift of Leadership*, Mark Levin states that "voluntary organizations have the ability to go beyond the training of people in various trades and professions." Through leadership in voluntary organizations, many political, business, and social leaders in the U.S. have "honed their skills and abilities in the leadership ranks of America's non-profit volunteer organizations." Virtually all business leaders, including pharmacy leaders, have been active leaders in their professional or trade association, and most rely on these experiences to add to their credibility as industry leaders.[6]

One of the most important roles associations can assume is to create successful volunteers. This can be accomplished by combining a volunteer's innate need to serve with the tools necessary for successful leadership. It requires that the association set specific goals for volunteer leaders, and provide recognition for a job well done. Within this framework, members are afforded the opportunity to excel at activities that they enjoy and that provide meaning and value for them and other members of the association. The payback for the volunteers is recognition by peers for work accomplished and the right to use this accomplishment as evidence of their expertise and leadership qualities.

Sustained leadership is essential to the long-term success of an association. Organizations can be reengineered by improving benefits, services, and operations, but leaders realize the need to reinstate or sustain the spirit that was the basis for the formation of the organization. Associations accomplish this by establishing organizational values and identifying a formal set of leaders' actions and behaviors that create the culture of the organization. The culture is strengthened and activated by setting a strategic plan, identifying and prioritizing tasks within the plan, and then communicating and reinforcing the mission, vision, and plan with members. The leaders must then model the culture by remaining enthusiastic, conveying positive messages to members, and encouraging them to take action, assessing the organization in a way that will fulfill their personal or professional goals.[7]

Steven Covey defines the three roles of a principle-centered leader or organization: pathfinding, aligning, and empowering.[1] The strategic plan represents the pathfinding for the organization. It ties together the culture (value system) and vision with the needs of the members. The organizational structure and system and operational processes must be aligned with the needs of the members so that they understand the mission, share the commitment to the vision, and appreciate the interdependent nature of associations. Alignment is then achieved when members are empowered to create and improve the structures and systems that will meet their needs. Organizations that model the roles of principle-centered leadership provide a forum for the successful creation of future leaders.

   Numerous skills can be developed through participation in association leadership positions. Examples include presentation and speaking, facilitation, negotiation, delegation, fundraising, recruitment, planning, and public relations skills. Such skills are particularly valuable to those who aspire to serve as members of the board or as presidents.[6] But they also apply to other aspects of members' lives, e.g., work, home, and other volunteer organizations.

Public service

Aside from public relations efforts that professional associations must undertake with members and other key constituents, many associations include educating and communicating with the general public among their primary goals. Benefits of public service programs are many.

   In pharmacy, promoting the profession to members of the general public is key to helping them understand the role of a pharmacist in drug therapy management. Few patients truly understand the benefit of establishing a relationship with their pharmacist, who can help them manage their drug therapy and share important information about their medications.

   Several years ago, the ASHP invested in a 3-year public relations plan to promote the role and value of health system pharmacists. The initial survey of consumers revealed that many did not realize that a pharmacist was involved in their care, but many expressed a desire to have a pharmacist visit with and counsel them on their medications. Since then, the ASHP has conducted several more targeted surveys and associated public relations campaigns to increase the promotion of the value of pharmacists. In 2000, the ASHP polled consumers regarding online health information. The survey of more than 1000 Americans revealed that consumers regularly use the Internet to find health information. Also, one out of three respondents said they do not believe that the supplemental materials that typically accompany prescriptions provide enough information about drug interactions. In addition, less than half (47%) strongly agreed that these information leaflets are helpful. In that same year, the ASHP launched a new Web site, www.SafeMedication.com, to help ensure that Internet users have a reliable online resource for up-to-date, accurate drug information. Other organizations have developed similar public health services. For example, the APhA houses a consumer information section called "Pharmacy and You" on its Web site (http://www.pharmacyandyou.org/) focused on patient information, the role of the pharmacist, and other consumer information needs.

   National and state pharmacy associations recognize National Pharmacy Week as an opportunity for promoting the value of pharmacist services. Public relations efforts include press releases, public display and information booths, community-based seminars, and health fairs. The target audience includes patients and other health care professionals. Associations such as the APhA and ASHP provide members with promotional materials and patient education information for use at hospital-based or other local events.

Several national pharmacy organizations have formed a coalition known as the Alliance for Pharmaceutical Care (see Table 22.3). One of its functions is to exhibit annually at the National State Legislators Conference, where groups of pharmacists representing participating organizations provide health screenings. The collaboration of these pharmacy organizations allows them to provide a popular service to legislators, who too are members of the public, at the same time educating them on the value of pharmacists in their individual health care.

A key public service of the JCAHO is a comprehensive guide to help individuals learn more about the safety and quality of JCAHO-accredited health care organizations and programs throughout the U.S. This guide, Quality Check™, includes each organization's name, address, telephone number, accreditation decision, accreditation date, current accreditation status and effective date, and its most recent performance report.

How do associations work?

Governance

Associations and professional societies are governed by a group of elected and appointed volunteer leaders whose responsibilities are directed by the associations' constitution and by-laws. According to Ernstthal and Jones, governance in associations is the participation of volunteer leaders in making crucial decisions regarding the operation and viability of an organization.[2] Responsibility for governance is held by the board of directors or a board of trustees, although the specific governance structure depends on the organization's size, resources, and the type of services and activities it carries out for members. Small organizations may appoint most or all of its members to the board, whereas large organizations usually appoint individuals who serve as a fair representation of the membership at large. Beyond the board of directors, several components in the structure of organization allow it to obtain input from members, which drives the policy-making process.

Many professional societies use a House of Delegates as the senior policy-making body. Members include representatives from geographic or other subdivisions of the organization, who meet usually once a year. The house considers policy recommendations from other sectors of the organization, sets policy, and makes recommendations to the board. Throughout the year, another decision-making body, typically a board of directors, makes interim decisions or performs specific managerial tasks.[2]

Throughout the year, organizational sectors, such as committees, councils, and special interest groups (SIGs), convene to discuss society matters and professional issues. Typically, the agendas for these organizational components are set in advance and driven by the strategic plan, a specific professional issue, or the policy-making or standards-setting process. Committees are usually appointed by the board and meet as often as necessary to accomplish their goals. They are responsible for designing and implementing a project or a member service or for making policy recommendations to the board or house.[2]

An organization may establish councils in addition to or in lieu of committees for making policy recommendations. Councils may meet only once a year, but can be called on as needed to consider an issue and make a recommendation. They are considered more strategic in their purpose, whereas committees typically function in an operational capacity.

SIGs represent a subsection of the membership that form on their own or are created by the board to address specific interests. Examples in pharmacy associations include SIGs for specialty practice areas, such as pediatrics, home care or home infusion, and management.

Management

Whereas the board of directors is responsible for setting direction and establishing policy, the chief executive and the staff carry out the operational activities of the association. Volunteers provide feedback and guidance to staff, and in some organizations are responsible for operational issues as well because the association has no staff. The relationship between a board and staff is delicate. It is important that the association president and board set very clear expectations for the chief executive and that the CEO provide continual updates and information to the board to assure successful decision making.

Policy-making infrastructure

A discussion of how associations work to set policy and implement member services will not be complete without discussing the four key elements that guide the governance and management of the association:

1. Culture and values
2. Policies and procedures
3. Processes and practices
4. Focus, direction, and structure

The elements provide the infrastructure that enables the organization to operate effectively under its volunteer and staff leadership.[3] Table 22.4 explains each of these elements.

Associations — "Your other life"

According to Billy Woodward, "Excellent professional leaders all seem to possess an ability to stay focused and act on their priorities while maintaining a balance between idealism and reality, as well as a sense of the future, while dealing with the challenges of today. The optimism shown by such

Table 22.4 Elements of Association Governance and Management

Element	Definition	Purpose
Culture and values	The common purpose, or set of values, held by the members and leaders.	Comprises the reason for which individuals choose to voluntarily associate with each other.
Policies and procedures	Policies define organization's position on external and internal issues; procedures are the corresponding steps or actions required to accomplish a desired endpoint.	Guides the organization in carrying out its strategic plan, operational agenda, and organizational decision-making.
Processes and practices	Processes are continual operations, made up of a set of procedures, required to accomplish a desired end, e.g., the recruitment of volunteers. Practices are tactics that often prove successful in similar situations to achieve common objectives or goals.	Established processes guide the ongoing operations of the organization to assure smooth transition from one leader to another and one board to another. Practices are typically viewed as industry standards that are commonly accepted means of accomplishing a task, e.g., the practice of surveying members to identify their priorities and preferences for association services. Practice may also be unique to one organization that has provided a consistent, desired outcome.
Focus, direction, and organizational structure	The culture of community that results from the identification and cultivation or members and their respective needs.	Help define and implement the vision, mission, and strategic and operating plan.

Source: Adapted from Secrets to achieving positive change: understanding the membership-based organization as a social system, Center for Excellence in Association Leadership Online Collection (www.cealweb.com), San Francisco, 2001.

leaders is based on a passion they possess to practice pharmacy to the best of their ability." Woodward believes this passion is kindled by "an unwavering lifetime dedication to the several important guidelines including standing on principles, engaging in continual learning, studying heroes, associating with winners, enjoy the journey of one's career, focusing on others and passing on the passion."[8] Associations provide a most unique opportunity to meet most, if not all, these challenges.

One of the goals of this chapter is to encourage pharmacy students to consider joining and becoming actively involved in an association. The choices are numerous, and so the final decision to select an organization and then to become actively involved requires an assessment of one's needs.

Step 1. Determine your career and self-development goals. Even if you are unclear about what direction your career will take, it is important to consider what options you wish to pursue, be it acute care, long-term care, ambulatory care, pharmaceutical industry, drug information, research, or a postgraduate degree. Some pharmacy organizations seek to represent pharmacists in all such practice settings whereas others focus on the professional development and policy or representation needs of specific groups.

Step 2. Identify the gaps in your current knowledge of (a) the profession of pharmacy, (b) the career path you have chosen, and (c) the skills you feel will be necessary to succeed. Many organizations provide not only professional pharmacy education but also seminars in personal development, covering topics such as résumé writing, interviewing, and professional speaking and writing. Associations can provide other knowledge and skills not found in pharmacy curricula and workplace settings. In the earlier example of legislative advocacy and the role of volunteers in the success of these efforts, organizations provide a unique opportunity for members to learn about and impact on the legislative and regulatory decisions that will affect their practices.

Step 3. Make a commitment to lifelong learning. Over time, many of us move away from membership or involvement in professional or civic volunteer organizations. The reasons are numerous, and might include a perceived lack of time, insufficient financial resources, a perception or belief that membership only benefits the active leaders, or a simple lack of interest. However, all professionals need continued learning. This is driven in part by the need to maintain licensure to continue praticing. More importantly, however, as professionals we have a moral obligation to maintain our knowledge of skills and abilities beyond the minimum legal requirement for licensure.

Step 4. Consider what you would lose if you were not involved. Membership
in a professional pharmacy association can be especially rewarding
to those who take an active role in the organization and their profession. All members, however, benefit from the services offered by their
professional organization.

The following is a list of features of membership in a pharmacy association. The list is not meant to be all-inclusive, but aims rather to help students
appreciate what benefits can be derived from membership and active
involvement in a professional pharmacy association:

- *Continuing education programs* are sometimes limited to members and
  are always available at discounted prices or even free to members.
- *Professional and legislative advocacy efforts* are most successful when
  fully supported by the membership. For many people, the experience
  is meaningful and provides a sense of professional satisfaction because they and their colleagues are able to make a difference for the
  profession or for patient care.
- *Official publications,* e.g., newsletters, journals, e-mail alerts, newslinks,
  and access to member-only information on the association's Web site,
  are features typically included with the cost of membership.
- *Recognition of professional achievement* through certification programs
  or award presentations instills a sense of accomplishment and pride
  in recipients. The latter, however, is limited to active members who
  have made significant contributions to the organization and the profession it represents.
- *Networking opportunities* abound in membership-based organizations.
  Membership databases are often available to members. Social and
  education events provide colleagues the opportunity to discuss and
  share ideas. Many pharmacy professionals who have achieved significant accomplishments in their careers are active members of an
  association. This active involvement benefits them in reaching their
  goals, and it continues to benefit other members who can learn from
  them.
- Most associations advertise *job opportunities* and a few allow members
  to post résumés online. Throughout the undergraduate experience,
  one is exposed to a number of career options. Deciding among these
  can be daunting at the very least. However, involvement in an organization, even as a student, can improve understanding of the various
  options and provide networking opportunities that are not apparent
  or available to nonmembers. Furthermore, several national pharmacy
  associations house information on postgraduate residencies and fellowships. Access to this information is afforded to members for free
  or at a discounted price. In fact, the ASHP, the official accrediting
  body for hospital and health-system-based residencies, conducts an

annual national match program for its accredited residency programs. The American College of Clinical Pharmacy (ACCP) has a process for peer review of research fellowship training programs. The APhA and the ASHP jointly administer the accreditation of community pharmacy residency programs.

- *Career advancement*, although not typically a stated benefit of membership, is likely one of the most beneficial reasons for a career-conscious member to be involved.
- *Skill building* is accomplished through active involvement.
- *Successful or enlightening research* can be shared through publication in the association's journal or through poster presentations or speaking engagements.

In his 1990 H.A.K. Whitney award lecture, David A. Zilz spoke about the increasing interdependence in pharmacy among clinicians, integrated private health care companies, and pharmaceutical companies. He said that associations and other organizations are often "created to bond individuals whose needs can best be met by becoming interdependent for the purpose of providing purchasing services, research networks, information support, and other activities that can no longer be carried out as successfully when those individuals act independently."[9] The movement toward interdependence is driven by advancements in communication technology; the explosion of new knowledge, which makes it difficult for an individual to stay current; and the creation of other interdependent structures, e.g., corporate mergers that force a paradigm shift in how members of the pharmacy community interact with one other. People should consider their own abilities to keep pace with each of these forces. How much easier would it be to obtain and share information from others while building your own career and practice if you were an informed member of a professional pharmacy association?

Where do I start?

Table 22.5 (at the end of the chapter) is a chart of national pharmacy and other related individual member and trade associations. The chart, although not all-inclusive, provides contact information, including addresses, Web sites, and phone numbers of many major pharmacy organizations.

Many of the national professional pharmacy associations foster the development of student chapters at colleges of pharmacy. Sometimes, these are combined with state affiliate chapters of the national association. Most school-based association chapters offer students the same privileges as those for active professional members, including access to publications, Web site resources, and information for career development and postgraduate pursuits.

State associations have student membership categories and are often the parent organization for the school-based chapter. Each state organization has chapters typically organized by geographic location.

After you become a member, the easiest way to become involved is to join a committee or seek opportunities to make contributions that are manageable and can be enjoyed. For example, consider writing a newsletter article, serving as a reviewer for a publication, or developing a student educational session in conjunction with local practitioners. Attending local meetings and interacting with other students and professionals provides the opportunity to market yourself and let others know your interests and strengths.

In addition to local (school-based) chapters, the national associations have student sections or forums designed to meet the unique needs of student members. Sections are managed by elected or appointed student leaders, providing them additional opportunities for personal growth and networking. Often, the national association's House of Delegates, the major decision-making body, reserves seats for student delegates who represent the interests of student members throughout the organization.

Regardless of the level at which you decide to become involved, individual members are responsible for knowing what they hope to achieve by joining and must be willing to contribute their time and talent to support the organization in its achievement of its vision and mission. Quoting Thomas Moore in his book *Care of the Soul*, William Zellmer, the 1996 recipient of the H.A.K. Whitney Lecture Award, defined having soul as having depth, value, relatedness, heart, and personal substance. During his Whitney lecture he noted, "The nature of our discipline (pharmacy) is the sum total of the inner drives — that is, the souls — of individual practitioners . . . Individually we can examine and adjust the focus of our own work. We can support and encourage our colleagues in the same pursuit. We can create and support, collectively, through our professional organizations, long-term efforts that build the soul of pharmacy."[10]

Career opportunities

Associations provide a unique opportunity to apply one's professional talents to the advancement of the profession. Many state and national associations hire professionals in the industry they represent. These individuals can guide the successful development and implementation of member programs and services by their practical experience and knowledge of the profession.

Applicable staff positions in associations include writers, professional associates, educational specialists, and association generalists. The last position is typically in association management, e.g., CEOs. Many pharmacist clinicians are hired to serve as writers and editors for pharmacy association journals. Professional associates use their pharmacy expertise to guide policy making on professional practice issues and serve as liaisons between members and other professional organizations. Educational specialists work with association staff to develop continuing education, certification, and training programs that best suit the needs of members in the management of their practice sites.

Like the pharmacy profession, associations provide experiential opportunities during which students are exposed various facets of the organization. The ASHP sponsors an 8-week rotation and a summer internship in association management for pharmacy students. In addition, the ASHP sponsors a 1-year postgraduate residency program. Many professional associations for association executives conduct student mentor and other training programs for students interested in becoming association executives. In addition, the ASAE administers a voluntary certification program designed to elevate professional standards, enhance individual performance, and designate those who demonstrate knowledge essential to the practice of association management.

State-based pharmacy associations are another resource for information on career opportunities in association management. Like their national counterparts, a few sponsor experiential clerkships for students interested in learning more about the management of an association. Job opportunities are posted on many association Web sites, e.g., the ASAE (www.asae.org) and many of its state and local affiliates.

Conclusion

Professional associations provide unique opportunities for networking, career advancement, and personal skill development. Individual contributions to an association in support of its mission assure advancement of the profession. As pharmacists we are obliged to contribute to our professional associations to assure continued success of the profession of pharmacy. This chapter serves as a resource for determining the best fit for you in your professional association of choice.

Table 22.5 Major National Pharmacy Associations

Academy of Managed Care Pharmacy (AMCP) 100 N. Pitt Street Alexandria, VA 22314-3134 Phone: (703) 683-8416 Fax: (703) 683-8417 Web site: www.amcp.org	American College of Clinical Pharmacy (ACCP) 3101 Broadway Kansas City, MO 64111-2446 Phone: (816) 531-2177 Fax: (816) 531-4990 Web site: www.accp.com
American Association for Homecare (AAHomecare) 625 Slaters Lane Alexandria, VA 22314-1176 Phone: (703) 836-6263 Fax: (703) 836-6730 Web site: www.aahomecare.org	American Council on Pharmaceutical Education (ACPE) 20 N. Clark Street Chicago, IL 60602-5109 Phone: (312) 664-3575 Fax: (312) 664-4652 Web site: www.acpe-accredit.org
American Association of Colleges of Pharmacy (AACP) 1426 Prince Street Alexandria, VA 22314-2815 Phone: (703) 739-2330 Fax: (703) 836-8982 Web site: www.aacp.org	American Foundation for Pharmaceutical Education (AFPE) 1 Church Street Rockville, MD 20850-4184 Phone: (301) 738-2160 Fax: (301) 738-2161 Web site: www.afpenet.org
American Association of Pharmaceutical Scientists (AAPS) 2107 Wilson Boulevard Arlington, VA 22201-3042 Phone: (703) 243-2800 Fax: (703) 243-9650 Web site: www.aapspharmaceutica.com	American Health and Beauty Aids Institute (AHBAI) 401 N. Michigan Avenue Chicago, IL 60611-4245 Phone: (312) 644-6610 Fax: (312) 321-5194 Web site: www.proudlady.org
American Association of Pharmacy Technicians, Inc. (AAPT) P.O. Box 1447 Greensboro, NC 27402-1447 Phone: (336) 275-1700 Fax: (336) 275-7222 Web site: www.pharmacytechnician.com	American Pharmacist Association (APhA) 2215 Constitution Avenue N.W. Washington, D.C. 20037-2907 Phone: (202) 628-4410 Fax: (202) 783-2351 Web site: www.aphanet.org
American College of Apothecaries (ACA) P.O. Box 341266 Memphis, TN 38184-1266 Phone: (901) 383-8119 Fax: (901) 383-8882 Web site: www.acainfo.org	American Public Health Association (APHA) 800 I Street N.W. Washington, D.C. 20001-3710 Phone: (202) 777-2742 Fax: (202) 777-2534 Web site: www.apha.org

Table 22.5 Major National Pharmacy Associations (continued)

American Society for Automation in
Pharmacy (ASAP)
492 Norristown Road
Blue Bell, PA 19422-2355
Phone: (610) 825-7783
Fax: (610) 825-7641
Web site: www.asapnet.org

American Society for Parenteral &
Enteral Nutrition (ASPEN)
8630 Fenton Street
Silver Spring, MD 20910-3803
Phone: (301) 587-6315
Fax: (301) 587-2365
Web site: www.nutritioncare.org

American Society for Pharmacy Law
(ASPL)
1224 Centre West Drive
Springfield, IL 62704-2184
Phone: (217) 391-0219
Fax: (217) 793-0041
Web site: www.aspl.org

American Society of Consultant
Pharmacists (ASCP)
1321 Duke Street
Alexandria, VA 22314-3563
Phone: (703) 739-1300
Fax: (703) 739-1321
Web site: www.ascp.com

American Society of Health-System
Pharmacists (ASHP)
7272 Wisconsin Avenue
Bethesda, MD 20814-4836
Phone: (301) 657-3000
Fax: (301) 652-8278
Web site: www.ashp.org

Board of Pharmaceutical Specialties
2215 Constitution Avenue N.W.
Washington, D.C. 20037-2985
Phone: (202) 429-7591
Fax: (202) 429-6304
Web site: www.bpsweb.org

Chain Drug Marketing Association, Inc.
(CDMA)
P.O. Box 995
Novi, MI 48376-0995
Phone: (248) 449-9300
Fax: (248) 449-9396
Web site: www.chaindrug.com

CIES — The Food Business Forum
7, rue de Madrid
75008 Paris, France
Phone: (1) 44 69 84 84
Fax: (1) 44 69 99 39
Web site: www.ciesnet.com

Consumer Healthcare Products
Association (CHPA)
1150 Connecticut Avenue N.W.
Washington, D.C. 20036-4104
Phone: (202) 429-9260
Fax: (202) 223-6835
Web site: www.chpa-info.org

Cosmetic, Toiletry, and Fragrance
Association (CTFA)
1101 17th Street N.W.
Washington, D.C. 20036-4722
Phone: (202) 331-1770
Fax: (202) 331-1969
Web site: www.ctfa.org

Drug, Chemical and Allied Trades
Association (DCAT)
510 Route 130
East Windsor, NJ 08520-0000
Phone: (609) 448-1000
Fax: (609) 448-1944
Web site: www.dcat.org

Food and Drug Law Institute (FDLI)
1000 Vermont Avenue N.W.
Washington, D.C. 20005-4913
Phone: (202) 371-1420
Fax: (202) 371-0649
Web site: www.fdli.org

Table 22.5 Major National Pharmacy Associations (continued)

Food and Nutrition Service (FNS)
3101 Park Center Drive
Alexandria, VA 22302-1500
Phone: (703) 305-2062
Fax: (703) 305-2908
Web site: www.fns.usda.gov

General Merchandise Distributors
Council (GMDC)
1275 Lake Plaza Drive
Colorado Springs, CO 80906-3583
Phone: (719) 576-4260
Fax: (719) 576-2661
Web site: www.gmdc.org

Generic Pharmaceutical Association
(GPhA)
1620 I Street N.W.
Washington, D.C. 20006-4033
Phone: (202) 833-9070
Fax: (202) 833-9612
Web site: www.genericaccess.com

Grocery Manufacturers of America, Inc.
(GMA)
1010 Wisconsin Avenue N.W.
Washington, D.C. 20007-3673
Phone: (202) 337-9400
Fax: (202) 337-4508
Web site: www.gmabrands.com

Health Insurance Association of America
(HIAA)
555 13th Street N.W.
Washington, D.C. 20004-1109
Phone: (202) 824-1600
Fax: (202) 824-1722
Web site: www.hiaa.org

Healthcare Distribution Management
Association (HDMA)
1821 Michael Faraday Drive
Reston, VA 20190-5342
Phone: (703) 787-0000
Fax: (703) 787-6930
Web site: www.healthcaredistribution.org

Institute for Safe Medication Practices
(ISMP)
1800 Byberry Road
Huntingdon Valley, PA 19006-3520
Phone: (215) 947-7797
Fax: (215) 914-1492
Web site: www.ismp.org

Institute for the Advancement of
Community Pharmacy (IACP)
9687 South Run Oaks Drive
Fairfax Station, VA 22039-2623
Phone: (703) 690-2559
Fax: (703) 493-9696
Web site: www.advancepharmacy.org

International Pharmaceutical Federation
(FIP)
P.O. Box 84200
2508 AE The Hague, the Netherlands
Phone: (70) 3021970
Fax: (70) 3021999
Web site: www.fip.nl

International Society for
Pharmacoeconomic and Outcomes
Research (ISPOR)
3100 Princeton Pike
Lawrenceville, NJ 08648-2300
Phone: (609) 219-0773
Fax: (609) 219-0774
Web site: www.ispor.org

National Association of Chain Drug
Stores (NACDS)
P.O. Box 1417-D49
Alexandria, VA 22313-1417
Phone: (703) 549-3001
Fax: (703) 836-4869
Web site: www.nacds.org

National Association for Retail
Merchandising Services (NARMS)
P.O. Box 906
Plover, WI 54467-0906
Phone: (715) 342-0948
Fax: (715) 342-1943
Web site: www.narms.com

Table 22.5 Major National Pharmacy Associations (continued)

National Association of Boards of
Pharmacy (NABP)
700 Busse Highway
Park Ridge, IL 60068-2402
Phone: (847) 698-6227
Fax: (847) 698-0124
Web site: www.nabp.net

National Association of
Wholesaler-Distributors (NAW)
1725 K Street N.W.
Washington, D.C. 20006-1401
Phone: (202) 872-0885
Fax: (202) 785-0586
Web site: www.naw.org

National Committee for Quality
Assurance (NCQA)
2000 L Street N.W.
Washington, D.C. 20036-4918
Phone: (202) 955-3500
Fax: (202) 955-3599
Web site: www.ncqa.org

National Community Pharmacists
Association (NCPA)
205 Daingerfield Road
Alexandria, VA 22314-2833
Phone: (703) 683-8200
Fax: (703) 683-3619
Web site: www.ncpanet.org

National Conference of Pharmaceutical
Organizations (NCPO)
c/o Healthcare Distribution
Management Association (HDMA)
Reston, VA 20190-5348
Phone: (703) 787-0000
Fax: (703) 787-6930
Web site: www.nacds.org

National Council for Prescription Drug
Programs (NCPDP)
9240 E. Raintree Drive
Scottsdale, AZ 85260-7518
Phone: (480) 477-1000
Fax: (480) 767-1042
Web site: www.ncpdp.org

National Council of State Pharmacy
Association Executives (NCSPAE)
c/o Iowa Pharmacy Association
Des Moines, IA 50322-2900
Phone: (515) 270-0713
Fax: (515) 270-2979
Web site: www.ncspae.org

National Council on Patient Information
and Education (NCPIE)
4915 Saint Elmo Avenue
Bethesda, MD 20814-6082
Phone: (301) 656-8565
Fax: (301) 656-4464
Web site: www.talkaboutrx.org

The National Council on the Aging
(NCOA)
409 Third Street S.W.
Washington, D.C. 20024-3212
Phone: (202) 479-1200
Fax: (202) 479-0735
Web site: www.ncoa.org

National Institute for Pharmacist Care
Outcomes (NIPCO)
205 Daingerfield Road
Alexandria, VA 22314-2833
Phone: (703) 683-8200
Fax: (703) 683-3619
Web site: http://www.ncpanet.org/
NIPCO/nipintro.html

National Institute for Standards in
Pharmacist Credentialing (NISPC)
205 Daingerfield Road
Alexandria, VA 22314-2833
Phone: (703) 299-8790
Fax: (703) 683-3619
Web site: www.nispcnet.org

National Pharmaceutical Association
(NPhA)
The Courtyards Office Complex
Cary, NC 27511-4434
Phone: (800) 944-6742
Fax: (919) 469-5870
Web site: www.npha.net

Table 22.5 Major National Pharmacy Associations (continued)

National Pharmaceutical Council, Inc. (NPC) 1894 Preston White Drive Reston, VA 20191-5433 Phone: (703) 620-6390 Fax: (703) 476-0904 Web site: www.npcnow.org	Pharmaceutical Research and Manufacturers of America (PhRMA) 1100 15th Street N.W. Washington, D.C. 20005-1763 Phone: (202) 835-3420 Fax: (202) 835-3400 Web site: www.phrma.org
The National Quality Forum (NQF) 601 13th Street N.W. Washington, D.C. 20005-6708 Phone: (202) 783-1300 Fax: (202) 783-3434 Web site: www.qualityforum.org	Private Label Manufacturers Association (PLMA) 369 Lexington Avenue New York, NY 10017-6506 Phone: (212) 972-3131 Fax: (212) 983-1382 Web site: www.plma.com
National Retail Federation (NRF) Liberty Place Washington, D.C. 20004-2808 Phone: (202) 783-7971 Fax: (202) 737-2849 Web site: www.nrf.com	United States Pharmacopeia (USP) 12601 Twinbrook Parkway Rockville, MD 20852-1717 Phone: (301) 881-0666 Fax: (301) 816-8525 Web site: www.usp.org
Parenteral Drug Association (PDA) 7500 Old Georgetown Road Bethesda, MD 20814-6133 Phone: (301) 986-0293 Fax: (301) 986-0296 Web site: www.pda.org	Western Association of Food Chains (WAFC) 825 Colorado Boulevard Los Angeles, CA 90041-1714 Phone: (323) 254-7279 Fax: (323) 254-6032 Web site: www.wafc.com
Pharmaceutical Care Management Association (PCMA) 2300 9th Street S. Arlington, VA 22204-2320 Phone: (703) 920-8480 Fax: (703) 920-8491 Web site: www.pcmanet.org	

References

1. Covey, S.R., Three roles of the leader in the new paradigm, in *The Drucker Foundation — The Leader of the Future: New Visions, Strategies and Practices for the Next Era*, 1st ed., Hesselbein, F., Goldsmith, M. and Beckhard, R., Eds. Jossey-Bass Publishers, San Francisco, 1996, chap. 16.
2. Ernstthal, H. and Jones, B., *Principles of Association Management*, 3rd ed., American Society of Association Executives, Washington, D.C., 1996.

3. Secrets to achieving positive change: understanding the membership-based organization as a social system, Center for Excellence in Association Leadership Online Collection (www.cealweb.com), San Francisco, 2001.

4. ASAE operating ratio report, 9th ed., American Society of Association Executives, Washington, D.C., 1994.

5. Joint Commission on Healthcare Organizations, Mission statement, www.jcaho.org/about+us/index.htm, accessed January 13, 2004.

6. Levin, M., *The Gift of Leadership: How to Relight the Volunteer Spirit in the 21st Century.* 3rd ed., BAI, Inc., Columbia, 1999.

7. The spirit of leadership: steps designed to influence positive change, Center for Excellence in Association Leadership, San Francisco, 1998.

8. Woodward, B., The journey to professional excellence, a matter of priorities, *AJHP* 55, 782, 1998.

9. Zilz, D., Interdependence in pharmacy: risks, rewards and responsibilities. Harvey A.K. Whitney Award Lecture presented at the Annual Meeting of the American Society of Health-System Pharmacists, Boston, June 1990.

10. Zellmer, W., Searching for the soul of pharmacy, H.A.K. Whitney Award Lecture presented at the Annual Meeting of the American Society of Health-System Pharmacists, San Diego, June 1996.

chapter twenty-three

Corporate compliance programs and pharmacy

Joshua J. Spooner

Contents

Introduction

A corporate compliance program is a wide-ranging strategy for organizations that is designed to facilitate compliance with regulations pertaining to its business activities. The Office of the Inspector General (OIG), part of the Department of Health and Human Services, defines a corporate compliance program — as it pertains to health care providers — as "effective internal controls that promote adherence to applicable federal and state laws, and the program requirements of federal, state, and private health plans."[1] An effective corporate compliance plan is further defined by the government as one "that has been reasonably designed, implemented, and enforced so that it generally will be effective in preventing and detecting criminal conduct."[2]

There are many reasons behind the increased interest in establishing and implementing corporate compliance programs in health care. During the Clinton presidency, the government stepped up the investigation and prosecution of health care fraud and abuse, making it the government's second highest priority (behind violent crime) as a law enforcement priority.[3] Funding and personnel for investigating health care violations were increased under the Health Insurance Portability and Accountability Act (HIPAA) of 1996.[4] Between 1992 and 1999, the number of health care fraud cases filed by the government increased from 83 to 506, and the number of convictions increased from 59 to 263.[5] Additionally, settlements between the government and the accused corporation frequently exceed $50 million, and reached $875 million in one case.[6] Although it is unclear whether future administrations will continue to pursue health care fraud to the extent that the Clinton administration did, there is a growing concern among health care providers that they might become the subject of a fraud and abuse investigation.

Additionally, the number of private qui tam lawsuits filed against corporations has increased over the last 10 to 15 years. A qui tam lawsuit is a suit filed by an individual on behalf of the government in an attempt to recover penalties under the False Claims Act. These suits are often filed by competitors, disgruntled employees, or former employees aware of federal health program violations; the people who bring these lawsuits are often referred to as whistleblowers. On reviewing the suit, the government decides either to proceed with the action (by taking over the suit and becoming responsible for its prosecution) or declines to take action. Even if the government declines to take action, whistleblowers retain the right to proceed with the suit on their own. Depending on the level of government involvement in the lawsuit, whistleblowers can receive between 15 and 30% of the settlement in addition to reasonable expenses and attorney fees.[7] These potential financial incentives strongly entice whistleblowers to report fraud.

The large financial settlements agreed to by corporations in order to settle fraud and abuse lawsuits help illustrate one of the many incentives for health care corporations to develop corporate compliance programs. This chapter reviews several statutes that are frequently cited in fraud and abuse cases, reviews the penalties for noncompliance with federal health care regulations, presents the seven steps to developing an effective corporate compliance program, presents case reviews of noncompliance with federal health care regulations, reviews the benefits of an effective corporate compliance program, and examines ways in which corporate compliance programs affect pharmacy and pharmacists.

Sources of regulation

Most of the recent regulatory enforcement activity by the government pertaining to health care has focused on violations of the False Claims Statutes, the Prescription Drug Marketing Act, or the Anti-kickback Statute.

False Claims Statutes

The False Claims Statutes were designed to prevent the government from paying for goods or services that were either not provided or not provided in compliance with government regulations. Federal and state False Claims Statutes make it a felony to:

> *Knowingly present, or cause to be presented, to the Government ... a false or fraudulent claim for payment or approval; knowingly make, use, or cause to be made or used, a false record or statement to get a false or fraudulent claim paid or approved by the Government; or conspire to defraud the government by getting a false or fraudulent claim allowed or paid.*[8]

Specific proof of intent is not required; in the act, "knowingly" is defined as having actual knowledge of the information or acting in deliberate ignorance or reckless disregard of the veracity of the information. Issues such as provider charges or claims for unreasonable costs; services not rendered; services provided by unlicensed or unapproved personnel; excessive or unnecessary care; and services not in compliance with Medicare and Medicaid regulations, cost reports, or other requirements are all specifically addressed by these laws.[9]

The Prescription Drug Marketing Act

The Prescription Drug Marketing Act (PDMA) is an amendment to the Federal Food, Drug, and Cosmetic Act, the chief food and drug law of the U.S. The PDMA was established to limit the threat to public health posed by prescription drug diversion and counterfeiting. The act specifically prohibits the following acts: reimportation of U.S.-produced prescription drugs by persons other than the manufacturer (except when authorized by the secretary of Health and Human Services for emergency use); sale, purchase, or trade of drug samples or drug coupons; counterfeiting of drug coupons; resale of prescription drugs by hospitals, health care entities, or charitable organizations (excluding group-purchasing organizations); distribution of drug samples (except as provided in the act); and distribution of prescription drugs in interstate commerce without a state wholesaler's license.[10]

The Anti-kickback Statute and safe harbors

In 1972, Congress enacted the Medicare and Medicaid Anti-kickback Clause as part of the Social Security Amendments Act. This law was designed to shield patients and federal health care programs from fraud and abuse by "curtailing the corrupting influence of money on health care decisions."[11] The Anti-kickback Statute makes it illegal, among other things, to solicit or receive:

> *Any remuneration (including any kickback, bribe, or rebate), directly or indirectly, overtly or covertly, in cash or in kind to any person in return for referring an individual to a person for the furnishing, or arranging for the furnishing, of any item or service for which payment may be made in whole or in part under a Federal health care program.*[12]

Other components of the Anti-kickback Statute address the purchasing, leasing, or ordering of goods, facilities, or services. Many states have enacted statutes that extend these laws to non-Federal programs.[13]

The term *remuneration* simply means payment or compensation. Court decisions addressing the Anti-kickback Statute have interpreted remuneration broadly; three cases provide guidance. In the 1985 case *United States v. Greber*, the court found that if any portion of remuneration was intended to induce the referral of business, the Anti-kickback Statute would be violated.[14] This was followed by the *United States v. Bay State Ambulance* ruling in 1989, which resulted in an overall view that when anyone with the ability to provide federal health program revenues to a second party receives something of economic value in return for a referral, both parties will be responsible for the liabilities resulting from the violation.[15,16] The *Bay State* ruling was weakened by the decision in *Hanlester Network v. Shalala* in 1995, where the court ruled that the government must prove that a defendant knowingly and willfully engaged in prohibited conduct with the specific intent of violating the Anti-kickback Statute.[17] Thus, violations of the Anti-kickback Statute are more challenging for the government to prosecute than violations of the False Claims Act.

The Anti-kickback Statute contains four common sense exemptions that prevent the subjects from being subject to criminal or civil prosecution. Discounts or reductions in price obtained by providers of services are permitted, so long as they are properly disclosed in the costs claimed or charges made by the provider. Compensation paid by employers to legitimate employees is exempt (so long as the payments are not made to induce referrals), as is the administrative fee charged by group-purchasing organizations. The statute also allows the waiving of Medicare Part B coinsurance payments in connection with specific federally qualified health centers.

Additionally, the statute exempts any practice recognized as a regulatory safe harbor. Created by the Department of Health and Human Services (DHHS) in 1987, the safe harbor regulations identify certain payment and business practices that are allowed without the parties being subject to prosecution. There are currently 22 federally recognized safe harbors (Table 23.1). To be protected from prosecution under the Anti-kickback Statute, an arrangement must meet all the elements of a safe harbor regulation. However, failure to fully comply with a safe harbor regulation does not necessarily mean that the action is per se illegal. The OIG has stated that it will use prosecutorial discretion when determining whether to pursue a case.[18] Those who are unsure whether their particular arrangement qualifies for safe harbor protection can contact the OIG and request an advisory opinion.

Consequences of noncompliance with federal health care regulations

Following the discovery of noncompliance with federal health care regulations, the Department of Justice and the OIG consider the seriousness of the

Table 23.1 Regulatory Safe Harbors Exempt from Anti-kickback Statutes

- Investments in large, publicly held health care companies
- Investments in small health care joint ventures
- Space rental and equipment rental
- Personal services and management contracts
- Sales of retiring physicians' practices to other physicians
- Referral services
- Warranties
- Discounts
- Employee compensation
- Group-purchasing organizations
- Waivers of Medicare Part A inpatient cost-sharing amounts
- Increased coverage, reduced cost-sharing amounts, or reduced premium amounts offered by health plans to beneficiaries
- Price reductions offered to health plans by providers
- Investments in underserved areas
- Practitioner recruitment in underserved areas
- Obstetrical malpractice insurance subsidies for underserved areas
- Sales of practices to hospitals in underserved areas
- Investments in ambulatory surgical centers
- Investments in group practices
- Referral arrangements for specialty services
- Cooperative hospital service organizations
- Ambulance restocking arrangements

violations and the culpability of the organization when determining the level of sanctions, penalties, and exclusions that will be imposed.[19]

The government can seek multiple penalties against health care organizations found to be noncompliant. Violations of the False Claims Act can result in a penalty of $5,500 to $11,000 per claim, plus up to three times the amount of damages the government sustains.[8] Consider the average number of claims the typical physician or pharmacist makes yearly. Violations of the False Claims Act can, and have, quickly added up to millions of dollars. Further, the effect of the fine on the financial viability of the company has not been a significant concern of the government.[20] The government also retains the right to bring criminal charges against the executives of a company accused of wrongdoing.

Violations of the PDMA are felonies punishable by a fine up to $250,000 or a 10-year prison sentence, or both. Manufacturers can face escalating fines of up to $1 million per conviction if their representatives have received three or more convictions for illegally selling or trading drug samples within any 10-year period.[21]

Each violation of the Anti-kickback Statute carries the potential for a $25,000 criminal fine, a civil fine, or up to 5 years imprisonment, or all of these.[22] The court may also impose repayment of the amount of losses sustained by the government. Additionally, exclusion from participation in all Medicare and Medicaid programs is required for individuals or corporations convicted of violating the Anti-kickback Statute.

In addition to the monetary settlements, the OIG often imposes corporate integrity agreements on health care providers as part of a health care fraud investigation settlement. Through these agreements, the government implements its own compliance programs with companies alleged to have violated fraud and abuse laws.[23] These compliance measures help ensure the integrity of federal health care program claims submitted by the provider. The more comprehensive integrity agreements include the following requirements: hiring a compliance officer or appointment of a compliance committee, developing written standards and policies, implementation of a comprehensive employee training program, auditing billings to federal health care programs, establishing a confidential disclosure program, restricting employment of ineligible persons, and submitting a variety of reports to the OIG.[24] Each corporate integrity agreement is designed to address and subsequently correct the specific activities in violation of federal regulations, and is designed to meet the capabilities of the provider. The typical term of a comprehensive corporate integrity agreement is 3 to 5 years.

The OIG must exclude any person or corporation convicted of a felony relating to health care fraud from the Medicare program.[25] The law mandates minimum periods of exclusion from 1 to 3 years, depending on the basis for exclusion. For many corporations, it is this debarment from federal programs (more so than any criminal fine) that causes the most fear, as the loss of Medicare and Medicaid patients could ultimately cause the business to fail.

A provider can usually avoid conviction and debarment from federal health care programs by reaching a financial settlement with OIG and entering into a corporate integrity agreement with the government.

Lastly, the damage sustained to a company's reputation is immeasurable. An example is the case of National Medical Enterprises (NME), a multistate for-profit healthcare system. In 1994, NME paid $379 million in fines, penalties, and damages for alleged Medicare billing violations. Negative publicity generated from the settlement decreased NME's market value and made it a less attractive partner for a merger during a time of rapid consolidation in the hospital industry.[26]

Corporate compliance programs

The OIG has provided final compliance program guidance to nine segments of the health care industry, including hospitals, clinical laboratories, and home health agencies. The purpose of the compliance program guidance is to "assist the organization … in developing effective internal controls that promote adherence to applicable federal and state law, and the program requirements of federal, state, and private health plans."[1] The documents emphasize the benefits of establishing a voluntary compliance program and review the elements found in effective compliance programs (outlined later). Although the OIG has not developed any program guidance for establishing compliance programs for pharmacies, it has targeted hospital outpatient pharmacies as an area for future review.[27]

Establishing voluntary corporate compliance programs

There are seven basic steps to designing and implementing an effective voluntary corporate compliance program (Table 23.2). These steps are designed to ensure that precautions are taken to prevent or minimize the impact of fraud and abuse on the organization as a whole. To be successful, the organization must provide the necessary time and resources to properly design, implement, and monitor each of the following seven steps.

Table 23.2 Seven Steps to an Effective Voluntary Compliance Program

- Designate a chief compliance officer and a corporate compliance committee
- Write standard policies and procedures
- Educate and train affected employees
- Develop effective lines of communication to receive reports of suspected violations
- Develop an auditing process to monitor compliance
- Ensure consistent enforcement and discipline
- Investigate and remediate identified problems

Designate a chief compliance officer and a corporate compliance committee

The first step in developing a compliance program is to designate a chief compliance officer to serve as the focal point for compliance activities. The chief compliance officer is responsible for developing, implementing, and monitoring the corporate compliance program, and also for making periodic revisions to the compliance program based on the organizations' needs and in respect to changes in federal law. Another key responsibility of the chief compliance officer is to ensure the development of training programs and that employees and independent contractors have been made aware of the requirements of the organization's compliance program.

Chief compliance officers should be familiar with reimbursement issues and the laws regarding corporate compliance; experience in areas such as quality assurance and risk assessment is also helpful. One of the key attributes of chief compliance officers is their independence. For this reason, the OIG recommends that the chief compliance officer be someone other than the company's general counsel or chief financial officer in order to establish a system of checks and balances.

In addition, a corporate compliance committee should be formed to work with the chief compliance officer on all compliance activities. The corporate compliance committee should be composed of people from all of the key operating units in the organization, including finance, billing and coding, auditing, medical staff, nursing staff, pharmacy staff, legal, and human resources. The corporate compliance committee should meet on a regularly scheduled basis; the committee can meet more frequently when violations are detected, federal regulations are changed, or if the organization has become the target of a fraud and abuse investigation.

Write standard policies and procedures

Under the direction of the chief compliance officer and the corporate compliance committee, each organization should develop written compliance policies that pertain to the organization's practices that may be at risk for noncompliance. The policy should clearly delineate the organization's commitment to comply with all federal and state standards, with an emphasis on preventing fraud and abuse. The compliance plan should address, at a minimum, the False Claims Act, the Anti-kickback Statutes, physician self-referral laws, and laws regarding bribery and improper gifts. Once the plan is developed, it should be reviewed and approved by the organization's board of directors.

The practices relevant to pharmacy include billing for items or services not actually rendered, duplicate billing, false cost reports, and acceptance of gifts by employees. Policies about appropriate pharmacy billing practices and acceptance of gifts from manufacturers should be developed and communicated to all affected employees, including nurses, billing clerks, pharmacists, and finance department officials.

Pharmacists should be aware of the extent to which only a few violations can put the entire institution at significant risk for charges of fraud and abuse. For example, Medicare requires documentation that medications that are billed for are actually administered to patients. Medicare typically makes payments based on the bill submitted by the institution and relies on the integrity and accuracy of the hospital billing system. Hospitals that bill for medications based on pharmacy dispensing records are at greater risk for noncompliance.[28] This risk exists because of the potential for inaccurate documentation by nurses, inaccurate crediting of unadministered (or borrowed) medications, and wasted medications charged to the patient. Although Medicare does not withhold payment because of lack of documentation, it requires settlement if a pattern of overbilling is detected during an audit. Pharmacy departments should monitor the accuracy of patient billing records to assure that unintentional overbilling does not occur.

Educate and train affected employees

Once compliance standards have been established by the corporate compliance committee, the committee must work to develop education and training programs to ensure that employees are made aware of any new policies and procedures. It is probably in the best interest of the institution to educate all employees about the broad compliance program, along with instructions to report all violations to the chief compliance officer. Employees whose responsibilities include areas that can cause the most problems with compliance (such as billing and coding personnel) should undergo a more intensive training program regarding the standards that apply to their position. Lack of knowledge of a process or policy is not an acceptable argument against sanctioning.

Corporate compliance officers and managers depend on all employees to report any potential for fraudulent practice. For example, employees might not be in a position to commit fraud directly, but in the course of their job, might become aware of a violation occurring elsewhere in the organization. With their knowledge of good corporate compliance practices, they can alert the chief compliance officer.

Develop effective lines of communication to receive reports of suspected violations

The ability of the compliance officer to receive complaints from employees is vital to an effective compliance program. An effective reporting system alerts the corporate compliance committee to violations before the government discovers them or they become the subject of a qui tam lawsuit. Any employee who recognizes the possible occurrence of fraud and abuse should have a means of reporting the violation without fear of repercussions. To facilitate this, written confidentiality and nonretaliation policies should be developed and distributed to all employees. To enable the reporting of suspected violations, an employee should be able to lodge a complaint in several ways, including an anonymous voice-mail box, a suggestion box, via e-mail, and even a meeting with the chief compliance officer. The compliance officer or a designee should document the receipt of the complaint and note any response made by the organization in regard to the complaint.

Develop an auditing process to monitor compliance

To ensure that the compliance program is effective in deterring fraud and abuse, the corporate compliance committee should periodically audit records and documents that could subject the organization to criminal or civil liability. The audit should include a review of employment agreements, agreements with physicians or other potential referral sources, third-party arrangements, marketing materials, and nonemployee consultant arrangements.[29] The organization can either delegate this task to internal employees familiar with the systems being audited or hire an outside legal firm familiar with health care audits. The OIG also recommends that the program itself be reviewed at least annually to ensure that all elements are being met.

Ensure consistent enforcement and discipline

An effective compliance program should include a policy statement explaining the disciplinary actions that will be taken against individuals found to violate the organization's corporate compliance plan. Appropriate enforcement of disciplinary action is essential against individuals found committing an offense. The OIG suggests that sanctions should be significant enough to punish the offender and discourage others from following in their footsteps.[30] Employees found to be intentionally or recklessly noncompliant should face the most significant sanctions, up to and including financial penalties and termination. Furthermore, the consequences of noncompliance should be incorporated into the compliance training program and consistently enforced when an offense is identified.

Investigate and remediate identified problems

If problems are detected, the chief compliance officer and the corporate compliance committee are responsible for ensuring there is a full investigation of the source and causes of the problem. Detected but uncorrected problems leave the organization in a terrible situation: the government can contend that the organization knew that it was in violation and chose to do nothing about it. The sanctions imposed by the federal government tend to be stiffest in these cases. Therefore, particular attention should be spent on resolving issues for which past violations have been detected.

A component to this process might be the use of outside legal counsel or auditors to assist with the investigation. The investigation might include review of appropriate records and interviews with employees. Meticulous records of the investigation must be kept to ensure that the process was both complete and fair. Once a problem is confirmed to be a violation of the corporate compliance program or federal law, or both, the compliance officer is obligated to take appropriate steps, including disciplinary action, correction of the conduct in violation, and referral to appropriate criminal or civil enforcement agencies.

Case reviews of corporate compliance with federal regulations

A review of several cases will help illustrate the points examined so far. One of the largest health care fraud and abuse investigations conducted by the government focused upon the activities of The Healthcare Company (HCA, formerly Columbia/HCA), the largest for-profit hospital chain in the U.S. Notified about violations of the False Claims Act by over 25 individual whistleblowers, the government conducted a 7-year investigation into HCA's billing practices.[31] The government uncovered evidence of several different types of Medicare and Medicaid fraud, including billings for laboratory services not medically necessary and not ordered by physicians, upcoding of diagnostic codes to increase reimbursement payments, and the disguising of marketing and advertising costs as community education services and receiving reimbursement for those education services from Medicare.[32] To avoid trial, HCA agreed to plead guilty to the charges and pay over $840 million in criminal fines, civil fines, and damages. As part of the civil settlement, HCA entered into a comprehensive corporate integrity agreement with the government for 8 years. This agreement requires HCA and independent review organizations to conduct audits and reviews of inpatient coding, laboratory billing, and outpatient billing methods and HCA's financial relationships with physicians.[32] The agreement calls for HCA to provide the OIG with annual reports detailing the effectiveness of the compliance program.

The OIG has also recently completed several investigations into so-called partial-fill prescriptions dispensed by community pharmacies. A partial-fill prescription situation arose when a pharmacy did not have the full amount of the requested medication on hand to complete the order. The common industry standard was to dispense a partial amount of the prescription and ask the customer to return for the balance of the medication in a few days time. Pharmacies would often bill third-party payers such as state Medicaid programs for the full amount of the prescriptions in such cases, even though many of the patients never returned to the pharmacy to pick up the balance of their pills. A whistleblower notified the federal government that the chain pharmacy he worked for often failed to provide partial refunds to third-party payers for prescriptions wherein the partial fills were dispensed and the balance of the pills were never picked up by customers, a violation of the

False Claims Act.[33] The OIG and several state attorney generals determined the violations to be an industry-wide problem. The OIG and the Department of Justice made arrangements with many of the major chain pharmacies in this country to resolve the case; the chains agreed (individually) to pay between $1.7 and $7.6 million to settle each case, and several chains were also required to enter into comprehensive corporate integrity agreements with the government.[33–36]

Our last example examines a manufacturer seeking an OIG advisory opinion during the development of a patient assistance program (PAP). Before the year 2000, Medicare Part B provided coverage and payment for immunosuppressive drugs for up to 36 months following a transplant; Part B beneficiaries were required to pay a 20% copayment.[37] During this time, one manufacturer of immunosuppressive drugs operated a PAP for the financially needy. Through the program, the manufacturer provided the drug at no cost to financially needy, uninsured patients, including Medicare beneficiaries who had exhausted their 36 months of Part B coverage who met income criteria and lacked secondary insurance coverage. In the year 2000, Congress eliminated the 36-month limitation on immunosuppressive drugs, effectively creating lifetime coverage of the products under Part B.[38] Once the Part B coverage limitation was lifted, Medicare patients who received the drugs at no cost after 36 months of Part B coverage became ineligible for the manufacturer's PAP, and again became responsible for the 20 percent co-payments. The manufacturer wanted to modify its PAP to include financially needy Medicare patients who used the drugs. Instead of providing the drugs for free to these patients, the manufacturer wanted to reimburse patients their 20% copayment, leaving patients with no out-of-pocket costs associated with the prescription. The manufacturer submitted this proposed change in their PAP to the OIG for an advisory opinion. The OIG determined that the arrangement would be a clear violation of the Anti-kickback Statute, as the manufacturer would be paying the beneficiary (in the form of a copayment reimbursement) to use its products. The OIG also cited that the program would provide the manufacturer's products with an obvious financial advantage in the market, and that the arrangement could result in increased costs to the Medicare program by encouraging prescribing of the brand name drugs rather than lower-cost generic versions.[37,39] By seeking an advisory opinion from the OIG, the manufacturer learned that the proposed changes to their PAP would have violated federal health care regulations, which could have exposed the company to prosecution. With this knowledge, the manufacturer had the opportunity to modify its PAP to ensure that it did not run afoul of federal regulations.

Benefits of a voluntary corporate compliance program

Establishment of an effective voluntary corporate compliance program can bestow many benefits to a company. According to the OIG, an effective plan can reduce the potential liability of the provider. The central benefit of corporate compliance programs for the health care provider is to minimize or reduce the threat of a lawsuit and its attendant consequences. Providers with effective corporate compliance programs actively seek to weed out fraud, and as such are less likely to be seen as has having intended to commit the crime. Instead, the OIG (and the courts) would be more likely to see an act of fraud and abuse as a civil or administrative offense rather than a criminal offense, resulting in lesser consequences. The government examines the seriousness of the offense and the culpability of the organization when deciding punishment. The presence of a voluntary corporate compliance program making a reasonable effort to detect and avoid violations can significantly lower an organization's culpability score and the subsequent penalty.

In addition to the benefits in criminal proceedings, benefits can also be achieved in civil actions or personal liability cases, or both. Boards of directors can be held accountable through the federal sentencing guidelines for organizations when fraud and abuse occur. The government's decision to prosecute is often based on the desire to deter future misconduct.[40] If reasonable steps have been made to prevent improper activities, then there is little the government can gain from seeking criminal charges.

If a company is convicted of or settles a health care fraud and abuse suit, the presence of a voluntary corporate compliance program may allow the organization to avoid the imposition of a mandated corporate integrity agreement. These agreements are much more stringent and burdensome than voluntary compliance programs; corporate integrity agreements often include requirements for the submission of annual compliance reports to the government and allow the government the right to examine corporate records during unannounced audits and onsite visits. Clearly, a company would rather develop a voluntary corporate compliance program than have a corporate integrity agreement imposed on it as part of a settlement.

Organizations with effective compliance programs are less likely to be the subject of a qui tam lawsuit. Disgruntled employees and competitors would be less likely to bring qui tam suits because, if successful, a compliance program will have already identified and corrected many of the violations, leaving fewer (if any) things for a qui tam relator to report. Further, in the past, corporate executives who were aware of violations may have brought a qui tam lawsuit in the past to protect themselves from criminal and civil liability. A corporate compliance program gives them a place to bring known violations where they can be addressed constructively.

Cost: a barrier to corporate compliance programs

The major barrier to the implementation of voluntary compliance programs is cost. Health care organizations, especially hospitals, are asked to devote a significant amount of capital and resources to develop corporate compliance programs at a time when many are facing tightening budgets and reduced reimbursement rates. In 1999, the General Accounting Office (GAO) interviewed 25 hospitals regarding their corporate compliance program implementation status.[41] Of those that could provide cost data, a corporate compliance program was estimated to cost approximately 1% of total patient revenue. The expenses associated with operating a compliance program varied with the size of the hospital and the fastidiousness of the program. For example, one medium-sized hospital spent $15,000 annually to operate a corporate compliance program, where one employee spent about 10% of his time performing the duties of the chief compliance officer. In contrast, one large hospital system employed four full-time attorneys and associated staff; this program cost about $2.5 million annually. Despite the high costs associated with the development and maintenance of a corporate compliance program, organizations that have implemented these programs maintain that the benefits outweigh the costs.

Corporate compliance and pharmacy

In several ways, pharmacy can (and should) be an integral part of a health system's corporate compliance program. The most visible aspect of corporate compliance for pharmacy is the appropriate billing of pharmaceuticals. A hospital's director of pharmacy is responsible for ensuring that charges for medications are correctly submitted to Medicare, Medicaid, and other managed care organizations. If a nurse does not record a medication as being administered to the patient, a charge for it should not be processed. Doses that are wasted or diverted should not be billed for. Medication distribution systems that base billing on medications dispensed rather than medications administered have a higher potential for billing fraud claims.[28] Pharmacy needs to be particularly careful in situations where medications are dispensed from floor stock; examples include operating rooms, emergency departments, and intensive care units.

Similarly, billing Medicare or Medicaid for medications that were obtained as free samples or trial supplies from manufacturers would also be considered as fraud under the False Claims Act. Furthermore, pharmacies that receive medication samples and bills for them also violate the PDMA. The pharmacist must track the disposition of free samples and trial supplies and assure that they are not fraudulently billed for.

Although the issues surrounding the billing for pharmacist cognitive services have not been addressed by the OIG, the potential exists for

Table 23.3 Office of Inspector General Special Fraud Alerts

- Joint venture arrangements
- Routine waiver of Medicare Part B copayments and deductibles
- Hospital incentives to referring physicians
- Prescription drug marketing practices
- Arrangements for the provision of clinical laboratory services
- Home health fraud
- Provision of medical supplies to nursing facilities

increased scrutiny by the government as the profession expands this aspect of pharmaceutical care. Landrum and Williams described a hospital-based program for billing for pharmacist cognitive services.[42] While a review of their charges revealed that the overall reimbursement rate for their activities was 35%, the article did not mention whether the authors conducted an audit to determine whether the billed service matched the clinical service documented in the medical record. This will be an area of concern for pharmacists as billing for cognitive services grows.

Whereas inappropriate billing may represent an obvious fraudulent activity, other activities can also violate the Anti-kickback Statute, False Claims Act, or other laws and statutes. The OIG has designated seven areas as special fraud alerts (Table 23.3),[3] which guide providers in determining what activities may represent violations of one of the laws Two special fraud alerts warrant attention by pharmacy practitioners: (1) the routine waiver of Medicare Part B copayments and deductibles and (2) prescription drug marketing practices.

Routine waiver of Medicare Part B copayments

The regular collection of copayments or coinsurance from Medicare Part B enrollees is a required activity for health care providers who provide services to beneficiaries. With any copayment, patients consider the benefits of the goods or services they will receive relative to the amount of the copayment. In general, this process leads to a more knowledgeable and selective health care consumer and lower overall health care costs.[43] In terms of pharmacy, outpatient prescription services rendered to Medicare Part B recipients must be given in exchange for the appropriate copayment or coinsurance. The routine waiving of these copayments can be considered an unlawful inducement to patients to use a particular service or provider. However, the law does provide for the occasional copayment waiver for patients with significant financial hardship.

The Centers for Medicare and Medicaid Services (CMS) has issued new regulations regarding the billing of outpatient services for patients receiving Medicare Part B benefits.[44] This new reimbursement scheme, the Ambulatory Payment Classifications (APCs), revises some of the old coding schemes for medications and devices paid for by Medicare Part B. Pharmacists should be familiar with these new codes and should play a strong role in working with the financing department to ensure that the new coding scheme is both understood and properly utilized. This will be particularly important for community and health-system pharmacists if a Medicare prescription benefit is enacted.

Prescription drug marketing practices

One of the goals of prescription drug marketing is to influence providers to select a specific brand of medication for their patients. Pharmacists who influence the selection of a particular drug in exchange for something from the drug manufacturer or supplier are violating the Anti-kickback Statute. Specific examples provided by the OIG include product conversion activities, wherein pharmacists are paid to contact physicians and influence them to change a prescription from one brand to another. One manufacturer paid pharmacists money to call physicians and request that they change a prescription from Drug A to Drug B; the physician was unaware of the financial incentive provided to the pharmacist for the switch. In this case, both the manufacturer and the pharmacist were in violation of the Anti-kickback Statute.

In the current era of formulary restrictions and preferred product status, manufacturers' rebates to health plans and hospitals in hopes of improving their formulary positioning are commonplace. When appropriately documented and disclosed in the costs, these "gifts" are protected by one of the safe harbor regulations. However, without disclosure, these incentives may be subject to prosecution under the Anti-kickback Statute. Similarly, monetary gifts may be considered improper under this statute, particularly if the gift is made to a person in a position to generate business or is related to the volume of business. Although the concepts of upfront rebates and signing bonus payments have not been directly addressed in the area of pharmacy, the Chief Counsel to the Inspector General has rendered an opinion of this type of activity with respect to medical supply companies.[43] In essence, a manufacturer giving upfront rebates and signing bonuses to a purchaser (e.g., a hospital) raises serious issues under the Anti-kickback Statute. A health plan or hospital that receives money (or gifts) in exchange for improving a product's formulary status is likely to be in violation. Although one may consider this payment as a discount or a rebate and protected as a safe harbor, the Chief Counsel to the Inspector General views "such payments difficult to trace to ensure proper disclosure" and may interfere with the purchaser's usual ability to make appropriate purchasing decisions on behalf of federal beneficiaries.

Corporate compliance programs should involve the pharmacy department to ensure appropriate documentation and submission of medication-related claims. The idea of a pharmacy compliance officer serving as a member of the corporate compliance committee has been raised.[28] This pharmacist would be directly involved in writing policies and procedures for proper medication billing, developing a procedure for auditing of pharmacy billing practices, and assuring that practices related to pharmacy meet federal regulations.

In 2002, the Pharmaceutical Research and Manufacturers of America (PhRMA), the trade group for pharmaceutical and biotechnology companies, issued a new marketing code for its members.[45] Developed in response to concern that promotional activities were tarnishing public opinion about the pharmaceutical industry,[46] the voluntary code reinforces PhRMA's intention that interactions between representatives of the manufacturer and health professionals were to enhance the practice of medicine and benefit patients.

Three provisions of the code merit further attention. The code calls for a ban on all gifts to practitioners that are intended for personal benefit or do not primarily benefit patients or are not primarily associated with the practitioners practice; promotional activities such as a gas-and-go (wherein a sales representative details physicians while filling up their car with free gasoline at a local service station) or providing food for an office staff to gain a visit with the practitioner are not acceptable under the code. Informational presentations by manufacturers can no longer be done in conjunction with entertainment or recreational activities (such as a presentation preceding a sporting event), and any meals provided to attendees during a presentation must be modest by local standards. Additionally, the code prohibits financial support for the attendance of a health professional's spouse at educational or professional meetings.

Some have cited potential weaknesses of the PhRMA code, including the fact that it is a voluntary program without consequences for violations and that the code is vague, leaving each company free to interpret it differently.[46] A few months following the release of the PhRMA code, the OIG issued draft compliance program guidance for pharmaceutical manufacturers.[47] In the draft guidance, the OIG states that adhering to the PhRMA code is merely a "good starting point" that "will not necessarily protect a manufacturer from prosecution or liability for illegal conduct."[47] The OIG also recommended that manufacturers comply with the standards of the PhRMA code, and that arrangements that failed to meet the minimum standards of the PhRMA code were likely to receive increased scrutiny from government authorities.

Conclusion

The federal government has recently increased the investigation and prosecution of health care fraud and abuse. Federal laws such as the False Claims Act and the Anti-kickback Statute provide sufficient means for the federal government to detect and prosecute health care providers committing fraud and abuse. Corporate compliance programs and corporate integrity agreements guide health care providers in developing practices that decrease the occurrence of fraud and minimize its impact when it occurs. The development and implementation of a corporate compliance program will likely protect the organization from harsh penalties stemming from claims of fraud and protect the individuals responsible for the organization.

Although pharmacists have not been a specific target of the government's fraud and abuse investigations, several recent high-profile settlements between the pharmaceutical industry and the government highlight the importance of educating pharmacists on the principles of corporate compliance programs. Pharmacy is a growing player in the corporate compliance arena, and the utility for a pharmacy compliance officer within organizations should be considered. Further, with the current movement toward pharmacist billing for cognitive services, the potential for fraud and abuse of these services also exists. As practitioners develop programs by which they bill for cognitive services, they should pay particular attention to their billing practices to avoid compliance issues.

References

Note: Legal cases can be obtained at most law libraries or on the Lexis-Nexis database. Federal laws can be obtained at libraries housing federal documents.

1. The Office of the Inspector General. The Office of Inspector General's compliance program guidance for hospitals. www.hhs.govprogorg/oig/oigreg/cpghosp.pdf, accessed March 14, 2001.
2. United States Sentencing Guideline Manual §8A1.2 cmt. (3)(k) (1998).
3. Bellick P. In crackdown on health care fraud, U.S. focuses on training hospitals and clinics.*The New York Times*; December 12, 1995: A32.
4. Pub L. No. 104-191, 110 Stat. 1936, 1991–2021 (1996).
5. Steinhauer J. Justice department finds success chasing health care fraud. *The New York Times*. January 23, 2001, p. A19.
6. Anonymous. TAP to audit marketing documents related to top Lupron, Prevacid buyers. *The Pink Sheet* October 8, 2001: 3–4.
7. 31 U.S.C. §3730 (1996).
8. 31 U.S.C. §3729 (1996).
9. Anonymous. Regulatory control of providers' financial relationships. In *Health Law: Cases, Materials, and Problems*, 3rd ed., Furrow BR, Greaney TL, Johnson SH et al., (Eds.). St. Paul, MN: West Group, 1997.
10. Food and Drug Administration. Requirements of laws and regulations enforced by the U.S. Food and Drug Administration. www.fda.gov/opacom/morechoices/smallbusiness/blubook.htm, accessed March 26, 2001.
11. Office of Inspector General. Federal anti-kickback law and regulatory safe harbors fact sheet, http://oig.hhs.gov/fraud/docs/safeharborregulations/safefs.htm, accessed January 12, 2004.
12. 42 U.S.C. §1320a-7b (1)(A).
13. Self-referrals: effectiveness of state efforts to restrict referrals is questioned, 2 Health L. Rep. (BNA) 16, d3 (April 22, 1993).
14. 760 F 2d 68, cert. denied, 474 U.S. 988, 106 S.Ct. 396, 88 L. Ed. 2d 348 (1985).
15. 874 F 2d 20 (1st Cir. 1989).
16. Gosfield AG. The new playing field. *St. Louis Univ. L. J.* 1997; 41: 869.
17. Hanlester Network v. Shalala, United States Court of Appeals for the Ninth Circuit, 51 f.3d 1390; 1995 U.S. App.
18. 56 Fed. Reg. 35,954 (1991).
19. Brown JG. An open letter to health care providers. March 3, 1997. www.hhs.gov/progorg/oig/modcomp/ltrhcp.html, accessed February 26, 2001.
20. United States v. Eureka Lab., Inc., 103 F 3d 908, 914 (9th Cir. 1996).
21. Summary H.R. 1207 Prescription Drug Marketing Act of 1987. www.i3sfa.com/pdm.%20summary.pdf, accessed March 26, 2001.
22. Office of Inspector General. Federal anti-kickback law and regulatory safe harbors fact sheet.

23. Radinsky G. Making sense of the federal sentencing guidelines: how health care corporations can manage risk by adopting corporate compliance programs. *J. Hlth. Law* 1997; 30: 113.
24. Office of Inspector General. Corporate integrity agreements (CIAs) & settlement agreements with integrity provisions. http://oig.hhs.gov/fraud/cia/index.htm, accessed January 12, 2004.
25. 42 U.S.C.A. § 1320a-7 (A) (1) & (2).
26. NME pact illustrates increased DOJ leverage. DOJ Alert 2 (Prentice Hall) No. 14, August 1, 1994.
27. Department of Health and Human Services. Office of Inspector General projects: fiscal year 2001 work plan. www.oig.hhs.gov/reading/workplan/2001/hcfa.pdf, accessed May 30, 2002.
28. Shane R. Detecting and preventing health care fraud and abuse — we've only just begun [Commentary]. *Am. J. Hlth.-Syst. Pharm.* 2000; 57: 1078–1080.
29. Warnock TL. Corporate compliance programs: understanding the extent of an entity's exposure. *Tenn. Hlth. Law Update*, August 1995.
30. 63 Fed. Reg. No. 35, pp. 8797–8998 (1998).
31. Sniffen MJ. $840 million penalty: hospital chain pleads guilty in government fraud settlement. December 14, 2000. www.abcnews.go.com/sections/us/dailynews/hca_settlement001214.html, accessed April 30, 2001.
32. United States Department of Justice. HCA — The Health Care Company and subsidiaries to pay $840 million in criminal fines and civil damages and penalties. Press Release 2000–696, December 14, 2000.
33. Huntley H. Eckerd will pay to end prescription allegations. *St. Petersburg (FL) Times*, May 25, 2002.
34. Anonymous. CVS reaches settlement with states on partial fill prescriptions. January 9, 2003. news.findlaw.com/prnewswire/20030109/09jan2003155609.html, accessed March 14, 2003.
35. Anonymous. Rite Aid settles Medicaid partial Rx fill investigation for $7.1 mil. *The Green Sheet*, October 15, 2001: 3.
36. Anonymous. Walgreens settles lawsuit for $7.6 million. http://www.beloit-dailynews.com/999/2ill16.htm, accessed March, 2003.
37. Morris L. OIG advisory opinion no. 03-3. Department of Health and Human Services, February 3, 2003.
38. 42 U.S.C. § 1395x (s) (2) (J) (Supp. 2001).
39. Anonymous. Novartis Neoral patient assistance proposal violates kickback laws, IG says. *The Pink Sheet*, February 17, 2003.
40. Kowal SM. Corporate compliance programs: a shield against criminal liability. *Food Drug L. J.* 1998; 53: 517–526.
41. General Account Office Report. Medicare: early evidence of compliance program effectiveness is inconclusive. GAO/HEHS-99-59, 1999.
42. Michalets EL, Williams E. Reimbursement for pharmacists' cognitive services in the inpatient setting. *Am. J. Hlth.-Syst. Pharm.* 2001; 58: 164–166.
43. Office of Inspector General. Publication of OIG special fraud alerts. December 1994. http://org.hhs.gov/fraud/docs/alertsandbulletins/121994.html, accessed January 12, 2004.
44. Centers for Medicare & Medicaid Services. Hospital outpatient prospective payment system. August 2000. http://cms.hhs.gov/regulations/hopps, accessed March 13, 2003.

45. Pharmaceutical Research and Manufacturers of America. PhRMA code on interactions with healthcare professionals. www.phrma.org/publications/policy/2002-04-19.391.pdf, accessed January 10, 2003.
46. Ross W. New rules, new roles for the sales force. *Med. Market. Media* 2002; 11: 39–48.
47. Office of Inspector General. Draft OIG compliance program guidance for pharmaceutical manufacturers. September 2002. http://www.oig.hhs.gov/fraud/docs/complianceguidance/draftcpgpharm09272002.pdf, accessed March 13, 2003.

chapter twenty-four

eHealth

Jacob Mathew and Diana Papshev

Contents

Introduction

The use of emerging information and technology, especially the Internet, to improve or enable health or health care is known as electronic health or eHealth. eHealth is the intersection of medical informatics, public health, and business, delivering health services and information through the Internet and related technologies. It combines both the clinical and nonclinical sectors and includes individual and population health-oriented tools. In the broader sense, it represents a commitment for networked, global thinking to improve health care locally, regionally, and worldwide by using information and communication technology.

The current health care system is fragmented and not connected. Lack of connectedness and continuity among various stakeholders reinforces each segment of the industry to function in a silo mode. For example, pharmacies are not interconnected to prescribers or laboratories, and prescribers are not interconnected to payers or hospitals. The fragmentation of the current prescription management makes the process expensive, unsafe, inefficient, and dissatisfying to customers. The U.S. spends more on health care than any other country does. Health care spending, approximately $1.1 trillion (13.5% of gross domestic product, GDP) in 1998, is projected to reach $2.2 trillion (16.2% of GDP) by 2008. About a quarter of this expenditure may be attributed to administrative inefficiencies and waste. In addition, between 44,000 and 98,000 people may die every year as a result of medical errors (Kohn et al., 1999), and variations in medical practice may result in uneven patient outcomes. Current pharmacy management is flawed with inefficiencies and redundancies. At the time physicians provide care to their patients, their access to critical information is limited by time and resources. Patient medication history, clinical references, and formulary rules are not typically available. Once the prescription reaches the pharmacy, many issues arise related to illegible prescriptions, clinical interactions, and formulary restrictions. To resolve these issues, the pharmacist embarks on a barrage of phone calls to either the physician or the insurer. The calls sometimes are not made until after hours, so the physician might not return the call until the next business day. Often, a single prescription can go through a number of loops between a prescriber, a pharmacy, and an insurer before the medication reaches the intended patient.

The cost of drug-related problems, including medication errors, inappropriate prescribing, and drug interactions, soared from an estimated $77 billion in 1995 to an estimated $177 billion in 2000. There are also administrative costs due to ineffiencies in the prescription process. Approximately 50% of physician office calls are pharmacy related, with pharmacists calling nearly 150 million times a year. Patients are frustrated with formulary-related barriers and delays in obtaining a prescription, in addition to the long waits at physician offices. The current process is unsafe, inefficient, and costly; the need for a new system is clear and justified. It has been proposed that technology can resolve many of these flaws by improving the existing process. Although implementation of technological improvements has many associated issues, many stakeholders in the health care industry are beginning to consider and adopt these technological solutions.

The Internet

In January 2001, approximately 168 million people, or 60% of the U.S. population, had access to the Internet at home or work, and 86% of adult users of the Internet accessed health-related information. The number of health-related Web sites available is unknown, but it is believed that the more than 19,000 health sites indexed in May 2001 on Yahoo!, Inc. represent only a small fraction of the universe of eHealth sites. Internet use has been lower in populations that are underserved, but the profile of the Internet user community is shifting from one comprised initially of white, educated, young men to a much more diverse group of users. Also, the Internet has always been less prevalent in lower-income families, but they now represent the fastest growing segment of recent users and computer purchasers. However, a digital divide may still persist as newer, more expensive technologies become available, such as broadband access. Compared with other industry sectors, such as finance and commerce, the use of Internet in the health sector is unfolding more slowly.

As with most other Internet-related sectors, the eHealth field is driven primarily by for-profit eHealth companies. At present, many of the most recognized eHealth companies are consumer-oriented portals (WebMD) that seek to be one-stop shops for health information and health-related products. The most common focus of larger eHealth companies seems to be on providing tools, solutions, products, or services that support some aspect of clinical care, including administrative transactions, clinical information systems, telemedicine and telehealth, and sales of health-related products. Although the promise of applying emerging and cutting-edge information and communication technologies to improve health and health care is substantial, it is critical that there be an understanding of what technology can and cannot do. Major potential risks associated with the widespread use and adoption of eHealth tools include fraudulent online activities and poor quality resources, violations of privacy and confidentiality, unintended errors from inadequately tested or complex tools, potential misuse of applications, increasing social isolation from online activities, and widening the socioeconomic divide.

Origins of eHealth

The concept of eHealth began with the need to provide and support care from a distance. Call centers were an example of a solution. The basic function of call centers is to provide information or services at a distance, a concept used in many industries. To date, many types of call centers are used in the health care industry. The following are examples related to pharmacy:

- Poison control centers
- Drug information centers
- Pharmacy help lines
- Home care centers

These centers use phones to provide medical information related to certain conditions or drugs (e.g., drug information center), demand management for patients or health care providers seeking help (e.g., poison control center), or remote care (e.g., home care centers).

Emergence of eHealth

As the Internet was evolving in the late 1990s, entrepreneurs and venture capitalists invested heavily in the notion of widespread use of information technology. eHealth companies emerged everywhere. Some aided physicians and health care providers with clinical information, billing, and office management services. Others focused directly on patients, giving them new access to information about their specific problems and concerns. All these ventures used the new Internet medium to deliver products and services that they hoped would revolutionize health care. Examples of these sites included DrKoop.com, Drugstore.com, and PlanetRx.com. These sites promised an information-intensive and prototypical service industry; however, many predictable yet unforeseen challenges and obstacles caused a collapse in the Internet sector as a whole. An analysis of first-generation eHealth companies identified four critical strategic factors that tend to predict success or failure: a compelling value, an unambiguous revenue model, competitive barriers to entry, and an organizational structure for cost control. None of the first-generation companies had all four criteria for success, which led to the downfall of many sites. The potential for eHealth to streamline and improve medical care remains excellent despite the widespread failure of eHealth and other dotcom companies following the burst of the Internet bubble in 2000. A new, stronger generation of eHealth companies is emerging and benefiting from the mistakes of earlier pioneers.

Domains of eHealth

There are currently five emerging domains of eHealth that are in development, with constant modifications and reinventions: content, commerce, computer technology, connectivity, and care.

Content

The content domain is represented by Web sites providing health-related information online; it promises to deliver convenient access to information. An example of a consumer content Web site is WebMD and that of a professional content Web site is Medscape. The major challenge that the eHealth domain faces is the credibility of the posted information. Many of the established sites are credible; however, caution must be taken when viewing a new site. The author and sources of information must be evaluated.

Health on the Net (HON) (www.hon.ch) is a nonprofit organization designed to aid nonmedical Internet users to reliable and valid information on health-related issues. Web pages that meet the standards set forth by HON can display its HON code logo, indicating that such high standards are met. This symbol can provide the layperson a reasonable sense of certainty that the information provided on the site is credible.

Commerce

The commerce domain is based on the principles of eCommerce. This domain is well exemplified by Internet pharmacies. Once a novel method of drug distribution, now Internet pharmacy capabilities are available for practically every retail chain. At present, traditional brick and mortar pharmacies either partner with existing Internet pharmacies or create their own Web counterparts, which illustrates the increasing importance of business on the Internet. Retail giant CVS pharmacy acquired the Internet pharmacy soma.com and changed the name to reflect the new ownership. Walgreens launched an upgraded, full-service Internet pharmacy to compete more successfully in the pharmacy industry. It is estimated that currently over 400 businesses operate on the Internet that dispense prescription drugs. In 2001, Internet pharmacies generated about $1.4 billion in sales and are expected to generate over $15 billion by 2004. Examples of popular current Internet pharmacies are Drugstore.com (partners with Rite-Aid), walgreens.com, cvs.com, eckerd.com, and medco-health.com (a large pharmacy benefit management firm). These sites promise convenient access to information and patient satisfaction. Some sites offer online prescription refills and other convenient services. Although these sites cater to the patient needs, they face some obstacles and challenges.

Initially, when Internet pharmacy practice emerged, no regulations specifically applied. For example, regulations of which state or entity should cover an Internet pharmacy site that gathers prescriptions written by Pennsylvania physicians, processes them in Texas, and fills them in Arizona? What if the site is registered outside the U.S. and prescriptions are dispensed without a requirement of a prescription? This practice is now closely watched by many regulatory sectors, such as the Food and Drug Administration (FDA), the National Association of Boards of Pharmacy (NABP), and state boards of pharmacy. The main reason for initiating this new layer of regulation was the public concern about unsafe pharmacy practices and the need to coordinate state regulations. Some sites that are registered and located in the U.S., in order to get around the prescription requirement, provide services of on-staff physicians for a separate fee. This practice of prescribing merely for the purpose of dispensing is considered unethical and illegal. The primary industry response to Internet pharmacy growth has come from two sources: the NABP and a newly formed broad-based coalition. The NABP was established in 1904 to assist state licensing boards of pharmacy in developing, implementing, and enforcing uniform standards to protect public health. In the spring of 1999, the NABP established the Verified Internet Pharmacy Practice Sites (VIPPS) program in response to increasing public concern about the safety of Internet pharmacies. The VIPPS program establishes a good housekeeping type seal of approval that Internet pharmacies can display on their homepages. Pharmacies displaying the VIPPS seal have demonstrated to NABP compliance with VIPPS criteria, including patient rights to privacy, authentication and security of prescription orders, adherence to a recognized quality assurance policy, adherence to regulations of all states involved in the prescription processing and fulfilment process, and provision of meaningful consultation between patients and pharmacist. The first action by the federal government was in 1999 when the FDA added information to its Web site in order to assist consumers safely purchasing drugs over the Internet. On August 5, 1999, Representative Ronald Klink (Dem.-PA) introduced House Resolution 2763, the Internet Pharmacy Consumer Protection Act. To deal with the growth of internationally based Internet pharmacies illegally selling prescription drugs, the FDA has begun to issue cyber warning letters transmitted electronically to Web sites the FDA has identified as selling drugs illegally. Other challenges encountered in this eHealth domain include ensuring privacy and confidentially related to transfer of highly sensitive patient information. In addition, consumers must be confident in the site's ability to provide for a secure payment process as with other eCommerce Web sites.

Computer technology

Another emerging domain in eHealth is computer technologies, which can be defined as facilitating provision of health services, both clinical and administrative, through computer applications. Examples include ePrescribing, smart cards, and electronic medical records. ePrescribing, or electronic prescribing, is a term that applies to automation of the prescription writing process (e.g., using a PDA or a PC to generate a prescription). Smart cards have an embedded computer chip, which can store patient medical records and insurance information. Smart cards can help patients create a link among their health care providers. Because of the fragmented status of the U.S. health care system, many health care providers managing the same patient are not aware of each other's actions. For example, a patient's primary care physician might not be aware of the diagnostic procedures and prescription medications ordered for the patient by the cardiologist. If such information were stored on a smart card, each physician would be able to review each other's treatment plans. Similar to smart cards, electronic medical records store comprehensive patient medical information in a central repository, but instead of a card computerized databases are used.

These technologies promise to improve quality of care, influence prescribing behavior, decrease drug spending, and decrease administration burden. They attempt to improve quality of care by reducing medication errors related to illegible handwriting, inappropriate prescribing, and medication noncompliance. Many reports postulate that ePrescribing can decrease drug-related problems by as much as 50%, based on hospital experiences with computerized physician order entry. Therefore, if ePrescribing reduces the cost of drug-related problems by 50%, the impact will be $88.7 billion.

A more conservative estimate of even a 2% reduction in drug-related problems can result in savings of $3.55 billion. Computer technologies also deliver the opportunity to influence prescribing behavior at the point of care. Health care professionals can view clinical and administrative information, such as insurer formularies, at the point of care; this information can influence the medication prescribed to the patient. There is the possibility of a decrease in drug spending because of the improvement in formulary compliance and increased generic substitution. Several ePrescribing pilots reported that when formulary information is displayed at the point of care, generic prescribing reaches up to 55%, a 10% increase from the current market rate of 45%. Reduced administrative burden will result from an increased usage of computer technologies, which will eliminate the need for redundant phone calls and manual chart reviews. If pharmacy follow-up calls are reduced by one third, the industry might save approximately 1.9 million pharmacist hours, nearly a $66 million cost savings.

Implementation of these technologies is associated with several challenges. The most significant challenge is that of implementation costs. If ePrescribing were to be implemented in the entire ambulatory market for at least 1 year, the cost could easily approach several billion dollars. Implementation of electronic medical records would be significantly more expensive. Because these technologies affect many stakeholders (i.e., physicians, pharmacies, insurers, hospitals, pharmaceutical industry, patients), it is unclear how the cost burden should be shared. In other words, who should pay and how much? Another challenge is the slow adoption rate. A very small number of providers are currently using these technologies. Slow adoption rates are mainly due to high implementation costs and providers' resistance to change.

Connectivity

The connectivity domain of eHealth involves connecting participants in the provision of health care services. There are several examples of connectivity in the health care industry currently. One example is an extension of ePrescribing Currently, some electronic prescribing products print the prescription in the office only. Other products take the prescription-writing process one step further and electronically deliver a prescription directly to a pharmacy. Currently, most products offer this option by transmitting prescriptions through a satellite network or over telephone lines to a fax machine in the pharmacy. Some products can transmit prescriptions to the pharmacy's computer terminals directly through the process of electronic data interchange. Two organizations, RxHub and SureScripts, created by pharmacy benefit managers and retail pharmacies, established an electronic system that would connect all parties in the ePrescribing process.

Another example of connectivity extends to the pharmaceutical industry and the practice of physician detailing by pharmaceutical sales representatives. There are attempts to virtually detail physicians by electronically connecting physicians with sales representatives. For example, some companies use video–audio conferencing to execute eDetailing. In an environment where pharmaceutical companies face fierce competition and saturation of the detailing market, the Internet can also be used to continue promoting drugs. Yet another example of connectivity is online patient communities, which allow for peer-to-peer and person-to-person messaging, information exchange, emotional support, and community building. For instance, the Cancer Survivors Network provides such an opportunity for patients suffering from cancer.

Care

Unlike other domains, the care domain, also referred to as telemedicine, is directly involved in provision of patient care. Telemedicine uses communication and information technology to deliver health care services over large and small distances. It is a process whereby a patient and a health care provider are connected at the point of care in a timely manner. The interaction can take place by telephone, fax, e-mail, Internet, biometric sensors, or even by the Cadillac Northstar operator in one's car. The telehealth industry encompasses practices, products, and services that bring medical care and health information to any location. It extends the arm of the health care system for people at home, work, at play, at school, or anywhere the care is needed or desired. For example, a patient with a heart condition can have the heart electrostimulator adjusted over the Internet by a physician located hundreds of miles away. Telemedicine promises improved access to care and education, increased efficiency in diagnosis and treatment, reduced cost of providing services, and improved productivity. However, high costs are associated with telemedicine. Further, the depersonalization of care, along with legal and legislative restriction, and provider resistance limit the use of this technology.

Conclusion

What does the future hold for eHealth and what can we expect in the future? In forecasting the future, predictions of implementation, adoption, and resolution of challenges need to be included. As the Internet becomes truly global, increasing numbers of eHealth resources will be developed overseas and for global audiences. Thus, issues such as communication barriers, cross-cultural factors, and international quality assurance mechanisms will be increasingly important. The emergence of broadband Internet service and access makes it likely that future eHealth applications will increasingly provide multimedia content, including full motion video. Clinical eHealth services, such as real-time medical consultations, will be in high demand with an increase in broadband and as traffic congestion issues resolved. The number of people worldwide with wireless Internet access is expected to grow from 6 million in 2000 to 484 million in 2005. The trend toward handheld devices, Web-enabled phones, and interactive television will encourage eHealth developers to cater to wider audience segments and spur development for a variety of access devices and formats. With patients frequently turning to the Web for medical information, health care players need to understand how important eHealth is for communicating with patients and educating them to participate in decisions regarding their care. Many challenges and questions arise when we look into the future of eHealth. How long will it really take to become relativity paperless in health care? How many new, serious errors will be caused by information systems as their use increases in health systems? What are the policy, ethical, and legal issues around these emerging technologies? With the new patient privacy guidelines, who will assure secure and confidential sharing of information for access to the right stakeholders? Who will pay for it, and how much? For widespread implementation of eHealth concepts, all of these questions must be addressed.

Bibliography

Angaran DM. Telemedicine and telepharmacy: current status and future implications. *Am. J. Hlth.-Syst. Pharm.* 1999; 56: 1405–1426.

Eng, TR. The eHealth landscape: a terrain map of emerging information and communication technologies in health and health care. Princeton, NJ: The Robert Wood Johnson Foundation, 2001.

Eysenbach G. What is e-health [editorial]. *J. Med. Intern. Res.* 2001; 3(2): e20. http://ww.jmir.org/2001/2/e20/.

Focus Group on Telepharmacy. *Am. J. Hlth.-Syst. Pharm.* 2001; 58: 167–169.

Green EJ. Update on the increasing regulation of Internet and online pharmacies. *Drug Ben. Tr.* 1999; 11(9): 27–28.

Kohn LT, Corrigan JM, Donaldson MS, Eds. To err is human: building a safer health system. Washington, D.C.: National Academy Press, 1999.

Internet Healthcare Coalition. eHealth code of ethics, 2000. http://www.ihealthcoalition.org/ethics/ehcode.html, accessed February 19, 2003.

Medicom International. Internet pharmacies: opportunities and challenges, 1999. http://www.medicomint.com, accessed January 29, 2001.

Medscape TechMed. The rise and fall of e-health: lessons from the first generation of internet healthcare, 2002. http://www.medscape.com/viewarticle/431144_print, accessed January 28, 2003.

Medscape TechMed. The future of e-health: looking for signs of life after the internet bubble, 2002. http://www.medscape.com/viewarticle/438135_print, accessed January 28, 2003.

Oliver A. Internet pharmacies: regulation of a growing industry. *J. Law Med. Eth.* 2000; 28: 98–101.

Papshev D, Peterson AM. Electronic prescribing in ambulatory practice: promises, pitfalls, and potential solutions. *Am. J. Manag. Care* 2001; 7(7): 725–736.

Peterson AM. A survey of selected Internet pharmacies in the United States. *J. Am. Pharm Assoc.* 2001; 41: 205–212.

The Institute for Safe Medication Practices. A call to action: eliminate handwritten prescriptions within 3 years!, 2000. http://www.ismp.org/MSAarticles/Whitepaper1.html, accessed October 1, 2001.

Von Knoop C, Lovich D, Silverstein MB, Tutty M. Vital signs: e-health in the United States, 2002. http://www.bcg.com, accessed February 19, 2003.

chapter twenty-five

Pharmacist Workforce Challenges: Exploring Today's Manpower Shortage

Katherine K. Knapp

Published by Cardinal Health, 12/01. Reprinted with permission.

Contents

Foreword

Understanding our workforce

There is no doubt that manpower is a top of mind issue for virtually all pharmacy managers, irrespective of practice setting. Recruitment of new staff requires a great deal of time and energy. Training to the level of competency we require today requires substantial effort and resources. Vacancies are a tremendous burden on existing staff who must, often without choice, staff those shifts that are open, including evenings, nights and holidays. The smart manager needs to devote as much time and attention to the retention of staff as to recruitment. Yet, turnover is inevitable and minimizing it is essential for us to be successful in our manpower planning.

Knapp's work in this "Pharmacist Workforce Challenges" monograph is especially illuminating. She has compiled data from each segment of pharmacy practice and from virtually every perspective. This work is timely since other health professions are experiencing similar workforce issues, thus having created an industry wide problem.

Recent data from the American Health Association paint a bleak picture. Within the hospital sector, vacancies among pharmacists top out at 21%, radiological technologists at 18%, medical records coders at 18%, laboratory technologists at 12% and nurses at 11%.* Bidding wars for limited staffs in certain markets are common. Sign-on bonuses may attract candidates, but do they build loyalty to the hiring organization? An examination of where we can achieve synergies with other health professions, particularly with nursing, could prove fruitful.** Can we look comprehensively at the skills and knowledge base of nurses, physicians and pharmacists to determine where we can best deploy these scarce resources? Can we develop

---

* —. The hospital workforce shortage: immediate and future. http://www.ahapolicyforum.org/trendwatch/twjune2001.asp. Accessed November 1, 2001.

** Gouveia WA, Shane R. Establishing professional synergy with nursing. *Am. J. Health-Syst Pharm.* 2001;58(21).

multi-skilled technical staffs that can help facilitate the medication use system? Can we implement flexible information technologies that can support our professional staffs without taking even more of their time and attention than they now spend on information management?

Many of the issues that caused this pharmacist workforce shortage are positive. The transition to the all PharmD degree was long overdue. The increased use of prescription drugs has extended the lives of countless Americans, many of whom rely on chronic medication use to maintain health. Hospitals and their ambulatory centers are areas of intense and increasingly complex medication administration. The medication safety initiatives in which pharmacists are involved are essential to providing safe and appropriate medication administration. They are important to the public in restoring confidence in our work and in our profession. Pharmacists are integrally involved in implementing a number of medication safety initiatives and many organizations have a role for a pharmacist as medication safety officer, yet another extension of our workforce. Even the implementation and maintenance of computerized physician order entry will take increased effort by pharmacists to assure the success of these important systems.

A counterbalance to the positive roles that pharmacists play is the increase in the amount of time that we spend on reimbursement and payment issues. Pharmacists in ambulatory care play a role in adjudication of third party claims and often bring the news to patients that a drug ordered for them is not covered by their pharmacy benefit. This often places us in conflict with the patient and their physician in a system that is not our creation. The difficult financial condition of many hospitals places the pharmacist in roles of assuring reimbursement for pharmaceuticals for both inpatient and ambulatory care. The Ambulatory Payment Classification (APC) system is intricate and terribly complex and pharmacists must be directly involved in some aspect of the coding to assure payment. These roles do not represent the optimal use of our scarce manpower.

I have proposed the following as solutions to pharmacy's workforce crisis.*** First, that pharmacy managers make every effort to make the pharmacy work environment as satisfying as possible. Second, that we review each pharmacist position to determine whether all of the tasks performed require a pharmacist's skill and knowledge. The selective use of well thought out and implemented information systems and other technologies can help in this regard. Finally, in order to be successful in the first two efforts, we must make a commitment to retrain pharmacists, including those released from the performance of non-pharmacist duties, as part of position restructuring. Knapp's data and their analysis suggest that there will not be any quick fixes to the shortage in the pharmacist workforce. This is a long-term

---

*** Gouveia WA. Solutions to pharmacy's staffing crisis. *Am. J. Health-Syst Pharm.* 2001; 58(9):807–8.

problem that will require considerable energy and creativity, something we have used in advancing our profession.

William A. Gouveia, MS
Director of Pharmacy
New England Medical Center
Boston, Massachusetts

Executive summary

Background. The recent, intense interest in the pharmacist workforce stems from the perception that there are not enough pharmacists to fill open positions. A similar shortfall occurred over a decade ago and gradually resolved. Therefore, the initial reports of a new shortage in 1998 were not met with alarm. It was not until more than a year passed during which vacancies continued to mount across a variety of pharmacist employment settings that the possibility of a long-term workforce problem was considered. A Congressional report in 2000 characterized the pharmacist shortage as an acute event most strongly related to increased use of prescription medications and new healthcare roles for pharmacists. Both these factors increased the demand for pharmacists and pharmaceutical care services.

A New Model Describing the Pharmacist Workforce. Data characterizing the pharmacist workforce have improved over the last decade. In 2000, the Bureau of Health Professions published information about a new model that projects pharmacist number by gender and age through 2020. The model estimates there were 196,011 active pharmacists in 2000 and that pharmacist numbers will increase by about 1.4% per year through 2010. This rate of growth slightly exceeds the projected U.S. population growth of approximately 1% per year. The model also portrays an increasingly female pharmacist workforce with 46% women pharmacists in 2000 rising to 58% by 2010. Through 2010, pharmacists leaving the workforce by reason of death or retirement will be predominantly men. The model also estimates that about 314 pharmacists trained outside the U.S. will enter the pharmacist workforce each year.

The principal shortcoming of the new model is that the estimated headcount it provides does not factor in work patterns of pharmacists. Historically, women pharmacists have preferred to work part-time during child-bearing and child-rearing years and men pharmacists have tended to work more than a 40-hour week. If these patterns were to persist, the increasingly female pharmacist workforce would coincide with a continually decreasing work contribution for each pharmacist. Another work pattern observed in women pharmacists has been a preference for work in institutional settings such as hospitals. If the shortage persists, this preference could be problematic for pharmacist employers in non-institutional settings.

Recent Information about the Pharmacist Shortage. In 2000, the American Society of Health-System Pharmacists (ASHP) called attention to growing pharmacist vacancies using survey data from directors of pharmacy. Their report noted that more pharmacy directors (70%) were having difficulty filling positions requiring experienced practitioners than filling entry-level positions (40%). These findings were mirrored by survey results from The Lazarus Report, also from directors of institutional pharmacies. The Lazarus Report also documented rapidly rising pharmacist salaries in 2000. The National Association of Chain Drug Stores (NACDS), through surveys at six-month intervals, has reported continually growing vacancies in community pharmacies since 1998. *Drug Topics,* a trade journal, has tracked the rise in pharmacist salaries across both the institutional and community settings, an indicator of increased demand. The Aggregate Demand Index, a monthly report of the difficulty in filling open positions across the U.S., found that, since 1999, the highest unmet demand for pharmacists was occurring in Minnesota, California, Wisconsin, Kentucky, Iowa and Texas. The same survey found that only in Hawaii and Rhode Island were supply and demand for pharmacists in balance.

Sorting Out Causes of the Shortage. The 2000 Congressional report concluded that the principal reason for the shortage of pharmacists was the recent growth in the use of prescription medications. Prescription growth rates in the latter 1990s outpaced growth rates earlier in the decade and greatly outpaced the growth of pharmacists. Several factors contributed. As the 1990s progressed, the Baby Boomers, a large population segment, entered age groups where medication use is known to accelerate. At the same time, third party coverage increased from 44% of prescriptions in 1992 to 78% in 1999 and covered prescriptions are known to be more often filled and refilled. Direct-to-consumer advertising was also growing in the late 1990s further increasing the demand for prescription medications. Prescription medication use was also rising in the institutional setting although this phenomenon is more difficult to quantify. Overall, all these factors, occurring concurrently, increased the demand for pharmacists and their services beyond the available supply.

Further exacerbating the emerging problem has been the expansion of pharmacist roles in healthcare. ASHP surveys of the responsibilities of ambulatory care pharmacists in 1997 and 1999 showed pharmacists in integrated health systems were increasing their routine participation in nontraditional activities involving both patient care and management. At the same time, community pharmacies began offering immunization programs and programs that address common, chronic diseases treated primarily with medications (for example, asthma and diabetes mellitus). Screening programs coupled with patient education targeting, for example, osteoporosis and hypertension have also become more widespread. These new activities further increased the demand for pharmacists.

Looking Forward ... What Can Help? The supply of pharmacists can be increased but probably not enough to serve as a sole solution to the shortage problem. Since 1996, six new pharmacy schools have opened. Other schools have completed the transition to the Doctor of Pharmacy degree, a step that often reduces graduate numbers, at least temporarily. Support for increasing the supply of pharmacists must include steps to increase applications to pharmacy schools that have been failing since 1997.

Pharmacists already in the workforce can also contribute to solving the shortage. With the proper incentives, women pharmacists may change from traditional work patterns and work more. Incentives may also induce pharmacists to postpone retirement and remain in the workforce.

Broader use of pharmacy technicians is another avenue for coping with the shortage. It is estimated that there are about 200,000 pharmacy technicians in the U.S., about one technician for every pharmacist. Other data characterizing pharmacy technicians are sparse. By passing the Pharmacy Technician Certification Board examination, almost 90,000 pharmacy technicians have demonstrated competencies that give pharmacists and employers confidence in delegating responsibilities to them. With the recognition of medication errors as an unsolved, national problem, however, other steps such as additional training may also be necessary.

Legislation also impacts on the shortage situation. Legislation, generally at the state level, is required to change the allowable activities of pharmacy technicians and other aspects of delivering healthcare. California and Florida could increase the flow of pharmacists into their state by adopting the reciprocity practices of other states. State-based changes could also accelerate the rate at which students move into practice after graduation.

Automation and technology offer the strongest possibilities for moving the quality of the medication use process forward even if pharmacists are in short supply. Many advances in automation have, to date, been applicable mostly to large systems such as the Veterans Affairs system or the Kaiser Permanente system. In institutions, automated medication dispensing cabinets and bar coding can enhance safety as well as productivity. Physician use of electronic prescribing software could make the process of dispensing prescriptions safer and more efficient. The adoption of automation and technology solutions can be held back by cost, restrictive legislation and the fact that many advances are still applicable primarily to large systems while many pharmacy operations are relatively small. However, as recently pointed out in an Institute of Medicine report, the very limited application of technology to healthcare has been an obstacle to achieving quality. The pharmacist shortage may be a spur to the wider and better use of automation and technology in the medication use process.

Summary. It is widely accepted that the pharmacist shortage is a reality. Nevertheless, quality gains in the medication use process must move forward; and, therefore, multiple, partial solutions should be considered and implemented judiciously. These solutions should be built on the expectation that the demand for pharmacists and their services will continue to grow in the foreseeable future.

Background on pharmacist workforce issues

Over the past 20 years, there have been periodic shifts in the balance between the supply and demand for pharmacists. For example, in the late 1980s and early 1990s, when an unexpected shortage of pharmacists developed, employers, educators, the professional associations and researchers were perplexed. At the time, the principal source of information about health profession workforces was the Bureau of Health Professions (BHPr). This organization, which received federal funding to report to the Congress every other year about the status of health professions—including pharmacy—in the United States, had made no predictions about an impending shortage.

Although that shortage was never explained, one outcome of the mismatch between BHPr information and what was observed in the market place was the creation of the Pharmacy Manpower Project (PMP), a consortium of pharmacy organizations and the Bureau of Health Professions. The PMP organized and coordinated a national census of pharmacists that showed that in 1991 there were approximately 194,570 pharmacists in the United States and about 171,611 of these pharmacists were actively practicing. The PMP census count matched quite closely to BHPr estimates. The close match between the census count and the estimates from BHPr suggested that whatever was causing the pharmacist shortage was not a miscalculation on the part of BHPr about how many pharmacists there actually were in the United States.

Eventually, in the middle 1990s, the imbalance between supply and demand resolved, at least to the extent that retail employers were able to open new pharmacies and institutional pharmacies were not hampered by workforce shortages. Meanwhile, the efforts to understand the dynamics of the early 1990s shortage led to the realization that data collection on the pharmacist workforce was insufficient. Most available data about workforce issues related to supply while the ability to study demand issues was very limited. Unless both supply and demand data were available and could be compared, it was virtually impossible to reach defensible conclusions about the cause of a workforce imbalance. In response, the PMP committed to a broader collection of data about the pharmacist workforce including demand data. These efforts were hastened by evidence of another shortage of the latter 1990s.

In 1998, the National Association of Chain Drug Stores (NACDS), speaking on behalf of its member organizations, announced that another shortage of pharmacists appeared to be developing. Their alert was based on survey data collected at six-month intervals from member organizations, mostly chain pharmacy corporations. The surveys were showing more and more vacancies in pharmacist positions. From that point to today, there has been increasing evidence of a national, dynamic shortage of pharmacists. The situation has sparked reaction across many sectors from the federal government to pharmacy corporations to schools and colleges of pharmacy. In the remainder of this paper, we will examine this workforce situation from both supply and demand perspectives.

Available information about the pharmacist workforce

2000 Congressional report

In December 2000, the Health Resources and Services Administration (HRSA) released a Congressionally-mandated report about the pharmacist shortage. The report was titled *The Pharmacist Workforce: A Study of the Supply and Demand for Pharmacists.*[1] The full text of the report is available on the Web at www.bhpr.hrsa.gov. The principal findings of the report included the following:

- There was (in 2000) an acute shortage of pharmacists in the United States that was most strongly related to increased demands for pharmacists and pharmaceutical care services.
- The demand for pharmacists and their services was not likely to slacken in the next 10 years.
- The growth in demand was strongly related to increased medication use across all practice sectors that had outpaced the growth of pharmacists and the U.S. population.
- The shortage of pharmacists could hinder the important role pharmacists play in reducing medication errors in all practice settings.
- The shortage of pharmacists could hinder needed improvements in the medication use process—both in the care of patients and in the provision of cost-effective medication use.
- Despite the addition of 10 new schools of pharmacy since 1980 and near-completion of the transition to the entry-level Doctor of Pharmacy (PharmD) degree, pharmacy graduates were projected to grow at only 1.4% through 2010—a rate far below the need created by expanding roles of pharmacists and expanding medication use.
- The shortage had intensified the competition for pharmacists with post-graduate training. Those pharmacists with advanced training were critical to resolving the shortage and improving medication use through their roles as pharmacy faculty, as clinical practitioners with specialized skills and as researchers in the medication use process.

This report was particularly valuable in comparison to previous efforts because it included consideration of both supply and demand factors affecting the pharmacist workforce. The report looked at the dramatic, recent growth in the use of prescription medications and linked this growth to a pharmacist workforce not able to keep up with rising demand either through producing more pharmacists or through changing systems associated with medication use.

The new Bureau of Health Professions (BHPr) pharmacist supply model

Important to pharmacist supply considerations are the projections of a new pharmacist supply model put forth by the Bureau of Health Professions in 2000.[2] The new model supplanted an earlier supply model that had been used throughout the 1980s and 1990s to estimate the size of the workforce. The new model included several improvements to its basic structure, a structure that consisted of a base count of pharmacists drawn from PMP census data to which new graduates were added annually and estimates of pharmacists departing from the workforce for reasons of retirement and death were subtracted. The improvements included addition of actual graduates (as opposed to estimates) from the 1990s by gender and degree, a revision of the separation rates used to estimate departing pharmacists and the inclusion of international pharmacy graduates.

Figure 25.1 shows active pharmacists in the United States including the new model's projections of pharmacist numbers to 2010, at which time the model estimates 224,524 active pharmacists. In 2000, the model estimated there were 196,011 active pharmacists. The annual growth of the workforce from 2000 to 2010 is projected at about 1.4% per year, somewhat more than the projected rate of population growth, which is about 1%. Based on these estimates, the number of pharmacists per 100,000 population will rise slowly

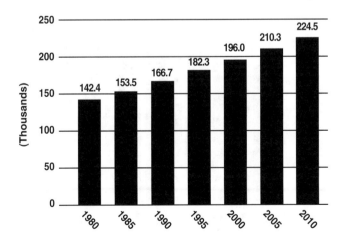

Figure 25.1 Active pharmacists in the U.S.: 1980–2010. (*Source*: BHPr Pharmacist Supply Model.)

to 75. However, as noted prominently in the 2000 HRSA report, the growth rates of both pharmacists and population lag substantially behind the growth of prescription medications (discussed later).

The new BHPr model also described the gender balance of the pharmacist workforce as shown in Figure 25.2. During the current decade, women pharmacists will become the predominant gender. Starting in 2000 when 46% of the pharmacist workforce were women, the percent women pharmacists will gradually rise to 58% by 2010. The significance of this shift rests on two established work preferences of women pharmacists. The first is a well-documented preference for part-time work, especially during child-bearing and child-rearing years, and the second is a preference for working in the hospital or institutional setting as compared to the community or retail setting.[3,4,5]

The loss of pharmacists through death and retirement, as portrayed by the BHPr model, is presented in Table 25.1. Each year more than 2% of the workforce must be replaced just to maintain constant numbers of pharmacists. Fortunately, BHPr estimates of new graduates exceed 7,000 each year so there is a net gain of pharmacists projected through 2010. Throughout this decade, those pharmacists leaving the workforce will be predominantly male by virtue of the fact that age is the principal determinant for leaving the workforce; and among older pharmacists, males are predominant. Table 25.1 illustrates the gender pattern of pharmacists leaving the workforce. Table 25.1 also illustrates that, over time, the gender balance of departing pharmacists gradually becomes less male and more female.

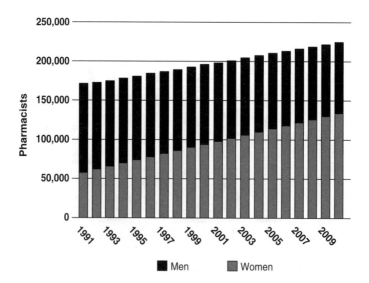

Figure 25.2 Changing gender ratios in the pharmacist workforce: 1991–2010. (*Source*: BHPr Pharmacist Supply Model.)

Table 25.1 Pharmacist Workforce Losses: Mostly Men

Year	Loss of Men	Loss of Women	Total Losses	Percent of Total Workforce
1995	4,338	902	5,240	2.9
2000	3,882	1,158	5,040	2.6
2005	3,711	1,578	5,289	2.5
2010	3,553	2,203	5,756	2.6

Source: BHPr Pharmacist Supply Model.

Estimates of international pharmacy graduates (IPGs), that is, U.S.-licensed pharmacists trained outside the United States, were also included in the new BHPr model. Unlike foreign-trained physicians, IPGs in the U.S. are relatively few in number; for example, only 358 IPGs passed the North American Pharmacy Licensure Examination (NAPLEX) in 1999, and this was the highest number of IPGs passing the NAPLEX in recent years. Likewise, in California, where there is a different licensure examination, only 51 IPGs tested successfully in 1999. The number of new IPGs annually, while small, has also been fluctuating with increasing numbers passing the NAPLEX and decreasing numbers gaining licensure through the California licensure examination. Thus, given these uncertainties, the BHPr model used a three-year average of 314 new licensees each year as its annual (unchanging) estimates of IPGs. This number is a small fraction of the over 7,000 annual graduates from U.S. schools.

There is uncertainty about the future numbers of IPGs and the role they might play in allaying the pharmacist shortage. Employers have made some efforts to recruit IPGs from some English-speaking countries with similar pharmacy training although recruitment is made more difficult by the requirement of a special immigration visa.[6] But generally, pharmacy programs outside the U.S. do not meet the increasing educational requirements of U.S. schools of pharmacy. Where international educational programs fall short, few U.S. schools have shown an interest in providing special programs to equalize coursework and particularly clinical experience. Thus, the uncertainty about IPGs' contribution to the future supply of pharmacists remains.

Next step ... refine the models

The BHPr model provides estimates of future headcounts of pharmacists—clearly a shortcoming in the sense that neither men nor women pharmacists contribute, on average, a single full-time equivalent (FTE) per person. Therefore, an important next step in more accurately predicting the size and character of the future pharmacy workforce is to overlay what is known about past and current work patterns of pharmacists on the BHPr model.

Table 25.2 outlines weekly hours worked by men and women pharmacists as recorded in a 2000 national survey.[7] The study found, as several

Table 25.2 2000 National Workforce Study: Hours Worked Per Week

Work Setting	Males	Females
Retail	42.6	37.4
Institutional	43.7	38.8
Non-Patient Care	43.3	35.7

Source: Pharmacy Manpower Project, National Workforce Study, 2000.

previous studies had, that men pharmacists in three principal work settings worked more than 40 hours per week and women pharmacists worked less than 40 hours weekly in the same settings.[7,8] This dichotomy in work patterns has implications on the *effective* size of the future workforce. Assuming that the women pharmacists continue to work, on average, less than 40 hours per week, as the workforce becomes more female, the average number of hours worked by each pharmacist will decrease. For example, in Table 25.2, in the retail setting, men pharmacists recorded 2.6 hours above a 40-hour workweek while women pharmacists worked 2.6 hours below the 40-hour workweek. As long as the workforce remains predominantly male—until about 2003—the total FTEs or the effective workforce will be greater than the headcount. Once women pharmacists are over 50% of the workforce, the headcount will be higher than the FTE count.

Table 25.3 presents a modification of BHPr estimates taking into account the changing gender balance of the workforce and corresponding weekly hours worked.[9] The table shows that, in 1991, for example, the effective workforce was about 1% greater than the headcount. By contrast, in 2010, the effective workforce will be about 3% less than the BHPr estimated headcount. The gap will continue to grow until a new equilibrium is reached and the gender balance of the workforce stabilizes. The growing gap between headcount and effective size of the workforce is not inevitable, however; for example, an increase in the percentage of male graduates in schools of pharmacy or an increase in the weekly hours worked by women pharmacists could reduce or nullify the gap.

Women pharmacists have also shown a preference for working in an institutional pharmacy setting—hospitals and medical centers—over a community pharmacy setting, and a recent study showedthat this propensity

Table 25.3 Headcounts Versus Estimated Full-Time Equivalents (FTEs)

	1991 (68% male)	2000 (54% male)	2010 (42% male)
Headcount	171,611	196,011	224,524
FTE*	173,581	193,412	217,709

*FTE = 40 Hours Per Week

Source: Presented at 2001 APhA Annual Meeting, San Francisco, CA (Gershon SK, Cultice JM, Knapp KK).

has persisted over many years.[3] In the context of a pharmacist shortage and an increasingly female workforce, this preference could result in greater difficulties for community pharmacy employers. This preference is, however, offset by another long-standing economic fact; that is, salaries are higher in the community sector (discussed later). If the pharmacist shortage persists, it is likely employers will use these competing motivations to vie for available pharmacists.

Surveys that shed light on pharmacist workforce issues

American Society of Health-System Pharmacists (ASHP)

The survey series described here is but one of several longitudinal surveys supported by ASHP. This survey series queried 432 directors of hospital and health-system pharmacies about the difficulty in filling vacancies in hospitals and health systems. Figure 25.3 shows the results of annual surveys in 1999 and 2000. The survey was not repeated in 2001. The figure shows the increasing difficulty experienced by those attempting to fill these positions between 1999 and 2000. Also reported was a higher level of difficulty in filling positions requiring experience than entry-level positions with 40% reporting "severe" difficulty in filling vacant entry-level positions while 70% reported "severe" difficulty filling experienced practitioner positions. The

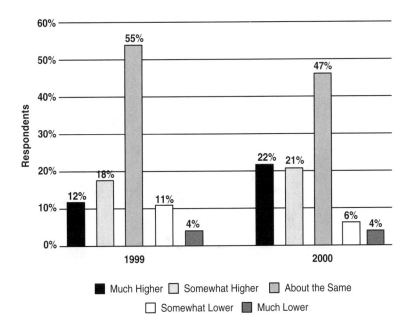

Figure 25.3 ASHP surveys: vacancies today compared to vacancies 5 years ago. (*Source*: ASHP Press Release, 7/25/00.)

results suggested that, over this time period, the market for experienced pharmacists was particularly and increasingly competitive.

The Lazarus Report

This survey series also addresses institutional pharmacy. Directors of pharmacy from 42 institutions throughout the United States regularly submit information about their pharmacy operations. Figure 25.4 describes a portion of the year 2000 and shows that from Spring 2000 to Fall 2000, there was some drop in the intensity of the pharmacist shortage nationally. Figure 25.5 shows the concomitant, rapid rise in mean entry-level salaries that perhaps contributed to the decline in open positions. The rapid rise in pharmacist salaries documented by this survey is one indicator of a demand for pharmacists in excess of available supply despite the addition of new graduates into the market place.

The National Association of Chain Drug Stores (NACDS)

The NACDS was the first pharmacy association to call attention to the emerging shortage of pharmacists. In surveys completed at six-month intervals, NACDS identified growing numbers of vacancies in community pharmacies. Figure 25.6 presents the results of a series of these surveys. Both full-time and part-time vacancies continued to climb throughout the period described.

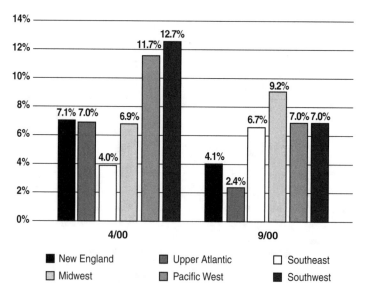

Figure 25.4   Lazarus Report 2000: vacancy rates in the institutional setting. (*Source:* The Lazarus Report, 9/00.)

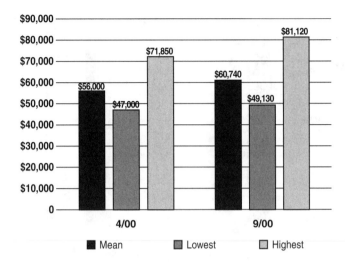

Figure 25.5 Lazarus Report 2000: entry level, annual salaries in the institutional setting. (*Source*: The Lazarus Report, 9/00.)

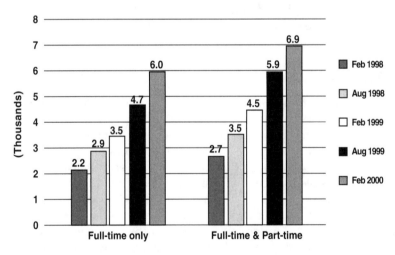

Figure 25.6   NACDS surveys: pharmacist vacancies in member drug stores. (*Source*: National Association of Chain Drug Stores Surveys, 1998–2000.)

Drug Topics

This publication is a trade journal that conducts several survey series addressing pharmacist salaries and other topics. The journal has been able to track the recent rise in pharmacist salaries. Figure 25.7 describes a 19.6% rise in chain pharmacy salaries between 1999 and 2001 and a 21.8% rise in hospital pharmacy salaries over the same period. While chain pharmacy

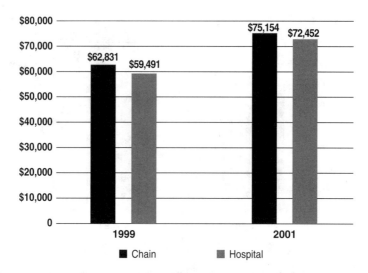

Figure 25.7 2001 *Drug Topics* salary survey: average annual salary. (*Source*: *Drug Topics*, 3/19/01.)

salaries remained higher than hospital salaries, the gap between them narrowed slightly. The dramatic salary rise over the two-year period is another indicator of the unmet demand for pharmacists.

The Aggregate Demand Index (ADI)

The Pharmacy Manpower Project has sponsored this national, monthly survey since August 1999. The data are provided by panelists who are directly involved in the hiring of pharmacists. Panelists submit monthly reports about the level of difficulty they have experienced in filling open positions. Specifically, panelists submit a difficulty rating for each state or states where they are responsible for keeping positions filled. The ratings are based on a 5-point scale where 5 = high demand: difficult to fill open positions; 4 = moderate demand: some difficulty filling open positions; 3 = demand in balance with supply; 2 = demand is less than the pharmacist supply available; and 1 = demand is much less than the pharmacist supply available. From these ratings, a mean rating or demand index for each state is determined. Then, using demand indices from all states and the District of Columbia, a population-weighted national index of the difficulty in filling open positions, the Aggregate Demand Index, is calculated. Population-weighted regional demand indices are also calculated. Figure 25.8 shows the ADI from August 1999 through July 2001. Except for the first survey in August 1999, the monthly demand levels have remained between 4 and 5 suggesting that there is an excess demand over available supply. The design and performance of the ADI project including details about the selection and composition of the panel and findings by geographic areas and type of position have been reported.[10]

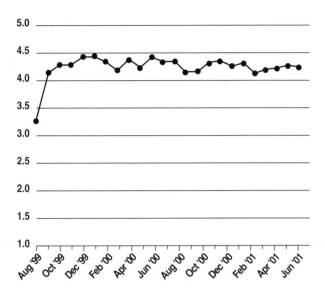

Figure 25.8 Aggregate Demand Index: August 1999–July 2001. (*Source*: Pharmacy Manpower Project, Aggregate Demand Index.)

The monthly results of the ADI project are posted on the Web (www.pharmacymanpower.com). The site can also be accessed using the key words "pharmacy manpower" on most search engines. To allow comparisons over time, the Web site for the project lists the ADI for the previous month and for the same month during the previous year. Regional and divisional indices convey the level of demand for pharmacist positions within smaller geographic areas. Information at the state level is maintained in the ADI database but not posted on the Web site at present. Data about demand levels that organizations face in filling types of pharmacy positions (primarily community positions, primarily institutional positions or both community and institutional positions) have also been tracked in the database but not posted on the Web site.

ADI data show that pharmacist demand levels vary substantially at the state level. From August 1999 through July 2001, the states with the highest demand level were Minnesota, California, Wisconsin, Kentucky, Iowa and Texas. The demand levels for these states averaged 4.5 or greater on the 5-point scale used by panelists signifying it was difficult to fill open positions. At the other extreme, Hawaii and Rhode Island were the states with the lowest demand levels; their average demand indices were less than 3.5 suggesting these states were in or close to balance with respect to the demand for pharmacists and the available supply. The remaining 42 states and the District of Columbia showed average demand levels between 3.5 and 4.5 indicating at least some difficulty in filling open positions.

The data from the ADI project can also be used to estimate the degree of exposure of the U.S. population to the pharmacist shortage. Based on state-level demand data, the percentage of the population living in states with varying levels of demand can be calculated; for example, in July 2001, 26% of the resident U.S. population lived in states where the demand level was greater than 4.5, 72% in areas where the demand level was between 3.5 and 4.5 and less than 2% in areas where the demand for pharmacists was in balance with available supply.

Some panelists from the ADI project can be described as hiring primarily community pharmacists (chain pharmacy organizations, independent pharmacies, supermarkets and mass merchandisers), others as hiring primarily institutional pharmacists (hospitals and medical centers) and others as hiring both community and institutional pharmacists (integrated health systems). From these, the ADI data yield demand information based on the type of organization. Figure 25.9 shows mean demand levels for the three types of organizations. From August 1999 through July 2001, organizations hiring both community and institutional pharmacists reported the highest difficulty in filling open positions (mean 4.7) followed by organizations with primarily institutional positions (mean 4.5) followed by organizations with primarily community positions (mean 4.0). The reasons for the varying levels of difficulty are not known.

Sorting out reasons ... and non-reasons ... for the pharmacist shortage

In the Congressional report cited earlier, invited public commentary about the cause(s) of the shortage yielded a variety of explanations. Some of these

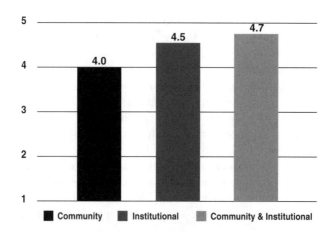

Figure 25.9 Demand index by type of organization: August 1999–July 2001. (*Source*: Pharmacy Manpower Project, Aggregate Demand Index.)

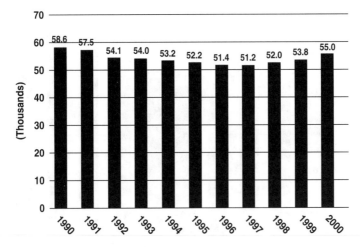

Figure 25.10 Licensed retail pharmacy outlets: 1990–2000. (*Source*: National Association of Chain Drug Stores, *Industry Profile 2001*.)

were supportable by evidence and others were not. In these sections, we explore some of the most commonly cited reasons for the shortage.

The growth of pharmacies

A popular conception is that the 1990s saw a vast expansion of community pharmacies. Indeed, many consumers and pharmacists alike have blamed the shortage of pharmacists on the "explosion" of community pharmacies. Actual counts of pharmacies portray a different story. Figure 25.10 shows total retail pharmacies from 1990 through 2000. The counts include independent, mass merchandise, supermarket and chain drug pharmacies. The data illustrate that pharmacy numbers in 2000 were over 3,000 fewer than in 1990. The decade saw significant contraction of the independent pharmacy sector, significant growth in the mass merchandise and supermarket sectors and modest growth in the chain drug store sector. While there are other issues such as store size, number of pharmacists per store and hours of operations, the data suggest that changes in the number of pharmacies do not explain the pharmacist shortage.

Prescription growth in the retail sector

The 1990s saw a tremendous growth in the use of medications, particularly prescription medications. In the main, patients acquire their prescriptions through community pharmacies (95%) or mail order pharmacies (5%). Figure 25.11 shows the growth of prescriptions in the 1990s. Through 1997, growth was averaging about 4% per year. Then in 1998 and 1999, growth rates of 7% and 9% respectively were observed. These years signaled the onset of today's pharmacist shortage. Although growth backed off to 5% in 2000, the

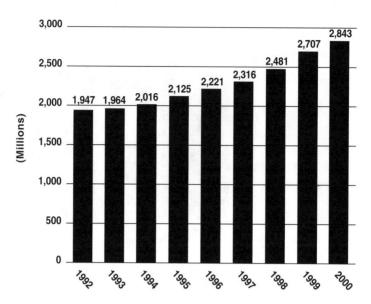

Figure 25.11 Retail prescriptions: 1992–2000. (*Source*: IMS Health; NACDS Economics Department.)

high numbers of retail prescriptions attained through the two years of rapid growth could be seen as maintaining pressure on a system being inundated with prescriptions.

The causes for the growth in retail prescriptions throughout the 1990s are easier to explain than the surge observed after 1997. The gradual growth of the over-65 year-old cohort of the U.S. population has driven increased consumption of prescription medications throughout the 1990s. Table 25.4 lists data showing how prescription use increases with age. There are two big jumps in per capita prescription usage: one as people move into the 45–65 year-old age group and the next when they move into the 65–74

Table 25.4 Annual Prescription Usage by Age Group and Gender

Age (Years)	Males	Females
0–4	5.6	5.2
5–17	3.3	2.4
18–24	3.2	5.7
25–44	4.0	8.0
45–64	10.4	16.5
65–74	20.5	21.1
75–84	23.3	23.2
85+	23.3	23.2

Source: Medical Expenditure Panel Study, 1996.

year-old group. The Baby Boomers, a large segment of the U.S. population, are moving through the 45–64 year-old consumption range and approaching the higher over-65 consumption rate—leading to increased prescription usage across the U.S.

A second cause for increased prescription consumption throughout the 1990s was the spread of prescription drug benefits, usually as part of health plans. In 1992, third party payers covered the cost of only 44% of prescriptions.**** By 1995, this percentage had grown to 62% and by 1999 to 78%. It has been established that prescriptions paid for by a third party are more likely to be filled and refilled; thus, the growth in prescription drug coverage promotes increased use of prescription medications. Other factors that could contribute are the growth in direct-to-consumer advertising that creates demand for prescription medications and the increase in prescribers—physicians and physician extenders such as physician assistants and nurse practitioners. Pharmacists also prescribe under protocol in some states.

Why was the system inundated by the rapid prescription growth? As shown in Figure 25.12, the numbers of pharmacists—including community pharmacists—were only growing at about 1.4% per year during the decade of the 1990s. The growth of pharmacists and the growth of retail prescriptions were mismatched. The situation becomes worse when we consider the overall growth in the use of medications as shown by the constant dollar value of medications in Figure 25.12. The rationale for using dollars to track overall medication use requires some explanation.

The problem with aggregating medication use across different practice settings is that units of measurement differ. For the community or retail setting, prescriptions provide a convenient measure of medication use. Hospitals and other institutional settings do not use "prescriptions" but rather "medication orders" as the basic unit for medication dispensation. The medication order can involve multiple and changing doses and, therefore, counting medication orders to measure medication use is not appropriate. Therefore, when combining settings to achieve an estimate of overall growth in medication use, dollars spent on medications, adjusted for inflation, become the best measure available. Dollars are still of limited value in describing medication use growth because of increases in medication costs, substitution of more costly medications for less costly ones and other reasons.

As shown in Figure 25.12, the rate of rise of the constant dollar value of medications was even higher than prescription drug growth. This suggests that not only were retail prescriptions growing but also the use of medications in hospitals, medical centers, long term care and other areas where pharmacists work. Thus, it is not surprising that pharmacists and pharmacies were eventually overwhelmed, observable starting in about 1998, by the amount of medication to be delivered and managed.

**** IMS Health data provided by the National Association of Chain Drug Stores.

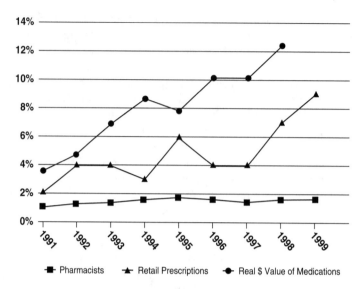

Figure 25.12 Relative growth rates. (*Sources*: IMS Health [prescription and dollar value]; BHPr Pharmacist Supply Model [pharmacists].)

Managed care and societal expectations

Simultaneously with the increased use of medications, pharmacists have been moving into new healthcare roles. This movement is particularly apparent in services to ambulatory patients and well people in the community. The increased demand is related to the spread of managed care that emphasizes the reduced use of hospitalization and other forms of institutional care and promotes prevention and providing care through clinics and outpatient services. The American Society of Health-System Pharmacists (ASHP) began a survey series in 1997 to track the activities of pharmacists in ambulatory care settings.[11] The series has focused on integrated health systems including hospital-based systems. The 1997 survey inquired about routine pharmacist participation in 24 ambulatory care activities; by 1999, the prevalence of most of these activities had increased substantially.[12] Table 25.5 shows the growth observed for the most prevalent functions. Most of these activities would not be considered "traditional" pharmacist functions. Several were related to "population health," a new way of thinking about healthcare developed through managed care's concern about health maintenance, prevention and cost containment. Pharmacists, with unique knowledge and experience in the use of medications, were an increasingly valuable resource to health systems developing formularies and trying to contain medication costs. Pharmacists were also found to be valuable partners in clinics for patients with chronic diseases such as asthma, hypertension, hypercholesterolemia and diabetes mellitus where medications are the mainstay of therapy.

Table 25.5 Examples of Routine Pharmacist Participation in Ambulatory Functions in Integrated Health Systems

Functions Reported by Survey Respondents	1997	1999
Using pharmacoeconomic data for making formulary decisions	76%	82%
Conducting medication management programs (DUR and DUE)	76%	81%
Monitoring patient outcomes	71%	73%
Conducting wellness and preventive health programs	58%	61%
Conducting specialized clinics	33%	38%

Source: American Society of Health-System Pharmacists, 1999 Survey of Managed Care and Ambulatory Care Pharmacy Practice.

Pharmacists were tapped also to play a role in oncology and anticoagulation clinics. The survey data did not show how many pharmacists were working in these new areas but the prevalence of the activities throughout integrated health systems suggests that the numbers were great enough to add demand for pharmacists to an already stressed system.

In addition to the expanding pharmacist roles documented by the ASHP surveys, there have been other new roles, although the documentation for these has not been as thorough. For example, pharmacists play an important role in medication error reduction. The awareness of medication errors as an important cause of morbidity and mortality was heightened by a 1999 report from the Institute of Medicine.[13] The report emphasized the need for better surveillance of the medication use process and the need for change where situations increased the likelihood of errors. The new emphasis on these activities—frequently involving pharmacists—came at a time when the pharmacist shortage was already established resulting in further pressure on pharmacists and their employers.

Another area of role expansion has been observed in community pharmacies. Responding to public health initiatives for higher levels of immunization and also an opportunity for a new source of revenue, pharmacists began to offer immunization programs in community pharmacies widely in the latter 1990s. Disease management services aimed at common, chronic diseases such as asthma and diabetes mellitus started appearing in community pharmacies during the same period. Screening programs coupled with patient education components targeting, for example, osteoporosis and hyperlipidemia are becoming more widespread. These activities have provided a new energy and enthusiasm for community practice even where revenue enhancement has been modest, and this has contributed to their continued growth. Thus, while these programs have increased the demand for pharmacists, they have also, with the continued shortage of pharmacists, offered a competitive advantage to employers in this practice sector.

Responding to the current workforce challenges

The several events that have driven the demand for pharmacists and their services upward have shown little tendency to abate. And yet, there is a commitment to continue improving the medication use process in which pharmacists play a key role. The next sections briefly explore solutions. Each of these is considered in the context of continuing the pursuit of the highest quality medication use process whether or not the current shortage of pharmacists persists.

Generating more pharmacists: pharmacy school applications, enrollments and graduates

Pharmacy school enrollments, like all professional program enrollments, have shown fluctuations since the 1980s as external conditions such as the national economy, the interest level in science, the prospects of healthcare careers and other variables have shifted. As noted in the 2000 report to Congress, a downturn in pharmacy graduates in the early 1980s potentially "cost" between 16,000 and 23,000 pharmacists for the workforce going forward.[1] This event is portrayed in Figure 25.13 which shows actual graduate numbers and potential graduates under two alternate scenarios: one where graduates remain constant from 1980 onward (resulting in about 16,000 more graduates) and another where graduates theoretically grow at the rate of the U.S. population over the period, slightly less than one percent annually (resulting in about 23,000 additional graduates). The two scenarios emphasize the importance of attention to the "pipeline"—that is, applications, numbers of students enrolling and numbers of students graduating. The impact of smaller graduating classes lasts literally for multiple decades.

The application pool size is an indicator of the level of interest in pharmacy careers. Figure 25.14 illustrates the application history for pharmacy schools during the 1990s. There was a strong upward trend in the early to middle 1990s followed by a sharp, downward trend after 1996. Between 1996 and 1999, there was a drop of 30% in applications. The reasons for the upward and then downward trends are not known; nevertheless, the downward trend of the late 1990s was ominous in that the need for more pharmacists was already apparent. Market factors that would tend to increase interest in pharmacy and therefore applications include solid prospects of employment after graduation and rising salaries. Both these factors are present in today's economy giving hope that the application pool will begin to grow again.

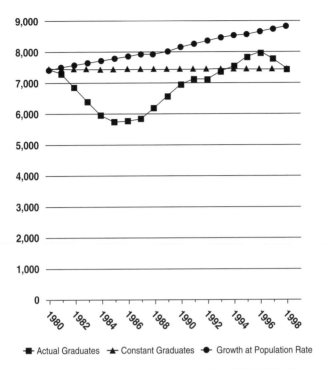

Figure 25.13 Actual graduates and alternate scenarios: 1980–1998. (*Source*: American Association of Colleges of Pharmacy [actual graduates].)

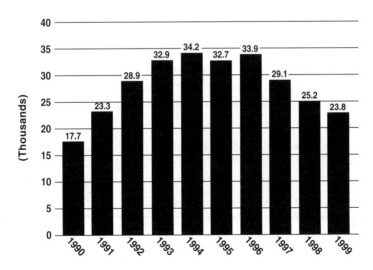

Figure 25.14 Pharmacy school applications: 1990–1999. (*Source*: American Association of Colleges of Pharmacy.)

New schools

During the 1990s, pharmacist graduate numbers, as shown in Figure 25.13, were held back somewhat by the transition to the entry-level PharmD degree and enhanced by the graduates from three new schools founded in 1987 (2) and 1992 (1). From 1996 to the present, six more schools were established that are already graduating pharmacists; and other schools are in various stages of development (Table 25.6). According to a survey of deans of pharmacy schools reported in the 2000 report to Congress, other schools and colleges of pharmacy are planning to expand class size in the near future.[1] Whether these actions will result in graduate numbers exceeding the estimates of the Bureau of Health Professions model which projects the addition of three new schools each decade with an average 100-person class in each remains to be seen. Should expansions and new schools exceed the anticipated 1.4% annual growth rate in graduates, this could impact beneficially on the shortage.

International graduates

The expanded recruitment of international pharmacy graduates has been suggested as an avenue to reduce the pharmacist shortage. There are significant barriers to this solution mostly related to educational equivalency issues that will only become more problematic when the PharmD becomes the sole entry-level degree in the United States in 2003. Nevertheless, special programs to bring international graduates into educational equivalency could be developed if demand were sufficient.

Staying in the workforce ... longer

The pharmacist workforce would increase in size if pharmacists postponed retirement and instead continue to work either full-time or part-time. Likewise, the size of the workforce would be increased if fewer pharmacists

Table 25.6 New Pharmacy Schools: Anticipated Class Size and Program Type

School/College of Pharmacy	Year	Class Size	Program
Lake Erie College of Osteopathic Medicine	2002	78	Accelerated
Nevada	2001	40	Accelerated
Palm Beach Atlantic	2001	45	
University of California, San Diego	2002	25	
University of Nevada	2003	40	
University of New England	2001		Accelerated
University of Oklahoma	2001		Accelerated

Source: Drug Topics, 3/5/01.

changed to other types of work. A recent study showed that, in 2000, pharmacists were not leaving practice in greater numbers than in 1990 despite the shortage and its pressures.[7] Thus, it is unlikely that these avenues would substantially impact on the shortage.

Expanding the pharmaceutical care team: pharmacy technicians

Pharmacy technicians assist pharmacists under supervision; they contribute particularly to the medication distribution process. Laws and regulations about the use of technicians vary from state to state, and there has been pressure to expand the use of pharmacy technicians as the pharmacist shortage has persisted. Unfortunately, there has been a paucity of published data about pharmacy technicians. The 2000 report to Congress estimated that there were about 200,000 pharmacy technicians in 2000, a ratio of approximately one technician for every pharmacist.[1]

Most parties knowledgeable about pharmacy issues agree that pharmacy technicians have become more important in recent years in delivering pharmaceutical care and have the potential to aid in addressing the pharmacist shortage. The expanded use of technicians is not, however, without problems. On one hand, proponents of broader responsibilities for technicians argue that pharmacy technicians can relieve pharmacists of many tasks that do not require their professional judgment and free them for other activities where their professional training is required. On the other hand, those focusing on medication safety—including many pharmacists—point to the uneven training of pharmacy technicians and to incidents where serious errors involving technicians have occurred.[14,15] A national certification program for pharmacy technicians, offered through the Pharmacy Technician Certification Board (PTCB), has been a major advance in the standardization of technician competencies and skills. The program has been widely and increasingly embraced by individual states. As of September 2001, 89,620 pharmacy technicians had passed this certification examination, close to one half the estimated number of technicians nationally.[16] The number of certified technicians has risen rapidly as only 47,973 technicians were PTCB-certified in 1999.

Increased productivity

There are several ways that the pharmacist workforce could become more productive. For example, an immediate gain in productivity would be observed if women pharmacists worked more hours weekly. A comparison between a 1990 survey and a 2000 survey showed that women have indeed increased weekly work hours but have still averaged less than a 40-hour workweek.[4]

Re-engineering the pharmacy work place has also been suggested to increase efficiency.[17] Previous studies of the activities of pharmacists have shown that handwritten prescriptions lead to lost productivity as pharmacists and physicians lose time clarifying handwriting.[18] A study sponsored by the NACDS showed that electronic communication problems between pharmacies and insurance programs reduce pharmacist productivity.[19] Respondents cited in the 2000 report to Congress noted that pharmacists and technicians do not work together optimally resulting in decreased productivity; they suggested that pharmacy students learn how to work with technicians as part of their training.[1]

Regulatory changes

As noted earlier, the continuing shortage has led to the introduction of state-level legislation to broaden the use of pharmacy technicians. Another avenue of possible regulatory change relates to licensure reciprocity. At present, California and Florida are the only two states that do not recognize pharmacist licensure achieved through passing the North American Pharmacist Licensure Examination (NAPLEX). Were these states to adopt reciprocity agreements similar to those that exist through the rest of the nation, the flow of pharmacists into these highly populated and high demand (according to the ADI project) states could be eased. It should be noted, however, that this measure would not increase the number of pharmacists. Other regulatory changes such as allowing students to take the NAPLEX during their final year of pharmacy school could accelerate the rate of entry of new pharmacists into the workforce.

Automation and technology

The expanded use of automation and technology probably offers the strongest possibilities for moving the quality of the medication use process forward even if pharmacist production is relatively slow growing. Automation for the preparation of prescriptions has been widely adopted in large, closed systems such as the Veterans Affairs system and the Kaiser Permanente integrated health system. Automated prescription filling in a central pharmacy facility that would act as a hub for clusters of community pharmacies, known as central fill, may speed prescription preparation while preserving opportunities for counseling and monitoring ambulatory patients. Within hospitals, the use of bar coding, highly sophisticated medication dispensing cabinets and automated medication preparation promote enhanced safety as well as productivity. Their wider adoption is likely if pharmacy personnel remain in short supply. Physician use of electronic prescribing software promises to reduce or eliminate problems related to illegibility of prescriptions and medication selection where a formulary is in effect. The processing of prescription claims could benefit from standardization, likely to be achieved through technology and resulting in better pharmacist productivity. Respondents cited in the 2000 report to Congress advocated the adoption of a universal prescription card to achieve this aim.[1]

The decision to expand the use of automation and technology may be a viable solution to address pharmacy staff shortages for some pharmacy operations; however, the adoption of automation and technology can be held back by cost, restrictive legislation and the fact that many advances are still applicable primarily to large operations while many pharmacy operations are relatively small. The 2001 report of the Institute of Medicine noted that the very limited application of technology to healthcare has been an obstacle to achieving quality.[20] The existence of a pharmacist shortage may, indeed, turn out to be a spur to the wider and better use of automation and technology in the medication use process.

Summary

The existence of a pharmacist shortage in the United States is an established fact. This situation has developed at the same time that national priorities for improved safety and quality in the medication use system have achieved wide support. Because it is unlikely that the number of new pharmacists can be greatly increased, the simultaneous implementation of multiple partial solutions should be considered. These solutions should be considered in the light of continuing progress toward a medication use system of the highest quality and a likely scenario that the demand for pharmacists and their services will continue to exceed the available supply.

References

1. Health Resources and Services Administration. The pharmacist workforce: a study of the supply and demand for pharmacists. Rockville, MD: Health Resources and Services Administration. December 2000.
2. Gershon SK, Cultice JM, Knapp KK. How many pharmacists are in our future? The Bureau of Health Professions project supply to 2020. J Am Pharm Assoc. 2000;40(6):757–64.
3. Walton SM, Cooksey JA. Differences between male and female pharmacists in part-time status and employment setting. J Am Pharm Assoc. 2001;41(5):703–8.
4. Mott DA, Sorofman BA, Kreling DH, Schommer JC, Pedersen CA. A four-state summary of the pharmacy workforce. J Am Pharm Assoc. 2001;41(5):693–702.
5. Quiñones AC, Mason HL. Characterizing pharmacy part-time practice. J Am Pharm Assoc. 2000;40(1):17–25.
6. Ukens C. The big lure: chains here courting foreign pharmacists to meet manpower shortages in their pharmacies. Drug Topics. 1999;43(23):48.
7. Midwest Pharmacy Workforce Research Consortium. National Pharmacists Workforce Survey: 2000. Alexandria, VA: Pharmacy Manpower Project. 2000.
8. Vector Research Inc. Census of Pharmacists. Alexandria, VA: Pharmacy Manpower Project. 1994.
9. Gershon SK, Cultice JM, Knapp KK. Further research on pharmacist supply trends: revised projections through 2020. Presented at the American Pharmaceutical Association Annual Meeting, San Francisco, CA, March 2001.

10. Knapp KK, Livesey JC. The Aggregate Demand Index: a report of the two-year performance of a tool measuring the balance between supply and demand for pharmacist positions. J Am Pharm Assoc. In press, 2001.
11. Reeder CE, Kozma CM, O'Malley C. ASHP survey of ambulatory care responsibilities of pharmacists in integrated health systems—1997. Am J Health-Syst Pharm. 1998;55(1):35–43.
12. Knapp KK, Blalock SJ, O'Malley CH. ASHP survey of ambulatory care responsibilities of pharmacists in managed care and integrated health systems—1999. Am J Health-Syst Pharm. 1999;56(23):2431–43.
13. Institute of Medicine. To err is human: building a safer health system. Kohn LT, Corrigan JM, Donaldson MS. Eds. Washington, DC: National Academy Press, 2000.
14. Hendren J. Pharmacy technicians: dispensing drugs at $6 to $12 an hour. http://sfgate.com/cgi-bin/article.cgi?file=/news/archive/2000/02/14/national1334EST0599.DTL&type=health. Accessed September 21, 2001.
15. Levine J. Study finds mistakes by pharmacist technicians: assistants' role in the spotlight. http://my.webmd.com/content/article/1728.55198. Accessed September 21, 2001.
16. —. Pharmacist Technician Certification Board. http://www.ptcb.org. Accessed September 21, 2001.
17. —. Re-engineering the medication use system: proceedings of a national interdisciplinary conference conducted by the Joint Commission of Pharmacy Practitioners. Am J Health-Syst Pharm. 2000;57(6):537–601.
18. Rupp MT. Value of community pharmacists' interventions to correct prescribing errors. Ann Pharmacother. 1992;26(12):1580–4.
19. Arthur Andersen LLP. Pharmacy activity cost and productivity study. Alexandria, VA: National Association of Chain Drug Stores. 1999.
20. Institute of Medicine Committee on Quality of Health Care in America. Crossing the quality chasm. Washington, DC: National Academy Press, 2001.

chapter twenty-six

Trends in marketing pharmaceuticals

Harold Glass

Contents

The U.S. health care market is experiencing profound stresses. As the cost of developing new drugs has risen substantially, with generally cited cost figures ranging between $500 million and $800 million, pharmaceutical prescription prices have increased at rates that are of major public concern to users, providers, and payers alike. According to IMS Health, the U.S. leads the world in the rate of spending growth on pharmaceuticals, having averaged a cumulative average growth rate of 14% over the last 10 years. This compares to 11% in other major markets of Europe and Asia. The U.S. pharmaceutical market has grown from $61 billion in 1993 to an anticipated $223 billion in 2003.

A number of reasons explain this increase. The average cost per day of care has increased as newer, more expensive drugs have replaced older ones.

0-8493-1446-1/04/$0.00+$1.50
© 2004 by CRC Press LLC

There have been price increases on many of the older drugs as well. In addition, the number of days a user takes a drug has also grown in recent years. Also, there has been an increase in the number of people taking prescription drugs. Drug consumption and prices have grown substantially and so has the attention devoted to these increases.

The market for pharmaceutical drugs is shaped by a number of trends, including an aging population, a changing economy, a slowdown in the Food and Drug Administration (FDA) new drug approvals, government reimbursement policies, and the uncertain role of managed care providers. Two drug-specific changes will have major impacts on the way people learn about and buy drugs: direct-to-consumer (DTC) advertising and switches of prescription drugs to over-the-counter (OTC) drugs. The U.S. is virtually alone in permitting DTC advertising of prescription drugs. Although allowed in the U.S. since 1980, DTC spending has exploded in recent years and shows every sign of continuing to do so. At the same time, there is a growing movement to switch certain types of prescription drugs to OTC status, offering new medical options and challenges for patients and heath care professionals.

Direct-to-consumer (DTC) advertising

Growth of DTC advertising

DTC advertising of prescription drugs has become a highly visible and even contentious issue. Although only the U.S. and New Zealand allow DTC advertising, this type of advertising has actually been in place in the U.S. for some time, beginning in 1980 with three printed ads for prescription drugs. First appearing in the popular magazine *Readers Digest*, these ads laid the foundation of what has become a multibillion dollar level of advertising expenditure.

In 1983, the FDA imposed a moratorium on DTC advertising to permit the collection and evaluation of evidence on the then new advertising tool. Mindful of potential first amendment arguments, the FDA lifted the moratorium in September 1985. Although the FDA commissioner at the time, Dr. Arthur Hull Hayes, personally felt that DTC was not in the public interest, the FDA concluded that the existing regulations were adequate to cover such advertising.

In the 1990s, DTC advertising increased dramatically. Technically, DTC advertising through electronic media had been legal since end of the FDA moratorium in 1985. In the 1997 Federal Food, Drug, and Cosmetic Act, the FDA required DTC advertisers to disclose major risks in using the advertised drug and to make adequate provision for "information in brief summary relating to side effects, contraindications and effectiveness."[1] Uncertainty existed though about what constituted "adequate provision."

In 1997 the FDA again addressed the definitional question, issuing guidelines to clarify what constituted adequate provision for broadcast advertising. Under the new guidelines, drug broadcasts had to refer the audience to four sources to obtain further information:

1. The doctor
2. A toll-free number
3. A Web site
4. Print advertisement

DTC spending increased rapidly from the mid-1990s. DTC expenditures increased over 200% from 1996 to 2000, with the total approaching $2.5 billion in 2000. The most rapid portion of the increased spending came from television advertising. In 1996, television spending represented more than a quarter of the total amount spent, with print and other advertising constituting more than 70% of DTC spending. By 2000, the relationship had changed completely: television represented 63% of all DTC advertising, whereas print and other form of advertising had declined to about a third.

The reasons for the large increase in DTC advertising are complex. The greater specificity of the 1997 FDA regulatory guidelines most certainly helped clarify the marketing landscape for DTC advertising. However, DTC spending had already begun to soar dramatically before the issuance of the guidelines. The clarity of the new guidelines probably facilitated additional DTC advertising. It is more likely that the guidelines were a response to the increased spending rather than the converse.

Many observers point to an increase on the part of consumers to be more involved in their own health care as a reason for increased DTC spending. Health care information sources have become more abundant and accessible, the Internet being the most striking example. As one critic of DTC, Sidney M. Wolf, wrote, "During the past two decades, there has been an irreversible change in the nature of the doctor-patient relationship. Patients are seeking much more medical information and are actively participating in decisions affecting their health."[2] DTC advertising might have been partly a response by pharmaceutical companies to the changing outlook by consumers. Many consumers were responsive to more information about prescription drugs, and to some pharmaceutical companies, direct advertising seemed a timely response.

The growth of managed care and formulary compliance might also have played a role. This change in the health care landscape was perceived by many in the pharmaceutical industry as putting added downward pressure on drug prices. Direct appeal to health care professionals was not regarded by pharmaceutical companies as incrementally effective as it had once been. Promotions directly to consumers represented another way to reach the consumer.

DTC advertising as a strategy

For as topical as DTC spending is, promotion on professionals, especially free samples and office-based promotions, represents a much higher level of spending by pharmaceutical companies. Total pharmaceutical company spending in the U.S. for promotion to professionals rose from $8.4 billion in 1996 to $13.2 billion in 2000. Although not increasing as fast as DTC advertising, professional promotion remains a significantly higher proportion of marketing costs in the U.S. than does DTC advertising. DTC spending is increasing faster than other forms of promotion, often at the expense of these marketing and sales avenues.

DTC advertising has not represented incremental marketing spending by the pharmaceutical industry. Relative to product sales, total spending on marketing promotion of all types, including to health care professionals and DTC, has remained fairly stable since 1996, at 14 to 15% of sales (Table 26.1). Many pharmaceutical companies have decided to spend a relatively higher share of their marketing dollars on DTC advertising, often taking the increased spending from other marketing efforts.

DTC advertising is fairly restricted in application. Pharmaceutical companies follow a variety of marketing strategies for their various drugs, including the use of DTC advertising. However, DTC advertising has not been used as a marketing tool for many pharmaceutical products. The vast majority of drugs make little to no use of DTC advertising programs. In contrast, promotion to professionals can be used for nearly every brand name drug. Pharmaceutical companies employ some combination of office-based promotion, hospital-based promotion, professional journal advertising, and free samples for virtually every drug they sell. The relative importance of these more traditional marketing elements in professional promotion might vary, depending on the type of drug. In-patient indications, for instance, often receive a relatively more concentrated emphasis in hospital promotions than do other types of indications. However, almost every drug probably receives some level of marketing promotion to health care professionals. This is not the case with DTC advertising.

Table 26.1 Spending on Direct-to-Consumer and on Promotion to Health Care Professionals in the U.S. as a Percentage of Pharmaceutical Company Sales

	1996	1997	1998	1999	2000
Direct-to-consumer advertising	1.2	1.5	1.6	1.8	2.2
Promotion to professionals	12.9	13.8	13.7	11.8	11.8
Total	14.1	15.3	15.3	13.6	14

Source: From IMS Health presentation at the Pharmaceutical Business seminar, London, June 24, 2003.

The DTC tool is used more selectively. Some indications are advertised more than others, and some particular drugs are advertised more than others. Spending on DTC advertising is concentrated on a few products and will probably remain so. In 2000, only 20 prescription drugs accounted for almost 60% of all industry DTC spending (Table 26.2). Drug companies employ DTC advertising though for a variety of drug classes, including antidepressants, antihistamines, antihyperlipidemics, and anti-inflammatory agents. DTC spending differs by drug class and individual drug.

Some types of drugs have almost no DTC money spent on them, whereas other drugs receive substantially higher DTC spending. For example, in 1999, DTC spending constituted 6.1% of all pharmaceutical company sales spending for antihistamines and 11.6% of sales expenditures for nasal sprays. Other

Table 26.2 Direct-to-Consumer Advertising in 2000 on the Top 20 Most Advertised Drugs

Ranking	Trade Name of Drug	Type of Drug	Spending on DTC Advertising (Million $)
1	Vioxx	Anti-inflammatory	161
2	Prilosec	Antiulcer	108
3	Claritin	Antihistamine	100
4	Paxil	Antidepressant	92
5	Zocor	Antihyperlipidemic	91
6	Viagra	Erectile dysfunction	90
7	Celebrex	Anti-inflammatory	79
8	Flonase	Anti-inflammatory for nasal allergies	78
9	Allegra	Antihistamine	67
10	Meridia	Weight loss	65
11	Flovent	Antiasthmatic	63
12	Pravachol	Antihyperlipidemic	62
13	Zyrtec	Antihistamine	60
14	Singulair	Antiasthmatic	59
15	Lipitor	Antihyperlipidemic	59
16	Nasonex	Nasal allergies	53
17	Ortho Tri-Cyclen	Oral contraceptive	47
18	Valtrex	Antiviral for genital herpes	40
19	Lamisil	Antifungal for toenail fungus	39
20	Prempro	Hormone replacement therapy	38

Source: From IMS Health presentation at the Pharmaceutical Business seminar, London, June 24, 2003.

Note: All drugs listed are registered trademarks.

drug types receive DTC support, but at appreciably lower levels as a percentage of sales. A case in point is antidepressants, for which only 0.5% of sales were devoted to DTC advertising in 1999. DTC advertising may be a component of the marketing mix for a number of drugs; however, the importance of the piece varies by drug class.

Within a specific drug class, pharmaceutical companies appear to use DTC advertising for some drugs but not others. For example, in 1999, Paxil was the only antidepressant for which substantial sums were spent on DTC advertising. Yet the drug faced many competitors. Likewise, Prilosec was the only proton-pump inhibitor for which the sponsor company spent large amounts on DTC. In contrast, most nonsedating antihistamines were advertised to consumers. Some types of drugs lend themselves more easily to DTC advertising, but decisions on specific drug advertising programs appear to depend on the respective pharmaceutical company's marketing strategy.

There appear to be higher levels of DTC advertising spending on prescription drugs associated with low incidence, mild side effects. Also, drugs receiving DTC advertising support usually treat chronic conditions. It is not always clear why one particular drug in a class receives DTC support whereas others in that class do not. The decision to use DTC advertising for a particular drug may be traceable only to the specific individuals in a drug company pursuing a particular marketing strategy.

Often, DTC spending is higher for newer drugs or drugs with no generic competition. It should be kept in mind that although DTC advertising first appeared in the early 1980s, DTC advertising is fundamentally still a relatively new marketing tool. Pharmaceutical companies are continuing to learn about the tool and when it is most effective. For instance, products facing patent expiry seem to gain less from advertising. With patent expiry, these drugs often face stern price competition from generics, experiencing rapid drops in sales.

On the other hand, mature drugs, late in their product life cycle, might have been approved for new indications. Substantial DTC advertising campaigns might be used for these drugs' new indications as a way to differentiate the drugs from others in that drug class. An example again is Paxil, which began a significant DTC advertising campaign for a new indication, social anxiety disorder.

The effectiveness of DTC advertising is still being debated. Surveys of consumers lead to two initial conclusions. First, a large and growing majority of consumers are aware that there is advertising for individual prescription drugs. Second, about a quarter of consumers have discussed a particular drug with their doctor based on advertisements that they see. Relatively few consumers though, less than one in twenty, report actually asking for and receiving the drug they had discussed.[3] Many doctors also indicate having been asked by patients for specific prescription drugs by name, and high percentages of doctors indicate that they are willing to prescribe the brand requested if it is consistent with the medical needs of the patient. One survey found that nearly three-quarters of family physicians even believed that DTC advertising put pressure on physicians to prescribe drugs that they would not otherwise have prescribed.[4]

Concerted efforts are being made by supporters and opponents alike to understand the impact of DTC advertising on both the doctor and patient. The largest portion of drug marketing effort though will remain concentrated on the physician. DTC advertising will likely only increase, but DTC advertising is unlikely to replace physician-directed promotion.[3] Without a doubt, DTC advertising will remain a controversial, even contentious, issue.

The DTC advertising controversy

DTC is a very visible issue, perhaps for two reasons. Spending on prescription drugs is the fastest growing segment in the health care budget.[4] Policy makers, consumers, health care professionals, and pharmaceutical companies have focused extensive attention on the cost of prescription drugs in the U.S. It is not just the cost of drugs that makes the issue so topical. DTC advertising uses television extensively, so millions of people are directly aware of prescription drug advertising. Printed DTC advertising had been around since the 1980s. The use of television as an advertising medium significantly changed the intensity of the debate.

Proponents of DTC advertising assert that such promotion by the drug industry produces better-informed consumers and ultimately leads to improved health care. Some proponents draw on first amendment issues of free speech, arguing that consumers should have the right to be more informed about health care options. Opponents lament that DTC advertising encourages the use of expensive, wasteful medicines, ultimately distracting medical attention and harming the quality of health care. More severe critics argue against advertising in any form as a tool in medical care, and assert that pharmaceutical companies make excessive profits by getting consumers to spend money on unneeded or unnecessarily expensive drugs.

Opposition to DTC

Sidney Wolf maintains that many drug advertisements are not balanced or accurate and duped physicians might inadequately resist patients' exhortations to write prescriptions for drugs patients see advertised. The question is not whether consumers should obtain information about treatment options. No one, Wolf emphasizes, would dispute that. The real issue is whether drug advertising, whose sole aim is to sell the product, really provides information medical consumers can use to make informed decisions. The education of patients and physicians is too important to be left to the pharmaceutical industry. A dangerous marketing tool might be growing at a time when it can least be appropriately monitored. DTC advertising is increasing as the number of actions taken by the FDA to enforce advertising regulations is declining, down from 139 warning letters to companies or notices of violation in 1997 to less than an estimated 75 in 2001.[2]

Opponents of DTC advertising stress that research has raised issues with the content of advertising. According to studies cited by critics, a substantial portion of people believed that only the safest and most effective drugs could be advertised directly to consumers. Opponents conclude from many of these studies that advertisements contain a higher proportion of promotional material than educational material.[5,6] The purpose of DTC advertising, then, is to convince and not inform, they argue, raising fundamental questions about the value of DTC advertising. From this perspective, the pharmaceutical industry's goal in DTC advertising is to maximize the consumption of drugs, not necessarily enhance the health of individual patients.

Writing in the *British Medical Journal*, J.R. Hoffman and M.S. Wilkes declare:

> Extending the scope of already ubiquitous promotions about "post-nasal drip," "unsightly rashes," or "cures" for baldness has little to do with educating patients or relieving suffering. It will, however, inevitably drain healthcare dollars, dramatically increase unnecessary prescribing, and strain patient-doctor relationships.[7]

Advertising is not necessarily education. Limited training and knowledge might overwhelm the patient and result in demands for inappropriate treatment and unnecessary risks. Patients do not usually have the necessary clinical and pharmacological training to evaluate a medication's appropriateness. Valuable physician time might be wasted in dialogue with patients to disabuse them of misunderstandings about drugs the patients have seen advertised.

Opponents also feel that advertising actually creates a costly consumer demand. DTC advertising in many cases promotes unnecessary drug consumption and inappropriate care. Higher costs, higher insurance premiums, and unnecessary adverse reactions to medications will be the result.

Proponents of DTC

Supporters of DTC advertising see the situation in a very different light. According to the proponents of DTC, advertising can be educational, even if one of the purposes is to persuade. Ads inform patients about the existence of pertinent drugs. These ads provide a better match between patient and drug. Consumers will be more likely to bring important and relevant information to the physician's attention, information that might otherwise be overlooked in the treatment. Describing symptoms, for instance, becomes clearer and more precise when patients are more informed.

The inadequate treatment of underdiagnosed conditions is a major issue in the provision of health care in the U.S., ultimately leading to higher societal medical costs. Informed patients will also recognize symptoms of treatable conditions and seek treatment in a more timely fashion. Compliance with drug regimens will, in many cases, improve because the prescribed medication is better suited to individual needs. The patient will also be more likely to return to the physician if the treatment is not working. Increasing consumer awareness will help reduce undertreatment, helping to improve the quality of life for many and manage the overall costs of health care for society. Direct advertising greatly reduces the undertreatment of important illnesses. Better-informed and aware patients will seek help for their medical problems and receive a safe and effective prescribed medicine. Writing in *JAMA*, Alan Holmer of The Pharmaceutical Industry Trade Association maintains, "Direct-to-consumer advertising is an excellent way to meet the growing demand for medical information, empowering consumers by educating them about health conditions and possible treatments."[8] In any event, DTC supporters highlight that the real gatekeeper of drug prescribing is the physician and other medical professionals. Physicians will only write prescriptions for a drug when they are familiar with the drug and comfortable prescribing it. Through Web sites from scientific societies, publishing companies, universities, patient organizations, and drug companies, consumers have access to a wealth of information about individual drugs and therapies. But consumers are not free to use any drug they wish. The physician is the watchdog. DTC merely provides additional information to consumers.

Richard L. Kravitz sums up how to understand the net benefits and risks of DTC advertising as they are known at this point.[9] The research will be complex and difficult. The net public health gain or loss will be determined by three factors: (1) the current prevalence of undertreatment (the number of patients who should be receiving treatment but are not and the number of patients receiving incomplete care), (2) the amount of any inappropriate or harmful prescribing stimulated by these DTC ads, and (3) the degree of harm accrued to undertreatment compared with that of overtreatment. He concludes that DTC advertising is here to stay. The real issue is how to manage this consumer advertising for the medical benefit of the consumer and society.

Over-the-counter (OTC) switches

OTC usage

More than 700 OTC products have ingredients or dosages that were previously available only by prescription. In the last few years, pharmaceutical and consumer product companies have taken the process of using OTC products substantially further. These companies have begun a particularly strenuous effort to see what prescription products will be suitable to the consumer market. Many of these OTC-switch programs, i.e., switching prescription drugs to consumer products, have been successful. Some, such as those involving ibuprofen and H_2 blockers, have been highly successful.

Before 1951, it was basically up to the manufacturers to decide whether a drug should be available only through prescription. Legislation in 1951 set the statutory basis for distinguishing between prescription and OTC medicines. The thalidomide controversy in the 1960s renewed congressional interest in the issue. By 1962, Congress passed legislation requiring that all OTC products be reviewed by the FDA to assure safety and efficacy for the labeled indications. The FDA eventually completed a massive effort to review the OTC products on the market. As a consequence, many products were withdrawn from the market or reformulated because of insufficient evidence of effectiveness. The FDA mandated that a few medicines be switched from prescription medication to OTC. In 1975, the FDA formalized the process of OTC switching, designating three methods to begin a switch approval process:

1. As an individually initiated petition
2. As a supplement to a new drug application submitted by the pharmaceutical manufacturer
3. Through the OTC review process

Manufacturers have initiated most OTC switches, although a number of cold, cough, and allergy products were switched to OTC status through initiation of the panel review process. In a recent case, a health care management company initiated the switch process. Blue Cross of California petitioned the FDA in 1998 to have Claritan, Allegra, and Zyrtec switched to OTC. Many antihistamine products were already on the market, but these were second-generation drugs, considered to be more effective and with fewer side effects. After reviewing the data, the FDA Pulmonary-Allergy Drugs Advisory Committee recommended the switch of Claritan from prescription to OTC, although the manufacturer, Schering-Plough, publicly opposed the FDA recommendation. Over time, and with pending patent expiry, Schering-Plough withdrew its objection.

No formal FDA guidelines exist for OTC switch, but the FDA uses several evaluation criteria in the approval decision. The drug:

- Must be safe and effective without the supervision of a licensed practitioner
- Have a low potential for misuse and abuse
- Treat conditions that are common, benign, and self-diagnosable by the average person
- Have labeling instructions understandable to the average person who will use the product

The FDA looks for a potential OTC-switched product to have been marketed as a prescription product for at least 5 years in the U.S., though the period varies by geography. The European Union has no time frame for

OTC switches, whereas Japan requires six years. For the FDA, a marketed prescription drug should not have demonstrated an unacceptable level of adverse events, and these adverse events should not have increased over time.

The switch to OTC products has met with a strong resonance in the marketplace. OTC switches are increasingly popular with the belief that patients should play a more central role in the managing their own health care. In the U.S., most people attempt to treat their ailments without professional consultation, and most often with an OTC medicine.[10] Diagnosis is traditionally used to describe activities by physicians wherein superior medical knowledge is essential to make sound decisions and avoid costly mistakes. This is becoming less true as an increasing number of self-diagnosis kits become available and the public becomes more knowledgeable. Switching selected prescription drugs to OTC availability provides more means for a patient to treat a self-diagnosed malady.

Many support increased OTC switches as a means of reducing health care costs. European health care authorities have been supportive for some time of increased self-medication by patients. Studies in the U.S. point to potentially reduced health care costs from the use of OTC products. For example, in the U.S., it is estimated that people saved $1 billion in health care costs in the first 3 years after a topical hydrocortisone acetate was switched to nonprescription status. Similarly, the OTC availability of switched vaginal antifungal preparations substantially reduced the costs of prescriptions and physician services in an HMO. A managed care organization saved around 25% of the cost of caring for patients with nonsevere heartburn or nonulcer dyspepsia by using an OTC acid reducer.[11]

OTC switching of prescription products might have supporters in many professional, government, and business communities. Not all prescription drugs lend themselves though to a consumer version. From a pharmaceutical company perspective, OTC products should have been used in large volumes as prescription drugs, either by a large number of people or by a smaller number of people over an extended time. From a regulatory viewpoint, OTC products must be safe and effective. Several therapeutic areas appear most likely for OTC-switching efforts by pharmaceutical companies. For example:

- *Hypertension.* Nearly half of those with hypertension receive no treatment. Yet it is the chief cause of stroke in people under the age of 65. Direct medical expenses in 2000 exceeded $25 billion. Lost wages and decreased productivity contributed to another $8 billion.
- *Osteoporosis.* Most sufferers receive no or little treatment. Ninety percent of women and 99% of men receive no treatment.
- *Hypercholesterolemia.* Over 1.5 millions will die from myocardial infarction (MI) and many survivors will have serious morbidity issues. The prevention of coronary heart disease through lipid-lowering and

  hypercholesterolemia therapy has been clinically demonstrated to reduce cardiac morbidity and mortality.

- *Benign prostatic hyperplasia.* There are about 34 million sufferers, most with a severely compromised quality of life.
- *Mild asthma, arthritis, incontinence, insomnia, migraine,* and *obesity.*

The decision to switch a drug to OTC status

Research-based pharmaceutical companies follow several basic strategies in switching a prescription drug to the consumer market, usually before a patent expires on a potential OTC candidate. One approach is to replace an expiring drug with an OTC version. The other approach is a dual strategy to market both the existing prescription drug and the OTC product. A dual strategy uses the same molecule and the same brand name simultaneously in the prescription and OTC market, but with a different strength or indication from one another. Dual strategies have been more widely employed in Europe than in the U.S.

Patent expiry, however, forces major changes for a pharmaceutical company. When a prescription product patent expires, substantially cheaper generic versions of the same drug often enter the market, capturing a large portion of sales from the expired drug. The market loss might take years, or, as is more often the case, the market loss is dramatic, sometimes involving only weeks. The drug company loses market share as customers switch or are switched by health care providers and professionals to lower cost generic versions.

The average price of the generic prescription is usually substantially lower than the branded version of the drug. In the 1980s and 1990s, several pharmaceutical companies established their own generic subsidiaries as a way of dealing with patent expirations in the hope of capturing many of the prescriptions lost to generic competitors. But with the advent of a generic competitor, branded drugs sales decline substantially, whether the pharmaceutical company subsidiary or an independent generic company captures the prescription.

Eventually, most pharmaceutical companies withdrew directly from the generic business. A number of legal issues were involved, but, most importantly, research-based pharmaceutical companies realized that they could not operate their generic subsidiaries with a cost structure necessary for these subsidiaries to be profitable. Traditional generic companies proved to combine much lower operating costs with a production and marketing flexibility that research-based pharmaceutical companies could not match. Pharmaceutical companies eventually abandoned many of their generic subsidiaries and looked for other ways to extend the revenues of their drugs facing patent expiry.

Switching a drug to OTC status is a way, in some cases, for pharmaceutical companies to offer a product to the market as its prescription drug approaches the end of its patented life. The switch can offer a number of benefits to the pharmaceutical company. Successful OTC switches means additional revenues to the pharmaceutical company. Also, drugs that successfully change from prescription to OTC are eligible for an additional 3-year extension to their patent life. The 3-year extension protects the drug from generic competition and also provides time for the company to establish the brand name of the OTC product. Pharmaceutical companies have had a difficult time competing as generic companies. A successful OTC switch provides a valuable tool for research-based pharmaceutical companies.

The decision to switch a prescription product to the OTC market is a major one. It has taken 3.5 to 8 years from the time management decided to pursue a switch until the product, with approved labeling, was shipped to the market. A number of negatives for the pharmaceutical company need to be considered in adopting an OTC-switch strategy. The introduction of an OTC version of a product may accelerate losses in the product's prescriptions. The company must conduct costly clinical trials for stability, formulations, and packaging criteria. In addition, labeling changes are required. Ultimately, for all the effort, there is no assurance of success in the marketplace.

A successful marketing program for a switched OTC drug is usually a demanding effort. For many ethical pharmaceutical companies, OTC marketing is substantially different from prescription drug marketing. Prescription pharmaceutical companies have developed numerous joint ventures to consumer product companies to market the switched OTC drug. OTC medications basically have three types of product benefits: efficacy, safety, and ease of use. A successful marketing strategy requires the successful development and communication of an OTC product's benefits. These usually involve one or more of the following:

- **Efficacy benefits**
  More effective relief
  Fast or faster acting
  Effective on severe symptoms
  Long or longer lasting
  Prevents symptoms
- **Safety**
  No or fewer side effects
  No interaction with other medications
  Can be used in all conditions
- **Ease of use**
  Easy to swallow
  Pleasant tasting
  Easy to carry
  Can be taken without water
  Needs to be taken less often

The Pepcid® AC case

The Pepcid AC case illustrates many of the factors at work in the OTC-switch process. Pepcid AC is by almost every account one of the most successful examples of a prescription drug switched to a nonprescription OTC. The launch of Pepcid AC in the OTC market resulted from a 5-year strategy developed by Merck and Johnson & Johnson to market OTC versions of Merck's leading prescription drugs. Prescription Pepcid AC was to be the first case. Originally marketed as a prescription medicine for the treatment of ulcers, Pepcid AC was a reduced-strength version marketed to consumers for the relief of acid indigestion and heartburn.

Merck realized that Pepcid AC could cut in to sales of its higher dosage prescription Pepcid, which would not be off patent by the time Pepcid AC was launched. Merck made a strategic decision to follow a dual-product strategy and promote both the lower dosage Pepcid AC and the higher dosage Pepcid.

Merck believed that it lacked experience in the OTC market and in 1989 developed a 50–50 joint venture with the leading consumer products company Johnson & Johnson to become a major player in the OTC market. The joint venture, Johnson & Johnson/Merck Consumer Pharmaceuticals Co. (JJM), drew employees from both parent operations, acquiring scientific and regulatory expertise from Merck with marketing and sales expertise from Johnson & Johnson.

Pepcid belonged to a revolutionary class of prescription antiulcer drugs, H_2-receptor antagonists, or H_2 blockers, which blocked the production of gastric acid in the stomach. SmithKline and French introduced the first drug in the class, Tagamet®, in 1977. Glaxo's Zantac® followed in 1983, quickly overtaking Tagamet as the largest selling drug of any kind in the U.S. Pepcid appeared in 1986, whereas Lilly introduced a fourth drug in the class, Axid®, in 1988.

While most observers, including many in Johnson & Johnson and Merck, expected that Tagamet HB, the OTC version of Tagamet, would be the first H_2 blocker to receive FDA regulatory approval for the OTC market, Pepcid AC eventually received the first FDA approval. Work on Tagamet HB had begun some time before that on Pepcid AC. However, Tagamet HB had to overcome lingering FDA reservations about product safety and other drug interactions. Although Tagamet eventually met these FDA concerns, Pepcid AC had already entered the consumer marketplace. Other competitors were expected to follow. Glaxo had reached an agreement with Warner–Lambert, and Lilly an agreement with American Home Products, to develop and market OTC versions of their own H_2 blockers.

The Pepcid AC management team had made a monumental strategic drug development decision. A sense of urgency in the JJM camp had prompted it to begin a series of costly clinical trials in a simultaneous, rather than sequential, fashion. Although there was higher risk, the strategy provided JJM with the data necessary to be first to market when the FDA slowed the Tagamet HB approval.

Pepcid AC anticipated customers from two distinct but related markets: traditional OTC antacids and the prescription H_2 market. The overlap between the two categories was substantial, as physicians had increasingly prescribed H_2 blockers for the relief of GERD and heartburn, even when no ulcer symptoms were present.

JJM conducted extensive market research to prepare for Pepcid AC's OTC launch. Concept testing began in 1991 to develop a unique and sustainable positioning for the new OTC drug, differentiating it from Tagamet HB and other anticipated entrants. The second phase of the testing involved 2000 consumers selected to include representative subsamples of antacid users and nonusers. The research results in first year volume estimates for Pepcid AC for several different position strategies, two dosage forms, three pricing levels, and three alternative competitive conditions. For instance, two main positioning strategies, treatment and prevention, were tested. The treatment strategies examined the product benefits of convenience and long-lasting relief against other competitive products, in which Pepcid AC's performance was found superior. The prevention strategies concentrated on the drug's distinctive potential to prevent symptoms. Focus groups and additional concept development testing, involving hundreds of participants, continued through 1993 and 1995. JJM eventually decided on the prevention strategy.

In addition to consumer research, JJM conducted market research with physicians to determine their concerns and expectations. Particularly distinctive was research with pharmacists. The results of this work indicated that pharmacists felt ignored by the major pharmaceutical companies despite their desire to take more part in consumer education and advice. JJM concluded that pharmacists, in particular, had an understanding of the longer-term implications involved with an OTC switch. JJM decided to devote a major portion of is consumer products sales force to promote early awareness and enthusiasm for Pepcid AC among pharmacists.

Armed with published clinical data and extensive marketing research, JJM began an aggressive product launch effort, including 90% coverage of all retail outlets within 5 weeks of launch. The entire Merck and J&J sales teams detailed Pepcid AC to over 100,000 primary care physicians and gastroenterologists. Heavy spending on consumer advertising was initiated, with the following goals:

- Target women 35 years and more who are the key household purchasers of OTC antacids.
- Position Pepcid AC to emphasize prevention and highlight Pepcid AC a superior breakthrough product when compared with antacids in terms of prevention and duration of relief.

- Communicate the benefits of being able to "eat the foods you want" and "sleep through the night," benefits not pushed in the prescription heritage of Pepcid.

Detailed monitoring of the emerging H_2 competitors remained an important part of JJM's effort, consuming significant resources and management attention. Pepcid AC development and marketing touched on virtually every aspect of an OTC switch. Merck took the critical, and ultimately successful, decision, to dual market Pepcid and Pepcid AC. The joint venture took major financial risks in its clinical trial program. The product positioning and rollout program also represented a major marketing challenge. From actual product launch on June 4, 1995, Pepcid AC captured and maintained a large portion of the market.

Conclusion

The marketplace for prescription and OTC drugs has grown substantially in the last decade. For certain categories of drugs, the changes in how these drugs are marketed have been immense. The movements toward DTC advertising and OTC switch are in line with the growing emphasis on people being responsible for their own health care. The exploding number of information channels also presents drug consumers with a near-overwhelming volume of data. In many ways, DTC advertising and OTC switching are in their infancy. However, much DTC advertising and OTC switches have led to major shifts in the drug sales. The changes of the last decade may only be a preview of more profound changes in the coming decade.

References

1. Federal Food, Drug, and Cosmetic Act. S502 (1997).
2. Wolfe SM. Direct-to-consumer advertising: education or emotion promotion. *N. Engl. J. Med.* 2002; 346(7): 524–526.
3. Rosenthal MB, Berndt ER, Donohue JM, Frank RG, Epstein AM. Promotion of prescription drugs to consumers. *N. Engl. J. Med.* 2002; 346(7): 498–505.
4. Lipsky MS, Taylor CA. The opinions and experiences of family physicians regarding direct-to-consumer. *J. Fam. Pract.* 1997; 15: 495–499.
5. Stryer D, Bero LA. Characteristics of materials distributed by drug companies. *J. Gen. Intern. Med.* 1996; 11: 575–583.
6. Bell RA, Kravitz RL, Wilkes MS. Direct-to-consumer prescription drug advertising and the public. *J. Gen. Intern. Med.* 1999; 14: 651–657.
7. Hoffman JR, Wilkes MS. Direct-to-consumer advertising of prescription drugs: an idea whose time should not come [Editorial]. *BMJ* 1999; 318: 1301–1302.
8. Holmer AF. Direct-to-consumer prescription drug advertising builds bridges between patients and physicians. *JAMA* 1999; 281(4): 380–382.
9. Kravitz RL. Direct-to-consumer advertising of prescription drugs. *West J. Med.* 2000; 173: 221–222.

10. Lipsky, MS, Waters T. The "prescription to OTC switch" movement. *Arch. Fam. Med.* 1999; 8: 297–300.
11. Arundell E, Cistarnas M, Heaton A, Kunz K. Economic Implications of self-treatment of heartburn/nonulcer dyspepsia with non-prescription famotidine in a managed care setting. *J. Manage. Care Pharm.* 1996; 2(3): 263–272.

Index

A

ABC inventory control method, 179–180
Accounting, 139–140, 160
  and budgeting, 141
  cycle of, 149, 150
  data recorded in, 142
  definition of, 140
  equation of, 142–143
  financial statements in, 146–149,
      see also Financial statements
    interpreting, 149–160
  journal and ledger maintenance in,
      143–146
    chart of accounts, 145–146
    ledger postings, 144–145
  need for, 140–141
  principles of, 141
  system of, 142
Accounting entity concept, 140–141
Accounting equation, 142–143
Accounts receivable turnover, 155–158
Accreditation, 406–407
  defined, 372
Accreditation programs, pharmacy,
      369–373
  of American Association of Colleges
      of Pharmacy, 373–374
  for community pharmacies, 388
  continuing education requirements
      in, 375
  of health care systems, 382–388
  individual pharmacist advanced
      practice credentials in,
      379–382
  of JCAHO, 383–388
  for managed care organizations, 388
  for online pharmacies, 388–389

organizations sponsoring, 382–392
  pharmacist licensure and, 374–375
  pharmacy technician certification in,
      375–376
  postgraduate training in, 376–379
Accrediting organizations, 392
Acid-test ratio, 153–154
Adverse drug events, reporting, 191
Advertising
  direct-to-consumer, 354–355,
      488–495
  for recruitment, 69
Advocacy role, of professional
      organizations, 401–404
Affiliative style, of leadership, 62–63
Aggregate Demand Index (ADI),
      472–474
Alliance for Pharmaceutical Health
      Care, 412
Ambulatory care settings, pharmacists
      in, 478–480
Ambulatory Payment Classifications,
      441
American Association of Colleges of
      Pharmacy, accreditation
      programs of, 373–382
American Pharmaceutical Association
      (APhA), Code of Ethics
      (1952), 347, 348–349
American Society of Health-System
      Pharmacists, surveys of
      pharmacist workforce,
      469–470
Anti-kickback Statute, 430–431
Antibiotic utilization review,
      196–197
Anticoagulation care provider, certified,
      382